Mechanisms of Motor Skill Development

CENTRE FOR ADVANCED STUDY IN THE DEVELOPMENTAL SCIENCES

Mechanisms of Motor Skill Development

Edited by

KEVIN CONNOLLY

*Department of Psychology,
University of Sheffield, England*

Proceedings of a C.A.S.D.S. Study Group on "Mechanisms of Motor Skill Development" held jointly with the Ciba Foundation, London, November 1968, being the fourth study group in a C.A.S.D.S. programme on "The Origins of Human Behaviour"

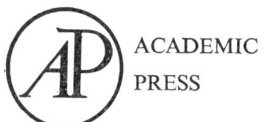

ACADEMIC PRESS

1970

LONDON
NEW YORK

ACADEMIC PRESS INC. (LONDON) LTD.
Berkeley Square House,
Berkeley Square,
London, W1X 6BA

U.S. Edition published by
ACADEMIC PRESS INC.
111 Fifth Avenue,
New York, New York 10003

Copyright © 1970 By THE DEVELOPMENTAL SCIENCES TRUST

All Rights Reserved

No part of this book may be reproduced in any form by photostat, microfilm, or any other means, without written permission from the publishers

Library of Congress Catalog Card Number: 75-141726
Standard Book Number: 12-185950-9

PRINTED IN GREAT BRITAIN BY
Adlard & Son Ltd., Bartholomew Press, Dorking.

Contents

Membership	ix
Developmental Sciences Trust	xi
Preface	xiii
Acknowledgements	xv

Introduction

Skill Development: Problems and Plans KEVIN CONNOLLY	3
Discussion	17

Reflex Mechanisms

Reflex Mechanisms and the Development of Prehension THOMAS E. TWITCHELL	25
Discussion	38
The Reflex Substrata of Voluntary Activity GENERAL DISCUSSION	47

Infancy: the Emergence of Skill

The Growth and Structure of Skill JEROME S. BRUNER	63
Discussion	92
Experience and the Development of Motor Mechanisms in Infancy BURTON L. WHITE	95
Discussion	133

The Experimental Analysis of Skill

Analysing Motor Skill Performance 139
   HARRY KAY

Discussion 151

Response Speed, Temporal Sequencing and Information Processing in Children 161
   KEVIN CONNOLLY

Discussion 188

The Analysis of Performance 193
   GENERAL DISCUSSION

Cognitive Factors in Skill Development

Sensory, Perceptual and Cognitive Factors in the Development of Voluntary Actions 207
   ARTHUR LEFFORD

Discussion 218

Vicarious Perceptual Actions: a Study of the Motor Components of Recognition, Immediate Memory and Thinking 225
   VLADMIR P. ZINCHENKO

Conditioning and Motor Control

Feedback Control of Covert Behaviour 245
   R. F. HEFFERLINE, L. J. J. BRUNO AND J. E. DAVIDOWITZ

Discussion 278

Animal Studies

The Development of Bird Song 287
   ROBERT A. HINDE

Discussion 296

Sensory-motor Integration

Learning to Draw 307
   M. L. J. ABERCROMBIE

Discussion 325

The Adaptability of the Visual–Motor System 337
   I. P. HOWARD

Discussion 351

Intersensory Integration and Motor Impairment 353
   GENERAL DISCUSSION

An Evaluation

Concluding Remarks 375
   KEVIN CONNOLLY

Author Index 383

Subject Index 389

Membership

Study Group on Mechanisms of Motor Skill Development held at Ciba Foundation, London, November 25th–29th, 1968

M. L. J. ABERCROMBIE
    Bartlett School of Architecture,
    University College,
    Gower Street,
    London, England.

J. S. BRUNER
(Chairman I)
    Center for Cognitive Studies,
    Harvard University,
    Cambridge, Mass., U.S.A.

K. J. CONNOLLY
(Chairman II)
    Department of Psychology,
    University of Sheffield,
    Sheffield

R. F. HEFFERLINE
    Department of Psychology,
    Columbia University,
    New York, U.S.A.

R. A. HINDE
    Sub-Department of Animal
    Behaviour, University of
    Cambridge, Madingley

I. P. HOWARD
    Department of Psychology,
    York University,
    Toronto,
    Canada

T. T. S. INGRAM
    Department of Child Life and
    Health, University of Edinburgh,
    Edinburgh,
    Scotland

H. KAY
    Department of Psychology,
    University of Sheffield,
    Sheffield

A. LEFFORD
    Department of Psychology,
    Yeshiva University,
    Bronx, N.Y., U.S.A.

H. F. R. PRECHTL
    Department of Developmental
    Neurology, University of
    Groningen, Oostersingel 59,
    Groningen, The Netherlands

T. E. TWITCHELL
   Department of Neurology,
   Tufts University Medical
   School, Boston, Mass., U.S.A.

B. L. WHITE
   Graduate School of Education,
   Harvard University,
   Cambridge, Mass., U.S.A.

V. P. ZINCHENKO
   Department of Psychology,
   Moscow State University,
   Moscow

Developmental Sciences Trust

The study group reported in this volume was organized by the Centre for Advanced Study in the Developmental Sciences in collaboration with the Ciba Foundation which kindly accommodated the group. It was held during the period when preparations were actively in progress to establish the Centre in its own premises near Oxford. Since then, however, it has unfortunately become necessary to abandon the project to establish that Centre owing to failure to obtain sufficient financial support. The description of the proposed Centre included in previous volumes in the present series therefore no longer applies.

The organization which undertook the planning of the Centre is the Developmental Sciences Trust. The demise of the Centre in no way affects the existence of this Trust which will continue to carry out its purpose by other means. This purpose is to promote the growth of knowledge about the development of human behaviour and the factors that influence it. More specifically, the Trust aims, first to stimulate and co-ordinate research in directions where it is most needed and to foster among scientists and teachers in these fields a developmental and multi-disciplinary perspective on human nature; second, to encourage the application of knowledge from the developmental sciences by those, in all sectors of society, engaged in coping with or preventing human problems.

The Trust is now being reorganized. In the meantime it will ensure that the proceedings of each of the five study groups already held as part of its initial programme will be published as planned.

TRUSTEES The Rt. Rev. the Lord Bishop of Durham
Lady Medawar
Sir Michael Perrin, CBE *Chairman*
Prof. W. H. Thorpe, FRS
Dr. G. E. W. Wolstenholme, OBE

EXECUTIVE COUNCIL Prof. B. M. Foss *Acting Chairman*
Dr. R. C. Mac Keith
Dr. C. Ounsted

DEVELOPMENTAL SCIENCES TRUST

ADMINISTRATOR Mr. W. M. F. Oliver

SCIENTIFIC   Dr. Jane Abercrombie (London)
ADVISORY PANEL Prof. M. Abercrombie (London)
                Prof. J. de Ajuriaguerra (Geneva)
                Dr. L. van Bogaert (Antwerp)
                Dr. J. Bowlby (London)
                Prof. J. Bruner (Harvard)
                Prof. R. Fox (Rutgers)
                Prof. D. A. Hamburg (Stanford)
                Prof. W. J. Hamilton (London)
                Prof. A. Heron (Melbourne)
                Prof. R. A. Hinde (Cambridge)
                Dr. T. T. S. Ingram (Edinburgh)
                Prof. M. Jahoda (Sussex)
                Prof. I. C. Kaufman (Denver)
                Prof. T. A. Lambo (Ibadan)
                Dr. E. Leach (Cambridge)
                Prof. L. P. Lipsitt (Providence)
                Prof. A. R. Luria (Moscow)
                Prof. J. Pfeiffer (New Hope)
                Prof. D. Ploog (Munich)
                Prof. H. F. R. Prechtl (Groningen)
                Dr. R. Robinson (London)
                Prof. J. M. Tanner (London)
                Prof. N. Tinbergen (Oxford)
                Prof. O. Wolff (London)
                Dr. P. H. Wolff (Boston)

Preface

The material presented in this volume is based upon the proceedings of an inter-disciplinary study group which met at the Ciba Foundation in London for five days to discuss "Mechanisms of motor skill development". The original plan was for fifteen scientists, representing biology, neurology, neurophysiology, paediatrics and psychology, to make up the group. Unfortunately, however, Professors Fog, Paillard and Zinchenko were prevented at the last moment from participating, their knowledge and individual viewpoints being greatly missed. It was particularly unfortunate that Paillard was unable to join the group because this robbed us of our only neurophysiologist.

The major portion of the meeting was devoted to discussion, the direction of which was left to the group to determine for itself as the week progressed. The book therefore contains material of three kinds. Nine papers were prepared before the meeting; those of Abercrombie, Bruner, Connolly (both papers), Hefferline, Hinde, Kay, Lefford and Twitchell. Since the meeting took place all the contributors have had an opportunity to revise their papers and most have made at least minor changes. Zinchenko, who was invited to prepare a paper for presentation to the group, sent it subsequently and it was not therefore discussed by the group. Howard and White both presented *ad hoc* papers at the request of the group and these have been more formally recast by their authors for publication in this volume. In addition to the formal papers there are discussions of two kinds. First there are the discussions which followed immediately after the presentation of papers and which primarily explore issues raised by the papers. In addition to these there were a number of general discussions three of which are published—"The Analysis of Performance", "The Reflex Substrata of Voluntary Activity" and "Intersensory Integration and Motor Impairment". These discussions centre around a short *ad hoc* contribution made by a member of the group.

All the discussions, which occupied most of our time, were recorded in full. They were extremely stimulating, often absorbing and most enjoyable. However, it is unlikely that they would be equally valuable when presented in a printed form and with some reluctance therefore I edited them severely. Inevitably some of the questions raised and problems pursued were situation specific and could only be appreciated within the group's immediate historical context. Whilst they might well serve to refresh the memories of the participants their value to the reader would be limited. A great deal of time was spent in discussing issues raised by two films, one presented by Bruner and the other by Kay. Although the problems explored were of great interest to the group I decided that without the benefit of the films these discussions would not be so engrossing or so valuable to the reader, they were therefore omitted. The order in which the papers and discussions are presented in the book is not that in which they were given at the meeting. The reader may therefore find in any one section a reference back to an earlier discussion which in the book is in fact a reference forward.

Much of the earlier literature on the development of motor skill is preoccupied with normative questions and with "developmental diagnosis"; in contrast the material reported in this volume is concerned with the growth of skill and with the mechanisms underlying its emergence in infancy and childhood. Some of the contributions report detailed experimental findings whilst others are primarily concerned with a consideration of the conceptual and empirical problems which their authors see as basic issues.

The approach is multi-disciplinary; contributions from experimental psychology, developmental neurology, experimental biology and paediatrics are offered. Personally I learned a great deal from the neurologists who contributed to the meeting and I hope that they in turn learned from the psychologists and biologists. Certainly at the end of the exercise I am all the more convinced of the desirability of an inter-disciplinary approach. I hope that collecting together in one volume contributions from different disciplines addressed to an area of common interest will encourage readers to explore beyond their own immediate specialist field.

It is a pleasure to thank Miss Isabel Gawler for her most valuable editorial assistance and in particular for her careful attention to detail which has been of immense help. I am grateful also to my secretary, Miss Kathy Gregory, who has typed quantities of often quite complex manuscript. The advice of the Director and staff of the Centre for Advanced Study in the Developmental Sciences is warmly acknowledged. On behalf of all the members of the group I should like to thank Dr. Gordon Wolstenholme and the Ciba Foundation for their hospitality and the excellent facilities which they made available for the meeting. Finally I wish to acknowledge the help of my wife Colette; her patience and skill with the English language have greatly improved the clarity and readability of the material. I must make it clear, however, that any errors which remain are my responsibility.

KEVIN CONNOLLY

Department of Psychology
University of Sheffield
June 1970

Acknowledgements

Illustrations are reproduced by kind permission of Dr. R. Held; *Journal of Nervous and Mental Diseases* (Copyright 1961, Williams and Wilkins Co. Baltimore); *Child Development* (Copyright 1964, Society for Research in Child Development); *Science* (Copyright 1963, 1965, American Association for the Advancement of Science); *Perceptual and Motor Skills* (Copyright 1968); *Merrill-Palmer Quarterly* (Copyright 1969, Merrill-Palmer Institute); Allyn and Bacon Inc. Baltimore (Copyright 1966); *British Journal of Psychology* (Copyright 1970, British Psychological Society); Pergamon Press (Copyright 1967); Spastics Society International Medical Publications and William Heinemann (Copyright 1964); *Journal of Experimental Analysis of Behavior* (Copyright 1963, Society for the Experimental Analysis of Behavior); *Transactions of the New York Academy of Sciences* (Copyright 1958, New York Academy of Sciences); Professor W. H. Thorpe and Cambridge University Press (Copyright 1961); Dr. Joan Stevenson and Cambridge University Press (Copyright 1969); Dr. Margrete Landmark; *Developmental Medicine and Child Neurology* (Copyright 1962, National Spastics Society); Dr. Marianne Frostig; Dr. Moya Tyson.

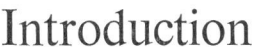

Skill Development: Problems and Plans

KEVIN CONNOLLY

University of Sheffield

IN THIS PAPER I shall attempt to evaluate critically some of the ideas and achievements in the field of motor development and indicate what appear to me to be enduring and fundamental problems. In no way is this intended as an exhaustive review.

Relatively little work has been undertaken in the course of the past quarter of a century in the field of motor skill development. Paradoxically enough, I think this is due largely to the great success of the earlier workers in providing answers to the questions which they posed. There are other reasons. Until recently experimental psychologists have not been interested in the development of young organisms: the behaviour of babies, infants and young children was regarded as essentially simple and remarkably uniform from one individual to another. The view that infant behaviour had little apparent meaning or purpose reflected inadequate models and experimental techniques.

The reappearance of interest in the field of motor development owes a good deal to seemingly remote advances which have been made in comparative psychology, and to the realization of the immense potential which the developmental approach has for elucidating the mechanisms controlling behaviour. As an area of scientific study, the development of skill has great theoretical significance. There are also important practical implications from the problems faced by handicapped children and children with various forms of neurological dysfunction. The striking advances in our understanding of adult skilled performance came from an importation of laboratory rigour into the field of industrial and military man-machine problems. There is no reason why similar advances cannot be made in the developmental sciences, particularly when an inter-disciplinary attack is made on a set of common problems.

I. THE MATURATION HYPOTHESIS

During the 1920's and 1930's much of the most vigorous research in child psychology was concerned with charting the course of motor development. One of the most substantial and sustained contributions to the field was made by Gesell, who was also the foremost proponent of maturation as the fundamental explanatory concept.

In reaction to the rather stark environmentalist position of the early behaviourists, Gesell argued that one of the principal objections to their approach stemmed from the fact that behaviourism explained too much and did not give due recognition to the inner controls and checks. Growth, being a property of the organism, was considered to be primarily controlled by the intrinsic physiology of development. As Gesell put it in 1929, "Growth itself is a process so intricate and so sensitive that there must be powerful stabilizing factors intrinsic rather than extrinsic, which preserve the balance of the total pattern and the direction of the growth trend. Maturation is, in a sense, the name for this regulatory mechanism". Although Gesell admitted to the importance of learning there is no doubt that he considered development during infancy to be primarily a function of maturation. "Development is a continuous process. Beginning with conception it proceeds stage by stage in orderly sequence, each stage representing a degree or level of maturity" (Gesell and Amatruda, 1947).

The ontogeny of behaviour was explained by Gesell (1954) in terms of a number of basic principles. The first of these, which represents the essence of the maturational framework, was the principle of individuating maturation. This was a statement to the effect that the growth impulse was endogenous rather than exogenous; environmental factors were seen to support and in certain circumstances to specify, but they did not engender the basic forms and sequences of ontogenesis. In other words, all individuals within a species will acquire certain motor patterns irrespective of the environment.

The basic statement of maturation as an endogenously controlled process was coupled with the principle of developmental direction. This was to the effect that development proceeds along the principal axes of the body in cephalo-caudal and proximo-distal directions. The stages were considered orderly and behavioural development was thought to follow continuous lines of ontogenetic sequence.

Gesell considered that mature behaviour was attained in a spiral rather than linear fashion and this was termed the principle of reciprocal interweaving. An example of this is provided by the alternation of extensors and flexors which permit walking. A similar idea is incorporated in the principle of self-regulatory fluctuation, which he developed to account for the oscillatory and more variable aspects of behaviour. It was considered a "process of reincorporation and consolidation, rather than one of hierarchical stratification". It permitted the coexistence of stability and variability as mutual complements.

As an individual develops, monolateral preferences emerge. In the neonate the tonic-neck-reflex undergoes gradual sequential changes from the asymmetrical fencing stance to the 6-month symmetrical posture with the head held in the midline position. The initial bilateral use of the hands leads eventually to the predominance of one in reaching and grasping. This inflection of the principle of reciprocal interweaving was termed the principle of functional asymmetry.

These principles expressing Gesell's maturation hypothesis were presumed to be synonymous with scientific laws. Although never subjected to an experimental test they were derived from repeated and meticulously detailed observations on the behaviour of babies and young children. Motor development, governed as it was by these basic laws of developmental morphology, provided the clearest example of the phenomenon of maturation. This approach focused on what were considered to be the fundamental issues of ontogeny. The important questions to which developmental psychologists and biologists addressed themselves concerned the presumed neurological changes associated with the observed behavioural changes. For McGraw (1945) the real issue of the maturation hypothesis was whether the neural organization formed the framework in which function took place, or whether function determined the neural organization?

Implicit in this approach is the view that behaviour emerges spontaneously with the maturation of the nervous system. It presents again a form of genetic predeterminism. Maturation is seen as an unfolding of gene-determined anatomical, physiological and behavioural patterns. An analogy is provided by what were called when I was a child "chinese paper flowers". These were tight little bundles of paper which, when placed in water, opened out into very pretty floral patterns. No matter what one did short of severe physical damage, they opened out in a predetermined way. If they were placed in a more viscous solution such as glycerol and water, it took a little longer but the pattern remained essentially the same. This represents to me Gesell's independence of the environment. We seem almost to be back with the nature/nurture controversy which bedevilled so much of the psychology of the first half of this century. However, advances in behaviour genetics have led to a radical reappraisal of this issue and to an abandonment of this oversimplified and misleading dichotomy (Fuller and Thompson, 1960; Hirsch, 1967).

Maturation as a process of unfolding was assumed by Coghill (1929), who ascribed behavioural development to the maturation of central nervous system tissues. Thus maturation determined the progression from generalized action patterns to specific local responses. This embodies another basic notion about motor development, namely the mass to specific trend. On the basis of observations on neonates and young children it was assumed that specific responses were progressively differentiated from gross movements of the musculature. Bousfield (1953) has offered a more sophisticated interpretation of this and similar trends in motor development in a theoretical rationale for behavioural development in early life. Coghill's (1929) generalizations about the patterns of behavioural development led him to postulate a process of "individuation" whereby the extremities of embryos (rat and cat) developed isolated movements. Carmichael (1934) and Bridgman and Carmichael (1935), working with foetal guinea-pigs at the stage when movements first appeared, obtained results which indicated that both generalized and localized movements may occur at this time. Windle (1940) reported specific movements preceding generalized ones. Subsequent studies by Windle (1950) appear to have resolved this dilemma by showing that any impairment of the embryo's respiratory condition abolishes reflexes and leads to the occurrence of mass movements. The mass to specific trend is also thought to apply to the development of behaviour in neonates and infants (Thompson, 1962). In a critical review Kuo (1939) argued that this was probably an oversimplification of the developmental process: certainly the newborn can exert only crude control over his legs, but he has a very fine control over oral responses. Kaye (1967) shows how sucking can be brought under stimulus control by the appropriate operant procedures. We should perhaps apply the notion of *ontogenetic organization* to these general trends—which systems are required by the infant and when. This, of course, is an evolutionary rather than maturational question.

The inadequacies of the traditional concept of maturation which viewed behavioural development as a purely endogenous unfolding of function have been discussed by Schneirla (1966). As he points out "... the dominance of this pattern of thought in scientific thinking has led to an almost conventional practice of overlooking, ignoring, minimizing, or misrepresenting the matrix of agencies contributed by the developmental medium to ontogenesis". He argues that the factors which contribute to ontogenesis must be re-defined to exclude the implications of the nature/nurture controversy and suggests that maturation be re-defined as ". . . the contributions to development of growth and tissue differentiation, together with their organic and functional trace effects surviving from earlier development". Experience he defines as ". . . the contributions to development of the effects of stimulation from all available sources (external and internal), including their functional trace effects surviving from earlier development". These definitions are objective and not based on a dichotomy between innate and acquired behaviour. The effects of maturation and experience cannot be separated. Experience here is not used synonymously with learning; rather it is defined broadly to denote any class of stimulus effects that result in functional changes ranging from biochemical and physiological processes to conditioning and learning. This of course is very different from the behaviourism which Gesell was reacting against.

The subtle ways in which the integration of maturation and experience may alter function in early development is seen in many studies of embryonic behaviour (Coghill, 1940, 1943; Hamburger, 1963). Functional integrations between rhythmical movements and voluntary responses to stimulation of the duck embryo have important consequences for the behaviour of the newly hatched ducklings (Gottlieb and Kuo, 1965). Self-organization and central patterning are important factors, the significance of the autonomous action of the nervous system independently of peripheral inputs is increasingly recognized (Lashley, 1951; Szekely, 1968). Bullock (1961) goes further: "Central patterning is the necessary and often sufficient condition for determining the main characteristic features of almost all actions, whether stimulus-triggered or spontaneous".

The notion of the essential unity between an individual's genome and his epigenetic system (Waddington, 1959) means that the relationship between genetic and environmental variables in the determination of behaviour is one of interaction. Genes must have a substrate on which to operate, and the nature of the substrate will influence their action.

II. THE SEQUENCE OF DEVELOPMENT

I have criticized the underlying conceptual framework of many of the early studies of motor development on the grounds that the maturation hypothesis, as previously stated, is an inadequate and misleading model. Theories apart, however, at a descriptive level there is a wealth of evidence supporting the generalizations which have been put forward.

The human new born is a motorically immature organism which tends to respond in a generalized fashion to stimulation. It is equally true that as development proceeds the response mechanisms become increasingly refined. For instance, a 3-year-old presents a much smoother performance when walking than does the child of 15 months who has just established independent locomotion. The changes leading to this relative smoothness of performance require explanation at several levels, neurological, psychological and neurophysiological. It must be remembered that these generalizations cannot be taken too far and they are not explanations.

A general criticism of stage dependent theories is that they lead to what is basically a survey or mapping of development. The descriptive or normative approach is an essential preliminary step prior to a definition of other parameters and relationships, but we must not stop at this juncture. In addition to asking the question *when*, we must also ask *how*; what are the processes underlying the observed changes which have been so elegantly described?

Investigators such as Burnside (1927), Bayley (1935), Ames (1937), McGraw (1941, 1945) and Illingworth (1966) have studied the development of prone progression, erect posture and walking in great detail. This kind of descriptive analysis has considerable predictive value in the clinical context and has become known in paediatrics as "developmental diagnosis", following Gesell and Amatruda (1947). One extremely important feature which emerges from these studies is an appreciation that common everyday behaviours, such as walking, are not single skills but rather a complex of delicately coordinated activities involving posture, balance and movement. The muscle groups involved in walking are not only those of the legs and feet, but also those of the arms, trunk and neck. Improvements in these activities will therefore depend upon the integration of information in many feedback loops. If too much attention is given to one source at the expense of another then the overall performance may suffer disastrously.

A short time ago I took my family to lunch in a restaurant, much to the delight of my 3-year-old daughter. When we reached the dessert she chose ice cream. There were no problems about transferring the ice cream from a sundae dish to her mouth via a spoon until her attention was caught by something on the other side of the room. As she gazed across the room the spoon, containing ice cream, which had remained poised halfway between the dish and her mouth, slowly turned over. It was from watching this performance that the idea of sub-routines occurred to me. Why could she not maintain a stable control over her arm and hand whilst directing her attention elsewhere? Using an analogy from digital computers we can think of the sub-units which go to make up everyday skills as sub-routines in a programme. The establishment of a fully functioning sub-routine would mean that a particular component of a given activity had been mastered. This implies that a child can select the appropriate signal from the array of internal messages. It implies also the existence of an error-detecting and correcting mechanism operating independently for a given sub-skill. In the case of my daughter and her spoon this was not an established sub-routine which could be run off; to maintain the ice cream on the spoon required some visual monitoring.

Until a child has reached a stage where some actions can be pre-programmed or until some sub-routines are established, he has to monitor signals as they arise and initiate responses to them. This means that the limit on control capacity is reached more quickly. Early one morning I met my 4-year-old daughter in the hall carrying from the drawing room to the kitchen a tray containing glasses and coffee cups. I asked her where she was going and received the terse reply, "Don't talk to me". She continued very slowly to the kitchen and put the tray down without mishap. Then she turned and explained that she was "helping Mummy". The feature about this which is particularly interesting is not merely that she could not cope with messages from me whilst engaged in this enterprise, but the fact that she knew she could not. Her response succeeded in reducing the information load.

III. MANIPULATIVE SKILLS

Manual skills are our chief examples of fine motor abilities; they are also characteristically familiar functions which have played an essential and distinctive role in man's evolution and cultural progress. Halverson (1933, 1937) made detailed studies of how an infant's reaching and grasping behaviour developed, and proposed no less than ten types of grasping arranged in a developmental sequence; running roughly from a crude, clawing type of hand closure to a precise index finger-thumb grasp, and from a primitive grasp reflex to a "voluntary" type of manipulation. The genetic sequence described by Gesell and Halverson (1936) was a significant step forward in our knowledge. The developmental sequence leading to voluntary grasping, reaching and manual manipulation appeared orderly and lawful. The sequence was also presumed to reflect stages of neurophysiological development which required a minimum of environmental interaction for mature development.

White, Castle and Held (1964) on the basis of a series of controlled observations have described the developmental course of visually directed reaching and relevant responses. A subsequent study by White and Held (1967) investigated the effects of experimental manipulations on the development of visuomotor behaviour in infants. Essentially what they demonstrated was that the appearance of prehension could be significantly accelerated by modifying and "enriching" the environmental conditions. This clearly has bearing on the maturation hypothesis.

From researches on the behaviour of embryos regarding the antecedents of patterned activity, both in structural and behavioural terms, a fundamental question arises as to how exteroceptive and proprioceptive stimuli take control of activity patterns. Similarly, at the level of manual skills, it may be asked how the transition from a reflexive to a "voluntary" grasp is accomplished? Twitchell (1965) considers the automatic grasping responses of the infant as the physiological substrata for the increasingly complex forms of prehension which emerge as development proceeds. It would seem likely that this transition is accomplished by an interaction of the organism with certain environmental factors. Hein and Held (1967), for example, have shown how important it is for an animal to view its own actively moving limbs if it is to make accurate visual placing responses. Reaching for and grasping an object requires some integration of perceptual-motor systems which may not be necessary for the elicitation of the initial grasp reflex.

IV. PERCEPTUAL-MOTOR INTEGRATION

The study of motor skill is concerned with the controlled spatial and temporal patterning of movements; a skilled response is one which is executed both rapidly and accurately. Much of the contemporary research on skill has attempted, for the purposes of analysis, to break down performance into input (perceptual functions), central processing (decision and command functions) and output (motor function). The work has shown quite clearly (Crossman, 1964) that an intimate connection exists between sensory and motor processes; the two interact and are not functionally independent. Let us consider a relatively simple example, reaching for an object. Picking up a pencil from my desk requires a series of operations which includes making an estimate of the distance and radial direction of the pencil from my body, taking account of posture, obstacles and other cues which are relevant for the movement; then finally initiating and monitoring a series of movements which will bring my hand to a particular spatial location. The establishment of connections between perceptual and motor functions and the integration of signals from an external source with those produced by my own movements is crucial. Information from different sensory channels must be integrated by the central nervous system and certain translation functions must develop.

Mammals show a surprising plasticity in the responses of their sensory-motor systems. Sensory deprivation or prolonged immobilization leads to a degeneration of performance on perceptual motor tasks (Freedman, 1961). Riesen (1958) has shown also that the young of primates and certain other mammals fail to develop normal, visually guided behaviour when deprived of visual contact with a stimulating environment. These findings suggest that the same mechanism may be involved in the development of sensory-motor control as with its maintenance and adaptation to changes in the perceptual world.

The concept of reafference developed by von Holst (1954) has been used by Hein and Held (1962) in constructing a model of visuomotor adaptation and development. Basically they suggest that the stimulus transforms which accompany a skilled movement are an important source of order. This order underlies and is essential for the organization and reorganization of plastic sensory-motor systems.

The difficulties which many young children have in copying two dimensional configurations are well known. Birch and Lefford (1963) studied the relationship between haptic, visual and kinaesthetic sense modalities for shape recognition. They found that the ability to make intersensory judgements improved with age and that this improvement could be described by a logarithmic growth function. In a subsequent monograph, Birch and Lefford (1967) applied these ideas of intersensory integration to an examination of the processes underlying voluntary motor control. Their various experiments led them to the view that ". . . improved intersensory organization is critical for the development of refined and modulated adaptation to the surrounding environment". If the young child is unable to interpret signals arising from his own responses, then the task will indeed be complex for him.

A further point in this context is that the intersensory discrimination of children may be poorer because the actual discrimination of any one sense mode may be inferior to that of an adult. Bryant (1968) has criticized some of the work on cross-modal matching on the grounds that it does not take account of this possibility. Recently, however, Connolly and Jones (1970) have investigated the relationship between intra- and cross-modal performance on tasks which involved estimating the length of straight lines. The results showed that cross-modal matching produced a higher variance than intra-modal matching but cross-modal matching improved significantly with age.

V. THE SPEED OF BEHAVIOUR

A distinction was drawn by Adams (1964) between the molar and molecular approaches to the analysis of skill. By far the largest volume of work has been cast within the molar framework, for example questions regarding the efficacy of "massed" versus "distributed" practice. Much of this work has been carried out within the context of S–R associationism and the primary focus has been on learning rather than performance. Over the past 20 years this imbalance has slowly been redressed. The ideas of Craik (1943), the development of cybernetics and the importation of engineering concepts into psychology have led to the emergence of the molecular approach with its emphasis on the analysis of performance. It is within this context that I want to consider the changes in the speed of behaviour which accompany development.

As long ago as 1892 Bryan used speed of tapping as a measure of the "speed of muscular movement" and found that the gain in speed as a function of age was approximately linear to the age of 16. Later studies by Goodenough and Brian (1929) and Goodenough and Tinker (1930) confirmed these findings. More recent work by Davol, Hastings and Klein (1965), Connolly, Brown and Bassett (1968) and Connolly (1968) has confirmed, using very different tasks, this observation regarding the substantial changes in speed which accompany increasing age.

A motor response takes time to initiate and lasts for a given period; a simple response may therefore be described in terms of the two parameters of latency and duration. More complex responses require, in addition, that certain sub-units be programmed into a particular temporal sequence. Accordingly there are, I think, three classes of variables which may, during the course of development, lead to the observed increases in speed of performance.

The first of these three classes may be conveniently termed "hardware" changes. I am here referring to some of the basic neurological and neurophysiological changes which accompany growth. The overall functioning efficiency of the central nervous system will be increased by improvements in its component parts. The myelination of axons adds to the size of the cortex and, although it is not necessary for function (the neonatal rat's central nervous system is almost completely lacking in myelinated fibres but the animal is nevertheless capable of some motor activity) it does serve to insulate fibres and appears to some extent to correlate with more mature electrophysiological responses (Eichorn, 1963). Langworthy (1933) studied the order of myelination in three widely differing mammalian species (opossum, cat and man) and found them very similar. In general, tracts become myelinated in order of their phylogenetic development which is also the order of importance in controlling fundamental activities, those most basic to the organism's life in the early stages develop first. In humans the process of myelination probably goes on into adolescence (Tanner, 1961). Clark (1958) has suggested that the myelin sheath has important effects on the transmission of impulses along the axon. It serves to accelerate the rate of conduction, the thicker the sheath the more rapid the conduction. Similarly, if an impulse is attenuated in the course of travelling down a non-myelinated fibre, the probability of firing subsequent synapses may be affected. Scheibel and Scheibel (1963), on the basis of their work with kittens, suggest that the facility of the young animal for discriminatory activity based on sensory cues is dependent on the development of short axon cells.

Fog and Fog (1963) argue that the development of cerebral inhibition is necessary for the acquisition of detailed discriminative control; associated movements as a measure of this continue to show changes with age to at least the 15-year level in normal children (Fog and Fog, 1963; Connolly and Stratton, 1968). Histological and biochemical changes in developing nervous tissue also suggest ways in which the component parts may become more efficient (Gruner, 1962).

Over and above these various changes in neural material, there may also be important mechanical developments; changes in the total mass of a limb, increases in muscle bulk and so forth. All of these factors, and others, could be implicated in speed of performance at various times in development.

The second class of variable may be termed "software". In addition to efficient hardware the functioning level of an organism, or a machine, will reflect the use made of it. There are usually more ways than one in which a given set of data may be analysed or a problem reduced to a solution. My mathematician friends aim not only at producing solutions to problems but at producing elegant ones. By elegance I understand them to mean, in part at least, parsimony in the number of assumptions or in the number of operations required. If one solution requires fewer assumptions and leads to the resolution of a problem in fewer operations, it is not only more elegant but also more efficient. In writing programmes for digital computers, the experienced programmer will probably produce one which requires the minimum number of operations, a feature which in turn will lead to a decrease in running time—faster performance. In a similar way children may increase their speed of performance by cutting out unnecessary operations (Connolly et al., 1968); they may well develop, for example, more effective selective filtering mechanisms (Connolly, 1970).

Thirdly, the speed of behaviour may also change by a compounding of these hard- and soft-ware factors. With the progressive establishment of organized neural networks, enriched continually by experience, the effective functioning size of the brain may be increased, and in consequence the capacity of the central processing machinery enlarged. This could permit, under certain circumstances, the parallel processing of information. The suggestion in a previous section of this paper regarding the establishment of "sub-routines" is perhaps an example of how this begins.

REFERENCES

ADAMS, J. A. 1964. Motor skills. *Ann. Rev. Psychol.* **15**, 181–202.

AMES, L. B. 1937. The sequential patterning of prone progression in the human infant. *Genet. Psychol. Monog.* **19**, 409–460.

BAYLEY, N. 1935. Development of motor abilities during the first three years. *Monog. Soc. Res. Child, Develop.* **1**.

BIRCH, H. G. and LEFFORD, A. 1963. Intersensory development in children. *Monog. Soc. Res. Child Develop.* **28**.

BIRCH, H. G. and LEFFORD, A. 1967. Visual differentiation, intersensory integration, and voluntary motor control. *Monog. Soc. Res. Child Develop.* **32**.

BOUSFIELD, W. A. 1953. The assumption of motor primacy and its significance for behavior development. *J. Genet. Psychol.* **83**, 79–88.

BRIDGMAN, C. S. and CARMICHAEL, L. 1935. An experimental study of the onset of behavior in the fetal guinea-pig. *J. Genet. Psychol.* **47**, 247–267.

BRYAN, W. L. 1892. On the development of voluntary motor ability. *Am. J. Psychol.* **5**, 125–204.

BRYANT, P. E. 1968. Comments on the design of developmental studies of cross-modal matching and cross-modal transfer. *Cortex*, **4**, 127–137.

BULLOCK, T. H. 1961. The origin of patterned nervous discharge. *Behaviour*, **17**, 48–59.

BURNSIDE, L. H. 1927. Coordination in the locomotion of infants. *Genet. Psychol. Monog.* **2**, 279–372.

CARMICHAEL, L. 1934. An experimental study in the prenatal guinea-pig of the origin and development of reflexes and patterns of behavior in relation to stimulation of specific receptor areas during the period of active fetal life. *Genet. Psychol. Mongr.* **16**, 337–491.

CLARK, W. E. LEGROS 1958. *The tissues of the body.* 4th edition. Clarendon Press, Oxford.
COGHILL, G. E. 1929. *Anatomy and the problem of behaviour.* Cambridge University Press.
COGHILL, G. E. 1940. Early embryonic somatic movements in birds and mammals other than man. *Monog. Soc. Res. Child Develop.* **5**, 25.
COGHILL, G. E. 1943. Flexion spasms and mass reflexes in relation to the ontogenetic development of behavior. *J. comp. Neurol.* **76**, 463–486.
CONNOLLY, K. 1968. Some mechanisms involved in the development of motor skills. *Aspects of Education*, **7**, 82–100.
CONNOLLY, K. 1970. Response speed, temporal sequencing and information processing in children. This volume.
CONNOLLY, K., BROWN, K. and BASSETT, E. 1968. Developmental changes in some components of a motor skill. *Brit. J. Psychol.* **59**, 305–314.
CONNOLLY, K. and JONES, B. 1970. A developmental study of afferent–reafferent integration. *Brit. J. Psychol.* **61**, 259–266.
CONNOLLY, K. and STRATTON, P. 1968. Development changes in associated movements. *Develop. Med. child Neurol.* **10**, 49–56.
CRAIK, K. J. W. 1943. *The nature of explanation.* Cambridge University Press.
CROSSMAN, E. R. F. W. 1964. Information processes in human skill. *Brit. Med. Bull.* **20**, 32–37.
DAVOL, S. H., HASTINGS, M. L. and KLEIN, D. A. 1965. The effect of age, sex and speed of rotation on rotary pursuit performance by young children. *Percept. mot. skills.* **21**, 351–357.
EICHORN, D. H. 1963. Biological correlates of behavior. In H. W. Stevenson (Ed.), *Child psychology*. Chicago: Nat. Soc. Stud. Ed. 62nd. Yearbook.
FOG, E. and FOG, M. 1963. Cerebral inhibition examined by associated movements. In M. Bax and R. C. MacKeith (Eds.), *Minimal cerebral dysfunction*. Spastics Society/Heinemann, London.
FREEDMAN, S. J. 1961. Perceptual changes in sensory deprivation: suggestions for a conative theory. *J. nerv. ment. Dis.* **132**, 17–21.
FULLER, J. L. and THOMPSON, W. R. 1960, *Behavior genetics*. Wiley, London.
GESELL, A. 1929. Maturation and infant behaviour pattern. *Psychol. Rev.* **36**, 307–319.
GESELL, A. 1954. The ontogeny of infant behaviour. In L. Carmichael (Ed.), *Manual of child psychology*. Wiley, London.
GESELL, A. and AMATRUDA, C. S. 1947. *Developmental diagnosis.* 2nd Edition. Hoeber Medical Division, Harper & Row, New York.
GESELL, A. and HALVERSON, H. M. 1936. The development of thumb opposition in the human infant. *J. Genet. Psychol.* **48**, 339–361.
GOODENOUGH, F. L. and BRIAN, E. R. 1929. Certain factors underlying the acquisition of motor skills by pre-school children. *J. exp. Psychol.* **12**, 127–155.
GOODENOUGH, F. L. and TINKER, M. A. 1930. A comparative study of several methods of measuring finger tapping in children and adults. *J. Genet. Psychol.* **38**, 146–160.
GOTTLIEB, G. and KUO, Z. Y. 1965. Development of behaviour in the duck embryo. *J. comp. physiol. Psychol.* **59**, 183–188.
GRUNER, G. E. 1962. Histological study of the maturation of the nervous system. *Develop. Med. child Neurol.* **4**, 626–639.

HALVERSON, H. M. 1933. The acquisition of skill in infancy. *J. Genet. Psychol.* **43**, 3–48.
HALVERSON, H. M. 1937. Studies on the grasping responses of early infancy. I. *J. Genet. Psychol.* **51**, 393–424.
HAMBURGER, V. 1963. Some aspects of the embryology of behavior. *Q. Rev. Biol.* **38**, 365.
HEIN, A. and HELD, R. 1962. A neural model for labile sensorimotor coordinations. In E. E. Bernard and M. R. Kare (Eds.), *Biological prototypes and synthetic systems*. Plenum Press, New York.
HEIN, A. and HELD, R. 1967. Dissociation of the visual placing response into elicited and guided components. *Science*, **158**, 390–391.
HIRSCH, J. 1967. (Ed.) *Behavior–genetic analysis*. McGraw-Hill, London.
HOLST VON, E. 1954. Relations between the central nervous system and peripheral organs. *Brit. J. Anim. Behav.* **2**, 89–94.
ILLINGWORTH, R. S. 1966. *The development of the infant and young child*. Livingstone, Edinburgh.
KAYE, H. 1967. Infant sucking behavior and its modification. In L. P. Lipsitt and C. C. Spiker (Eds.), *Advances in child development and behavior*. Vol. 3. Academic Press, London.
KUO, Z. Y. 1939. Total pattern or local reflexes. *Psychol. Rev.* **46**, 93–122.
LANGWORTHY, O. R. 1933. Development of behavior patterns and myelenization of the nervous system in the human fetus and infant. *Contrib. embryol.* **24** (139). *Carnegie Inst. Pub.* No. 443.
LASHLEY, K. S. 1951. The problem of social order in behavior. In L. P. Jeffress (Ed.), *Cerebral mechanisms in behavior: the Hixon Symposium*. Wiley, London.
McGRAW, M. B. 1941. Development of neuro-muscular mechanisms as reflected in the crawling and creeping behavior of the human infant. *J. Genet. Psychol.* **58**, 83–111.
McGRAW, M. B. 1945. *The neuro-muscular maturation of the human infant*. Columbia Univ. Press, New York. Reprinted 1963 with a new introduction. Hafner Pub. Co., London.
RIESEN, A. H. 1958. Plasticity of behavior: psychological series. In H. F. Harlow and C. N. Woosley (Eds.), *Biological and biochemical bases of behavior*. Univ. Wisconsin Press, Madison.
SCHEIBEL, M. E. and SCHEIBEL, A. B. 1963. Some structure-function correlates of development in young cats. In R. Hernández-Péon (Ed.), *The physiological basis of mental activity*. Electroenceph. clin. neurophysiol. Supp. **24.**
SCHNEIRLA, T. C. 1966. Behavioral development and comparative psychology. *Q. Rev. Biol.* **41**, 283–302.
SZEKELY, G. 1968. Development of limb movement: embryological, physiological and model studies. In G. E. W. Wolstenholme and M. O'Connor (Eds.), *Growth of the nervous system*. Churchill, London.
TANNER, J. K. 1961. *Education and physical growth*. London University Press.
Thompson, G. G. 1962. *Child psychology: growth trends in psychological adjustment*. Houghton Mifflin, Boston.
TWITCHELL, T. E. 1965. The automatic grasping responses of infants. *Neuropsychologia*, **3**, 247–259.
WADDINGTON, C. H. 1959. Evolutionary systems—animal and human. *Nature, Lond.* **183**, 1634–1638.

WHITE, B. L., CASTLE, P. and HELD, R. 1964. Observations on the development of visually directed reaching. *Child Developm.* **35,** 349–364.

WHITE, B. L. and HELD, R. 1967. Plasticity of sensorimotor development in the human infant. In J. Hellmuth (Ed.), *Exceptional infant*. Vol. 1. Special Child Publications, Seattle.

WINDLE, W. F. 1940. *Physiology of the fetus: origin and extent of function in prenatal life*. Saunders, Philadelphia.

WINDLE, W. F. 1950. Reflexes of mammalian embryos and fetuses. In P. Weiss (Ed.), *Genetic neurology*. Chicago: University Press.

Discussion

WHITE: There are a number of points which I should like to make. In offering a critique of the maturation hypothesis Connolly laid stress on the plasticity of development; this I agree is fundamental. In his writing Gesell claims to be interested in the environmental circumstances surrounding a child during development, but from his work this does not appear to have been considered an important variable. Many of us, in my country at least, cannot accept the notion that the course of development is inviolate and immutable. We need to know much more about how the genetic plan realises itself in development.

I have an intuition that one of the most interesting pay-offs from the study of the development of motor skills will not be so much in predicting subsequent motor capacity but rather changes in motivation. What I mean is this. Given a child who in his first few months of life shows well developed motor abilities then that child will be able to explore his environment more fully. This in turn may well lead to a child who is more zestful and more interested in things in general, especially in his proximal surroundings. This kind of thinking is consistent with the notions of Hunt and Piaget.

Connolly mentioned the tonic-neck-reflex. In the last few years I have heard a number of people suggest that the tonic-neck-reflex is not so paramount in the first few months as was once thought. I agree that the neonate does not usually show the tonic-neck-reflex, he shows fragments of it. On the other hand the 3–5-week-old infant invariably assumes this posture, indeed I think it almost lawful that the normal infant aged 1 month lies in a tonic-neck-reflex position when supine and I would date the achievement of symmetrical posture considerably earlier than 6 months. I should be interested to hear the observations of others on this question of the tonic-neck-reflex.

I think it is relatively easy and, of course, quite correct to show that there are holes in the notion of the "mass to specific" trend in motor development. This brings in my next point. Connolly said that we know when things occur but we do not know how they come about. I cannot agree with that; in my view much more is needed at the basic descriptive level. Let us do better in getting more solid methods for describing what is happening; let us take it out of the mind of the brilliant observer and get it out into the objective world. There is an enormous amount to be done and I am a little worried that we might start theorizing prematurely.

My last point concerns Connolly's concept of sub-routines and the question of parallel processing. These interested and attracted me very much. There is I think a relationship between these notions and some of our recent studies. Using relatively crude procedures we have been attending to whatever it is that the child seems to be doing from moment to moment. Our question (phrased rather loosely) was, what is the child's purpose at a particular moment? We started by looking at 4- and 5-year-old children and one of our interests was to see to what extent he could handle two tasks at once. We found instances where they could but these were not very frequent. An example I will mention is that of a child making imitation cakes from dough whilst at the same time holding a conversation with another child. My guess is that at the earliest this comes into ongoing behaviour around 3 and then only with very precocious children.

BRUNER: On your last point; I think you have to be very careful about the response system that you are looking at. I am going to try and convince you all in my paper that infants as young as 20 days can cope with more than one thing at once, to a degree that is, when tracking multiple objects.

CONNOLLY: On the question of description and explanation. I quite agree with White that we need much more descriptive work. He put this very prettily in one of his recent papers by saying that child development was a science without a natural history. Despite Gesell's enormous contribution I agree we are lacking this.

PRECHTL: Connolly mentioned babies aged 3 days showing generalized leg movements. I want to defend the newborn a little by saying that the generalized leg movements are, I think, an artefact. If you put a beetle in the supine position then you get very unco-ordinated movements, similar to those shown by the baby. However, if the baby is put into the prone position these unco-ordinated mass movements are gone and everything appears to be very skilful and co-ordinated. You get patterned locomotion, crawling movements, co-ordinated side to side movements of the head, head lifting and so forth. I think watching babies in the supine position may well be an artefact.

INGRAM: May I ask a question at this point? What happens when you put a newborn into water? McGraw did this, I think, and if my memory serves me correctly she found smooth and highly regulated swimming movements. This may support Precht's point.

PRECHTL: I tried to repeat this and make a film of it (Prechtl, H. R. F. 1953. *Die Entwicklung der frühkindlichen Motorik.* part 2, Gottingen). Compared with the same babies crawling, it appears to be exactly the same co-ordination. It is faster, but then there is not the same problem of inertia and friction from the surface that the baby is lying on.

BRUNER: Coghill in his discussion of *Amblystoma* again points out that you get the same serial order patterning for swimming movements and locomotor movements. The timing appears to be identical but there is a limited set of sub-routines, if I may use Connolly's term. May I just add at this point that when you hear my paper this afternoon I want to make it clear now that there was no collusion between Connolly and myself on terminology.

PRECHTL: On the question of myelination. We have to forget the idea that non-myelinated fibres do not function. This is just not true (Ullet, Dow and Larsell. 1944. *J. comp. Neurol.* **80,** 1). There is one relatively new point which has emerged, though it is still a bit hypothetical, concerning the main effect of myelination. You have a neurone, dendrites and then this myelinized sheet comes in. The spikes are generated from the area marked with an arrow in Fig. 1. With the myelinated sheets the firing frequency of the neurone increases because this area becomes more stable and can generate faster spikes. This increased speed of firing is, I think, one of the main effects of myelination.

CONNOLLY: And this may bear some relationship to rapid skilful movement.

PRECHTL: That I don't know, but it may well.

HINDE: May I make two rather general points. One concerns this question of description versus analysis. It has been said that the study of child development lacks a natural history. If I may speak as a biologist I would say that description is facilitated by the analysis which accompanies it. Indeed only by analysis can you learn the sort of things you want to describe. Therefore to say that we need one of these approaches, or must concentrate on one of them, seems to me to be quite wrong, they go hand in hand. If I may make another general point about Connolly's paper. He disposed very beautifully of the dichotomy of

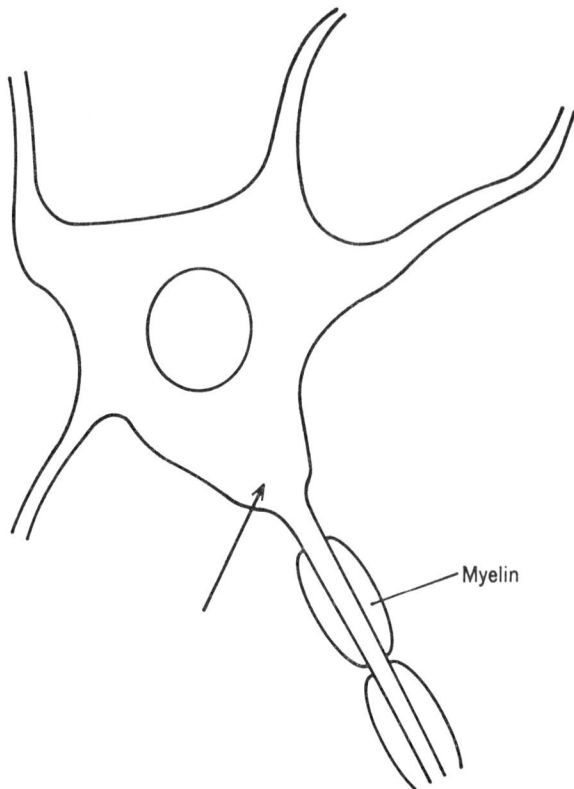

FIG. 1. Arrow indicates region on cell body where nerve spikes are generated.

behaviour into the innate and the acquired. Now there are other types of dichotomy which people make in this sphere. One, which we need not discuss at all in this context, is the dichotomy of sources of information which Lorenz uses and which is misleading in a number of ways. The third, which Connolly mentioned, is the dichotomy between maturation and experience; and he pointed out some of the deficiencies of this dichtomy. But then he seemed to me to undo the good that he had done by quoting Schneirla's slightly more sophisticated definition of maturation and implying that with these improved definitions we could get along a bit further with this dichotomy. I do not think this is correct. Schneirla did a great service by laying emphasis on the complexities involved in development, but he did not really formulate the simple-minded questions which have to be answered. This brings me to the fourth type of dichotomy, which is the dichotomy between differences. What is the difference between this behaviour and that behaviour due to? And I think if one focuses on differences (differences between this age group and that age group, between this individual and that individual) then I think one is much nearer to asking questions which are both harder-headed and more simple-minded, and which are therefore likely to prove more fertile.

TWITCHELL: I have never been impressed with the tonic-neck-reflex in the newborn and in the case of the neck reflexes which have been reported in the premature baby I assume these are passively imposed by moving the head in relation to the body. By 2–3 months I do not think the posture is easy to impose passively, I think it is more of a spontaneous movement. This brings up the question of the mechanism involved. The neck reflexes are very exaggerated in the case of a child with a congenital encephalopathy, but even then they are much more readily elicited by his own spontaneous head movements than those imposed passively by the examiner. I am told that Paillard has suggested that the joint receptors are facilitated by spontaneous movements and this could well be important in explaining the effect.

Environmental effects on maturation have been mentioned. We have observed this in regard to the appearance and "disappearance" of the neonatal stepping response. Paediatricians commonly note that the reaction cannot be elicited in many normal infants after several months. Some years ago we observed a segment of a population in whom the stepping response was present at birth but where there was no sign of its disappearance with maturation. These babies belonged to mothers who, characteristically in playing with them, made the baby step day after day. This suggested that there may be alteration or maturation of some of these reflex mechanisms by continuous environmental stimulation.

Russian work has shown that sucking is easily elicited after birth but the threshold rises in a day or so if the response is not continuously stimulated. Clearly we need more data on such changes as these.

Reflex Mechanisms

Reflex Mechanisms and the Development of Prehension[1]

THOMAS E. TWITCHELL

*Tufts University School of Medicine and
Massachusetts Institute of Technology*

IT HAS GENERALLY been held that reflex mechanisms play a role in the development of voluntary behaviour in the human infant. Thus, prehension is said to begin with some form of reflex grasping which gradually disappears during the first few months of life. This is followed by the appearance of crude voluntary grasping which becomes more dexterous as the infant matures.

Although a number of earlier studies have attempted to delineate the nature of reflex grasping, they have not defined the role that these reflexes might play in the genesis of voluntary prehension.

From our own studies the notion that voluntary grasping emerges from a primitive grasp reflex is clearly an oversimplification. First of all in an earlier paper (Twitchell, 1965), we noted that confusion both in terminology and in physiology had resulted from the failure of earlier investigators to define grasping reflexes precisely in terms of *adequate stimulus* and *response*. We then showed that there were actually three distinct types of reflex grasping in the infant rather than one, and that these were identical physiologically to the reactions described by Seyffarth and Denny-Brown (1948) in the adult patient with neurological disease. We therefore felt it appropriate to follow their terminology in describing the reactions of the infant.

Secondly, the important contribution of avoiding reactions in development of voluntary prehension is far more complex than previously suggested.

It is these aspects of the problem then with which we shall be concerned in this paper.

---

[1] The work described in this paper was aided by a grant from the John A. Hartford Foundation.

I. GRASPING REACTIONS

A. *Birth to 8 Weeks*

Proprioceptive dominance, flexor synergy, the traction response.

If an object is placed in the neonate's palm, the fingers, close around it and the grip tightens as one attempts to withdraw the object. Careful analysis of this reaction reveals several important features. First, the adequate stimulus is proprioceptive and not contact with the palm. Indeed it is not necessary to manipulate the hand at all to elicit the reaction, for a simple passive pull on the arm which stretches the flexor and adductor muscles of the shoulder suffices to elicit the response. Secondly, the response does not consist of finger flexion alone. Finger flexion occurs as part of a synergistic flexion at all joints of the limb in which flexion of the wrist is particularly striking, Fig. 1.

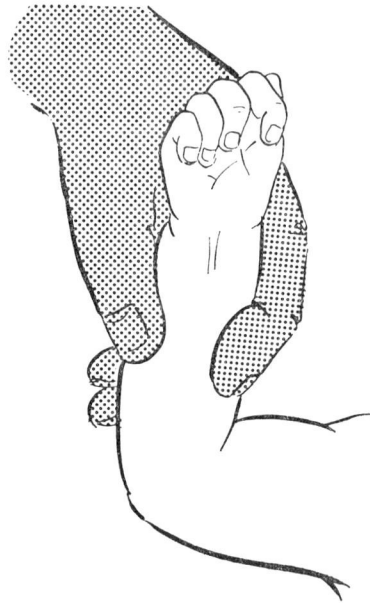

FIG. 1. Elicitation of the traction response.

Additional stretch of the flexor muscles at any joint can intensify the flexion at that joint: thus, if the finger flexors are stretched more during elicitation of the traction response, power of finger flexion is intensified.

This traction response is not a static reaction but from the time of birth can be facilitated or depressed by tonic-neck and contact body-righting reflexes and inhibited by concomitant contact stimulation of the dorsum of the hand. Essential modification of the reaction occurs soon thereafter.

B. *Two to 8 Weeks*

Beginning contact modulation of traction response, first phase of grasp reflex.

Between 2 and 4 weeks of age the traction response can be facilitated by contact stimulation of the palm. This requires a heavy pressing stimulus moving distally along the radial aspect of the palm. This stimulus elicits the synergistic flexion characteristic of the traction response.

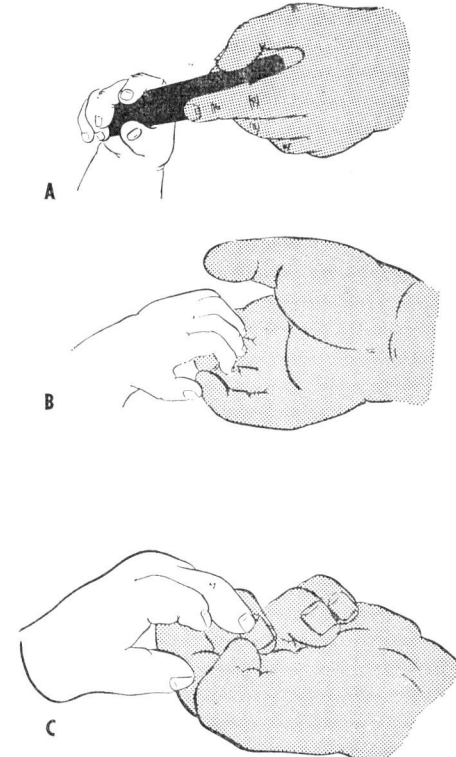

FIG. 2. The grasp reflex: (a) initial component, (b) fully developed, (c) fractionation showing flexion of index finger.

By 4–8 weeks of age a contact stimulus drawn out between the thumb and index finger will produce adduction and flexion of these digits, Fig. 2a. This "local reaction" is immediately followed by flexion at all joints of the arm (contact facilitation of traction response). The local reaction itself constitutes the first phase in the development of the grasp reflex.

Within the next few weeks the receptive field widens to include the entire radial aspect of the palm and volar surface of the proximal phalanges. Contact stimulation of the hand now causes all the fingers to flex, a sign of the final development of the grasp reflex.

C. *Eight to 20 Weeks*

Further conditioning of proprioceptive mechanism by contact, the grasp reflex, subsidence of flexor synergy.

The adequate stimulus for the full grasp reflex is a deeply pressing contact to the radial aspect of the palm moving distally out on to the proximal phalanges. The response consists of two phases. The immediate result of the contact stimulus is a sudden quick flexion of the fingers and thumb (catching phase). This flexion can now be sustained by traction on the fingers but only after they have been made to flex by the contact stimulus (proprioceptive holding phase), Fig. 2b. During the succeeding weeks, the grasp reflex is more easily elicited and the flexion becomes more powerful.

With the appearance of the grasp reflex, the ability to elicit the flexion synergy by either proprioceptive or contact stimuli declines. Nevertheless, an interrelationship between the grasp reflex and traction response can be demonstrated. We showed above how the synergistic flexion characteristic of the traction response could be elicited by a contact stimulus particularly during development of the initial component of the grasp reflex. Later during the early development of the complete grasp reflex, the holding phase may be further intensified if the pull against the fingers is sufficient to stretch also the other flexor muscles of the arm, thus facilitating the holding phase by a traction response mechanism.

Synergistic flexion at other joints is not a feature of the grasp reflex *per se*. The last vestige of traction response contamination of the grasp reflex is a concomitant flexion of the wrist and fingers following the adequate contact stimulus. When the grasp reflex is fully developed, dorsiflexion of the wrist accompanies the flexion of the fingers and adduction.

Neck and righting reactions are no longer so effective in altering limb posture but contact stimulation of the dorsum of the hand can inhibit the grasp reflex.

D. *Sixteen to 40 Weeks*

Digital independence, fractionation of the grasp reflex.

The grasp reflex itself undergoes progressive modification. During this period, if the contact stimulus is limited to the volar surface of one finger, that finger will flex alone, Fig. 2c. This fractionation of the grasp reflex can first be obtained in the index finger. Later, isolated flexion of the other digits can also be elicited by similar limited application of the stimulus.

E. *Sixteen to 36 Weeks*

Orientation of hand to contact stimulus, beginning of instinctive grasp reaction.

The next stage in the evolution of the automatic grasping responses is supination of the hand towards a light contact stimulus to the radial part of the hand, Fig. 3a. Some time later, stimulation of the ulnar part of the hand produces a corresponding pronation towards the stimulus. These orienting reactions become more and more facile during the next 4 to 8 weeks and are further modified to become part of a still more complex reaction.

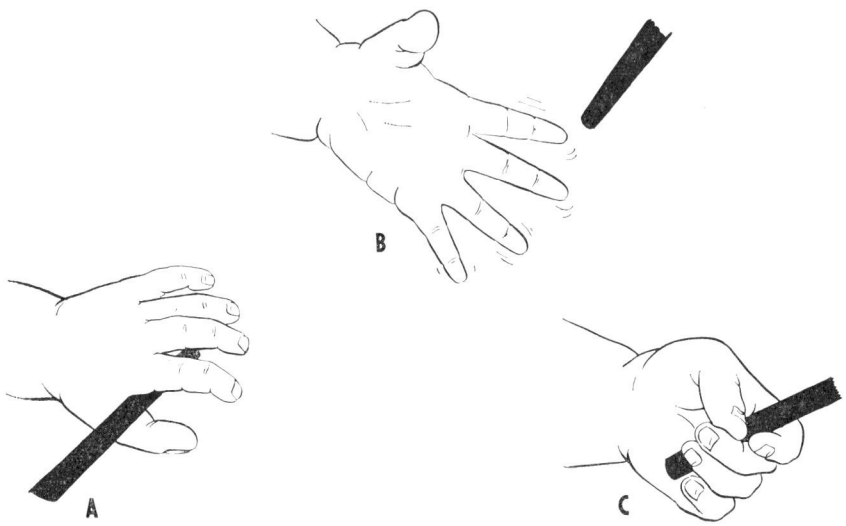

FIG. 3. The instinctive grasp reaction: (a) orientation, (b) groping, (c) final grasp.

F. *Twenty to 44 Weeks*

Exteroceptive dominance, final development of the instinctive grasp reaction.

Three to 4 weeks after the onset of orientation, contact stimulation of the radial or ulnar border of the hand elicits not only supination or pronation but also a slight palpating movement toward the stimulus as it is withdrawn (Fig. 3B). This contactual groping becomes more potent during the next few weeks. Eventually the hand not only gropes after a retreating contact stimulus but also adjusts to it and finally the finger closes around the stimulating object with a powerful grasp (trap reaction) (Fig. 3C). This documents complete development of the instinctive grasp reaction, the most complex of the automatic grasping reactions.

The instinctive grasp reaction initially can be obtained only from stimulation of the radial border of the hand. Within 2 to 3 weeks, stimulation of the ulnar border will also elicit the reaction. However, the hand then readjusts to grasp from the radial side.

The adequate stimulus for the instinctive grasp reaction when completely developed is a light stationary or moving contact to any part of the hand. It is to be emphasized that all of these groping and grasping reactions are obtained without the aid of vision.

Although the grasp reflex itself can be obtained while the instinctive grasp reaction is evolving, it becomes more capricious and difficult to elicit during the latter months of the first year of life. Some fragment of instinctive grasping in the form of slight flexion movements of the fingers following the adequate contact stimulus may normally persist throughout childhood into adult life.

II. AVOIDING REACTIONS

Contact stimulation of the hand can also elicit withdrawal or avoiding responses during infancy. Indeed, in the neonate the only response to a light contact stimulus is a slight withdrawl consisting of dorsiflexion and abduction of the fingers, Fig. 4. This withdrawal (avoiding) response is easier to elicit between 3 and 8 weeks of age. Now the fingers not only abduct and dorsiflex more widely, but the hand also pronates and the arm flexes to withdraw the hand from the stimulus. The avoiding response requires a lighter contact stimulus than the grasp reflex.

Between 12 and 20 weeks of age the avoiding response begins to show local signature. Now contact stimulation to the ulnar border of

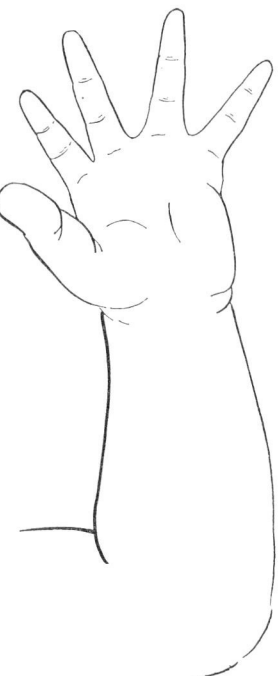

FIG. 4. Avoiding response.

the hand evokes pronation and adduction away from the stimulus; later, stimulation of the radial side of the hand produces supination and abduction. Within a few weeks, flexion or extension movements are added so that the hand begins to "avoid" contact with the stimulus rather than just "withdraw".

The instinctive avoiding reaction is fully developed by 24 to 40 weeks of age. Now light contact stimulation causes the hand in fact to avoid the stimulus by any number of adroit manoeuvres of flexion, extension, abduction, adduction, rotation, etc. One can actually "chase" the hand with a contact stimulus. As with the grasping automatisms described above, the avoiding reactions require only contact stimulation and do not depend on visual guidance.

Avoiding reactions are far more easy to elicit in the irritable infant when they dominate all activity and prevent elicitation of any of the grasping automatisms. Avoiding reactions normally may contaminate posture and movement through early childhood. A fragment of the instinctive avoiding reaction in the form of slight dorsiflexion of the fingers following their contact stimulus commonly persists throughout life.

III. THE ROLE OF GRASPING AND AVOIDING REACTIONS

Most studies of the development of prehension have concentrated on the guidance of the hand by vision. However, it is clear that the appearance and integration of the grasping and avoiding automatisms described above play an equally important role in this acquisition. Their importance is emphasized when development in a normal infant is contrasted with that in the infant with a congenital encephalopathy. During maturation these contact avoiding and grasping reactions evolve in overlapping fashion in an orderly sequence and profoundly affect posture and movement each step of the way.

At birth when the traction response dominates the scene, the infant's fingers are usually closed. An object may be placed in the hand at this stage and might be "held" for a second or so by utilization of this reaction. The object can be "held" for a longer time after a few weeks of age when the flexor synergy can be facilitated by contact stimulation of the palm.

By 3 to 8 weeks of age when the avoiding response has become facile, the fingers gradually begin to open more when the infant lies at rest. At this time, even though flexion of the fingers can be facilitated by contact with the palm, an object held in the hand is dropped if it touches the fingertips and activates the avoiding response causing the fingers to abduct and dorsiflex widely. Towards the end of this period, the infant may actively take an object placed in his hand. He begins to be attracted to brightly coloured toys and seems to desire to reach for them. However, there appears to be considerable flexor resistance to overcome (traction response and avoiding).

When the initial component of the grasp reflex appears, the fingers begin to flex and extend alternately, particularly when the baby is excited. This athetosis results from conflict between the opposing grasp reflex and avoiding response. Athetotic movements are common during the first year of life while these reactions are not yet in equilibrium.

Following development of the full grasp reflex, the hand may occasionally swipe at an object. Although the hand may be open at rest, it is frequently fisted during early swiping. The hand appears to be flung at an object and Halverson (1931) likened it to a "paw" at this stage.

This flinging enhances the traction response by stretch of flexor muscles, thus intensifying the flexion of the fingers and producing the fisted hand during these early swiping movements. As the grasp reflex becomes more facile and the flexor synergy effect subsides, the fingers are less flexed when they are projected towards an object. Attempts to reach them also become more and more frequent.

The object is initially approached from above and grasped only on contact with the palm. This initial prehension appears to be more accidental than intentional.

The emergence of the instinctive avoiding response at the time of these early attempts at voluntary prehension causes ataxia of reach and overpronation of the hand. The object is therefore grasped from the ulnar part of the hand. All the fingers close around it together (palmar grasp). The wrist may initially flex too much (final remnant of traction response effect).

Following the appearance of the early orientation phase of the instinctive grasp reaction (supination), the hand adjusts more easily to the object. Grasping is more dexterous and the object is directed to the radial part of the hand. Dexterous prehension is still impossible. A small object is particularly difficult for the infant to handle. He attempts to sweep it into the palm, all the fingers flex together. The required thumb-finger apposition does not appear until the grasp reflex can be fractioned during the second half-year of life.

Dexterous projection of the arm and precise orientation of the hand to an object follow development of the instinctive grasp reaction with its automatic palpating and adjusting response. Even at this stage the instinctive avoiding response can contaminate activity and the fingers may abduct or dorsiflex too much as the hand is extended towards the object.

The infant appears to be less dependent on visual control of prehension once the instinctive grasp reaction has evolved.

IV. DEVELOPMENT OF PREHENSION IN CHILDREN WITH CONGENITAL ENCEPHALOPATHY

The sequence described above is disrupted in infants and children with congenital encephalopathies. Common to their developmental history is a delay in the appearance of voluntary prehension. This almost universal feature among such patients may be surprising in that visual mechanisms appear to be intact, which leads me to inquire into the nature of the delay in prehension. This can be traced to a failure of integration of the reflex substrata described above (Twitchell, 1959).

The sequence of maturation of these reflexes can be derailed at any stage and the form of voluntary prehension which eventually appears is then reminiscent of that appearing in a comparable stage in the normal infant with an important qualification, which is that the residual reactions may hypertrophy and therefore become more exaggerated than their normal counterparts. Certain defects of prehension may be related to the persistence and exaggeration of these reactions.

When none of the grasping automatisms develop, prehension is impossible. Some abortive flexion and extension at proximal joints, based on labyrinthine and neck reflexes, may comprise the only available voluntary movements in the upper extremities.

If only the traction response develops, it may eventually be adapted to enable a crude form of voluntary prehension which, however, is long delayed in its appearance. Visual guidance of the reaction is essential. The hand is extended with difficulty and appears to be thrown at the target. It does not adjust or orient to the shape of the object. As the fingers close, the wrist also flexes thus weakening the grip by interposing a mechanical disadvantage to full flexion of the fingers (Twitchell, 1958).

When the traction response comprises the only substrate for voluntary grasping, the patient cannot flex one finger alone, for this ability normally requires the facilitation by the fractionated grasp reflex. Consequently, he cannot oppose his thumb and finger easily and his manipulation of objects is clumsy. Nevertheless some of these patients can be trained to make isolated movements. This can be accomplished by substituting proprioceptive facilitation for the natural contact, thus facilitating a reaction which has failed to develop (Lauretana et al., 1959). Even when the response is of a milder form, it may cause some ataxia with over-abduction and extension of the fingers as they approach an object. Some weakness of grip has also been attributed to avoiding response effects (Twitchell, 1958).

In the mildest degrees of disequilibrium in the development of these reflex substrata for prehension the defect may only be in terms of a certain clumsiness (Twitchell et al., 1966). The finer adjustments of the hand to an object and the orientation characteristic of the instinctive reactions do not appear. With certain movements some slight over-extension of the fingers, indicating a preponderant avoiding effect, may be the only evidence for imbalance of these reactions.

That a balance between these antagonistic reactions is required in the development of normal prehension is further evidenced by those rare instances in which a grasp reflex unopposed by an avoiding response occurs during maturation. In these cases movement is biased against extension: the fingers remain flexed and do not open enough; an object held is released only with difficulty.

V. DISCUSSION

The relationship between reflex grasping and voluntary prehension is not the simple one generally described. Reflex grasping itself is not a simple entity but comprises three distinct reactions which nevertheless appear to be closely interrelated during the maturation of the human infant.

The simplest reaction is the proprioceptive traction response. This is part of the contact body-righting reflex mechanism and is integrated at the brain stem level (Denny-Brown, 1962). Although the fingers flex simultaneously in this synergistic flexion response, isolated finger flexion can be obtained by proprioceptive facilitation (Lauretana *et al.*, 1959). Consequently, it may be assumed that the mechanism for isolated finger flexion is integrated at a brain stem level. However, it normally requires the contactual triggering of the grasp reflex for its elicitation.

With the appearance of the grasp reflex, the arm is freed from the constraints of the flexor synergy. Proprioceptive reactions now remain latent until triggered by a specific contactual stimulus, the grasp reflex, which when fractionated can facilitate isolated flexion of the fingers. The subcortical grasp reflex mechanism therefore acts as a facilitator of proprioceptive reactions.

Finally, with the appearance of the cortical instinctive grasp reaction, the exteroceptors dominate the scene and facilitate a highly discriminating projected reaction of the hand into the environment. Denny-Brown (1950) has suggested that the trap reaction may be the cortical modification of the grasp reflex and that the link between them may be the higher differentiation of sensory data necessary for the instinctive grasp reaction.

Equally important in the development of prehension is the equilibration of the avoiding responses with the grasping responses. This allows for further adjustment of the hand. The result of a defect in this equilibration is evidenced by the defective prehension of children with congenital encephalopathies.

Nor does voluntary prehension itself suddenly appear as a single entity. Its evolution is gradual and it appears as a further facilitation of the reflex mechanism appropriate for the given stage of development.

Each more complex form of voluntary grasping is anticipated by a more complex reflex substrate. Indeed the elements of any form of voluntary grasping can be obtained "experimentally", as it were, before the infant can adapt it to use, reflecting Carmichael's "principle of anticipatory maturation" (Carmichael, 1954).

The ability to project the hand into space and produce increasingly facile manipulative adjustments follows upon the development of the contact grasping reactions culminating in the development of the instinctive grasp reaction. The effect of disruption of these mechanisms is clear not only from the results of cerebral lesions which impair their activity, but also from the results of de-afferentation, which may selectively abolish them while leaving central nervous system and efferent pathways intact (Twitchell, 1954).

Although it is commonly stated that infantile reflexes disappear during maturation, we have shown that this is an erroneous impression (Twitchell, 1959). Indeed, disequilibrium of these reactions at any point in life can impair motor function.

This is, of course, not the whole story of the development of voluntary prehension, since we have omitted the important role of vision. In this regard Held and his co-workers have recently demonstrated the important role of actively induced movement in the development of visually guided behaviour. Thus, kittens reared in darkness but given passive transport when in light fail to perform tests of visually guided behaviour, while litter mates which were allowed to move actively under equivalent conditions accomplished the task readily (Held and Hein, 1963).

In other experiments it has been shown that the development of accurate visually guided reaching requires prior experience in viewing the limbs. Hein and Held (1967) reported on kittens which were reared without the ability to observe their forelimbs. When tested for visual placing, they could extend the limbs towards a horizontal surface but could not guide their paws accurately to the solid part of an interrupted surface. Thus visual placing could be dissociated into elicited extension which did not require prior viewing of the limbs and guided placing which did.

Held and Bauer (1967) have shown that a monkey raised from infancy without being able to see his hands during the first month of life does not reach accurately when the hand is first exposed. He fixes his gaze on to the novel object (his hand) as it enters into his visual field. He watches the movement of his hands in a manner reminiscent of the human infant during the early stages in the development of reaching (Piaget, 1952). Accurate visual guidance of prehension is then achieved gradually over the next few days.

Held and Bauer have suggested that visually guided reaching requires an integration of visuomotor control of head movement and nonvisual control of limb movement and that the achievement of such integration requires the viewing of the moving hand. The problem then is the "how" of the projection of the hand into the visual field. Some initial transient extensions may result from adaptation of labyrinthine and neck reflexes. We feel certain, however, that the contactual reactions described in this paper play the most important role not only in the projection of the hand but also in its manipulation. In this sense the integrity of these reactions is also an essential "ingredient" in the development of visually guided reaching.

Indeed, these visual and contactual mechanisms may be mutually facilitatory at a very early period of maturation as suggested by some of our studies now in progress. Thus contact and visual stimuli can combine to cause orientation, palpation and grasping at a time long before it can be elicited by either modality alone. This may provide the explanation for the remarkable acceleration of the development of prehension described by White and Held (1966) following visual and contactual enrichment of the infant's environment.

REFERENCES

CARMICHAEL, L. 1954. The phylogenetic development of behavior patterns. In *Proc. Assoc. Res. Nerv. Ment. Dis.* Williams and Wilkins, Baltimore.

DENNY-BROWN, D. 1950. Disintegration of motor function resulting from cerebral lesions. *J. nerv. ment. Dis.* **112**, 1–45.

DENNY-BROWN, D. 1962. The midbrain and motor integration. *Proc. Roy. Soc. Med.* **55**, 527–538.

HALVERSON, H. M. 1931. An experimental study of prehension in infants by means of systematic cinema records. *Genet. Psychol. Monog.* **10**, 107–286.

HEIN, A. and HELD, R. 1967. Dissociation of the visual placing response into elicited and guided components. *Science*, **158**, 390–392.

HELD, R. and BAUER, J. 1967. Visually guided reaching in infant monkeys after restricted rearing. *Science*, **155**, 718–720.

HELD, R. and HEIN, A. 1963. Movement-produced stimulation in the development of visually guided behavior. *J. comp. physiol. Psychol.* **56**, 872–876.

LAURETANA, M. M., PARTAN, D. L. and TWITCHELL, T. E. 1959. Rehabilitation of the upper extremity in infantile spastic hemiparesis. *Amer. J. Occup. Ther.* **13**, 264–267.

PIAGET, J. 1952. *The origins of intelligence in children.* Internat. Univ. Press, New York.

SEYFFARTH, H. and DENNY-BROWN, D. 1948. The grasp reflex and the instinctive grasp reaction. *Brain*, **71**, 109–183.

TWITCHELL, T. E. 1954. Sensory factors in purposive movement. *J. neurophysiol.* **17,** 239–252.
TWITCHELL, T. E. 1958. The grasping deficit in infantile spastic hemiparesis. *Neurology,* **8,** 13–21.
TWITCHELL, T. E. 1959. On the motor deficit in congenital bilateral athetosis. *J. nerv. ment. Dis.* **129,** 105–132.
TWITCHELL, T. E. 1965. The automatic grasping responses of infants. *Neuropsychologia.* **3,** 247–259.
TWITCHELL, T. E., LECOURS, A. R., RUDEL, R. G. and TEUBER, H. L. 1966. Minimal cerebral dysfunction in children: motor deficits. *Trans. Amer. Neurol. Assoc.* **91,** 353–355.
WHITE, B. L. and HELD, R. 1966. Plasticity of sensorimotor development in the human infant. In J. F. Rosenblith and W. Allinsmith (Eds.), *The causes of behavior.* Allyn Bacon, Boston.

Discussion

BRUNER: In talking about the neurological foundations of skill, Paillard uses imagery which comes from some of Guillaume's earlier work on the development of hand skills. He talks about an upper and lower motor neurone pattern, basically these are considered as a keyboard. The keyboard develops certain kinds of sequential patterns, the lower-keyboard which is the midbrain, brainstem, spinal type of thing, and the upper motor-neurone-keyboard which basically is tuned towards the modulation of the lower levels. He goes on to comment that a great many of the patterns which one gets in the lower motor-neurone-keyboard are organized in a form that has an antiphonic property to them. Of course you get responses which are in contrast to each other, like the avoidance response and the grasp response. Modulation in skill then is thought to be brought in from the upper motor-neurone-keyboard. The upper motor-neurone-keyboard develops later with the maturation of cortical centres. Paillard points out of course that you don't just have two of them, you have a whole series of these keyboards. This at least may give us a model to begin with, a way of conceptualizing our problem and it may have consequences from the point of view of predicting the sequence of responses. It is more than simply describing the behaviour; in so far as one can find conflicts, then one can predict that some new patterns are going to come in to resolve these conflicts.

I am very puzzled by the question of the visual guidance of responses. There are, I think, two kinds of visual guidance. One form of visual guidance has to do with guidance from the object towards which the behaviour is being directed, the other form has to do with looking at the hand itself. I am rather doubtful as to whether the subject's looking at his hand can be considered a form of visual guidance. One study carried out in our laboratory involved putting a plastic occluder on to a baby. It was rather difficult to get the baby to accept this but one of my students (James Alt) finally managed it. This meant that the infant could not see the hand on the ipsilateral side unless it came into the mid-field which was defined as $20°$ or so from the mid-line. The question of course was "What would the baby do when objects were placed in the mid-line; would there be any imbalance between which hand the baby would use?" In fact, would the hand ipsilateral to the occluder not be used at all? The results showed that there were no differences. It would appear that the object as such is sufficient to initiate hand operations. Once the baby makes contact with the object and he is looking at his hand, then a tremendous amount of activity is released, both visually guided and non-visually guided. However, to initiate an action towards an object in the visual field does not require perception of the hand. I think a particularly interesting point about this is in comparison with some of White's work (see paper by B. L. White in this volume). In one of his experiments White succeeded in drawing the infant's attention to his hands by putting a very attractive glove on the baby. However, this is not quite the same thing as having to look at the hand whilst the response is being guided, whilst in fact there is directed movement.

I am rather worried by results which have been obtained from shutting off a sense modality; putting a ruff on an animal and then taking an animal back into a normal situation and making inferences from this as to the course of development. My reason is as follows. If you study the literature on the restoration of sight following the removal of cataract, you will be struck by the number of people who simply cannot, after a certain point at about the age of 10 or so, get to use the visual field because they have built up so many response tendencies which do not depend upon the presence of visual information. My point is that when you remove the ruff from an animal (or whatever device is being used to temporarily cut out a sense modality or temporarily prevent the animal perceiving a limb) then it is not just the immediate removal of the deficit that we are looking at, rather a whole train of development which has been built around this deficit. So, in fact, the animal has to suppress a whole set of responses which he would be using without vision. The experiments are, of course, fascinating from a point of view of decomposing the different kinds of pathways into the nervous system, but I am rather dubious about taking them as a reflection of the nature of development as such.

TWITCHELL: What is the mechanism for first getting the hand into the visual field? We have already suggested that neck and labyrinthine reflexes may play a role. However, visual reactions themselves may be involved. In some patients, an object entering the visual field elicits an extension of the hand towards the object (without involving contact with it). If such a reaction occurrred during early development in the infant, it would provide a mechanism for getting the hand into the visual field. We have not looked for these mechanisms in normal infants as yet.

I have been impressed with Hein and Held's (1967, *Science*, **158**, 390) experiments with decomposition of what they call visually elicited extension and visual guidance. This appears to be similar to the relation between the grasp reflex and the instinctive grasp reaction. What they call visually elicited extension is a rather stereotyped reaction like the grasp reflex, and I think that this extension may be a visually triggered labyrinthine response. What they call visually guided reactions, however, are less stereotyped, more highly oriented kinds of reactions similar to the instinctive grasp reaction.

CONNOLLY: In the cat, can you elicit a placing response if you hold it around the torso and move it down towards a surface or just move it down indeed, in an undarkened room? I rather suspect you might.

TWITCHELL: There is a labyrinthine response causing extension of limbs as the animal is moved down in space. There is also the contact placing reaction elicited without visual contact. Hein and Held (1967, *Science*, **158**, 390) have differentiated labyrinthine from visual extension by moving the edge of the surface up to the cat so that the extension is a visually elicited rather than a labyrinthine response.

CONNOLLY: Was the response with the paws the same in both situations?

TWITCHELL: Yes. As far as we can tell you get exactly the same kind of thing.

CONNOLLY: Can you tell us anything about the hand reflexes and their emergence in blind babies? Have you looked at these at all?

TWITCHELL: No, we haven't. Often with blind babies as you know there is also some cerebral lesion. I have not seen very many, but there was one infant with cataracts whose brain function seemed to be pretty good and in whom the contactual reactions did develop at the appropriate period, although unfortunately we could not follow this infant after removal of the cataracts.

HINDE: I want to say just three qualitative things about monkeys. One is that the initial traction response is not in any way crude, it is beautifully adapted for holding on with. Secondly, in the position in which the young monkey lives nearly all the time, when its arms are groping they are nearly always in the mother's fur or face, because it can't really move its arms very much for the first few days of life without being in contact with its mother somewhere. When it is watching its hands, it is watching its hands moving over the surface of its mother's body. The third point is that at about 2 to 3 weeks, this visual reaching is a very characteristic thing, they hold on to the mother with one hand and grope about for objects with the other.

TWITCHELL: I don't believe the infant monkey has a pure traction response. I have examined a few infants and found what we call the grasp reflex present soon after birth. As I pointed out, this allows for more dexterous manipulation. Voluntary grasping based on adaptation of the traction response alone is pretty awkward. This is the kind of situation in either monkey or man with a pyramidal lesion.

HINDE: I thought that Hines (*Contrib. Embryol. Carneg. Inst. Wash.* **30**, 153–209) in her paper described something like this?

TWITCHELL: I think that what Marian Hines described was what we would call the grasp reflex.

BRUNER: Yes, I think she does speak of a "crude form of the grasp reflex".

ABERCROMBIE: May I ask what is perhaps a very naïve question. Some of you may know a great deal about this, but one of the things about visual control which has always puzzled me a great deal is that one of the most sensitive skills is imitating someone else's facial expression and one does not do this under visual control. A baby does this before it looks in a mirror, though I wouldn't like to say just how early it appears. Posture is an interesting one too, where children adopt "the way Daddy walks", "the way Daddy stands". It is rather difficult to imagine that they really know what they look like visually. The thought occurs to me that this might have something to do with Lefford's intersensory integration. I think it is very interesting that the feeding mechanism of human infants is so arranged that babies can watch the mother's face. As soon as the nipple is placed in the mouth, whether it is a bottle or a real nipple, the baby's eyes switch to engage with the mother's eyes. This is interesting in relation to the evolution of feeding because of the thoracic position of the breasts and because also of the fact that they have a great deal of redundant material. The size of the breast is not related to milk producing material and the size is often thought to be a secondary sexual characteristic but it also has the effect of keeping the baby's face sufficiently away from the chest to make it able to see the mother's face. So that at the same time that there are very vigorous feeding movements of the throat and tongue, both of which are essential for later development of speech, it will be able to see its mother's mouth move as the mother talks to him.

HINDE: You could argue that the breast being the size it is provides a reason for the nipple not needing to be as accessible as it is.

INGRAM: Morris (*The naked ape*. Weidenfeld and Nicolson, London, 1967) has suggested that breasts are just a substitute for big buttocks.

ABERCROMBIE: I don't think there is any reason to suppose that it is just one thing or only the other but it is a jolly convenient arrangement for the baby if it really matters that he sees the mother's face. When you think of the position that calves or piglets have, the last thing they can see is the mother's face.

CONNOLLY: I think it important to remember here that there are other ways than simply vision that children and adults use to establish motor control. Auditory feedback may be used to establish very skilful responses. Vision is a predominant modality but it isn't the only one which can be linked with proprioception and kinaesthesis. Blind children can make controlled movements and blind children are not late in speaking, if they are of average intelligence.

INGRAM: In cortical lesions causing hemiplegia with complicating athetosis, what is the pattern of finger movements?

TWITCHELL: The patient himself is usually unable to produce an isolated movement at all; he gets only a crude movement, flexion or extension of all the fingers together.

INGRAM: And doesn't it initiate the second finger use?

TWITCHELL: Maybe the first finger. Some of the patients do have what we call the initial component of a grasp reflex so that they are able to some extent, to employ a crude thumb-finger opposition.

PRECHTL: Providing the baby is in the right state, which is quiet and awake, and you play with a pin you can actually get single fingers stretched or flexed or you can get an adduction of the fist. When you give massive stimulation they always go together.

TWITCHELL: It seems to me that what you are describing may be a series of local reactions, but certainly they are integrated at still lower levels.

CONNOLLY: As you describe the spatial contactual response in the instinctive grasp reaction, once a child has got to the third stage can you still elicit the previous kind of reaction, can you still elicit the traction and can you still elicit the grasp reflex?

TWITCHELL: One can elicit some of the traction response at around five months but it isn't very easy. However, it is possible to elicit a grasp reflex in any of us here. It requires that the individual's attention be diverted in some way. It may be more easily elicited after mild sedation. Under natural conditions you usually elicit just a fragment of the avoiding or grasping reaction, the finger tips may slightly dorsiflex or slightly palmarflex.

PRECHTL: I am a little worried that we are inferring too much from adult pathology to the normal course of development. Things look similar but they are not really comparable.

TWITCHELL: It seems to me that at both stages you can give the same adequate stimulus, and get the same response. What you see in the adult, however, is this complicating factor which we call release. The adult response is always more exaggerated and sometimes tonically sustained.

CONNOLLY: How often do these responses, such as the grasp reflex, occur spontaneously? From watching babies I would say that the fisting which you describe is present at 3 or 4 days of age. The athetoid movements of the fingers similarly are frequently observed. Now, if you do look at a child of about 2 months of age do you see these things happening when you are not stimulating him?

TWITCHELL: Sure.

CONNOLLY: Frequently?

TWITCHELL: Now, when you say "happening" I'm not quite sure what you mean.

CONNOLLY: Do you see the infant making the grasp reflex occasionally?

TWITCHELL: I wouldn't say that the infant makes the grasp reflex without the adequate stimulus. I would say that the fingers may close but I cannot say that this is related to a reflex rather than some other mechanism.

CONNOLLY: Yes, this is the point about a reflex, it is necessary to have an input to elicit the reflex. But can you, in fact, distinguish the spontaneous response?

TWITCHELL: Yes, I think so. The responses are quite different. In the grasp reflex (as we use the term) the fingers actually flex with a quick snapping movement following the adequate contact stimulus. On the other hand, you can put your finger in a baby's hand and he might make spontaneous opening and closing movements. These are slower and

more deliberate, and one has to search further for their physiologic nature.
BRUNER: Visually-guided reaching begins, that is when the widespread banana-type hand goes out for an object, after the swiping stage. Where does it come from? Is it related to the reflex substrata in any way, this wide stretched kind of hand?
TWITCHELL: That is a posture which we have always related to an exaggeration of the avoiding reaction.
BRUNER: You think of it then as a hyper-avoiding reaction?
TWITCHELL: This is not an easy problem at all. You see, the grasping and avoiding reactions are unfolding together during maturation and at this time are in unstable equilibrium. This instability is really the basis for athetosis. During this period of disequilibrium of responses, overextension (dorsiflexion) of the fingers may occur as the hand is extended towards an object.
BRUNER: Even when they have overcome it, in the sense that they are reaching for an object, do you think of it as a hyper-avoidance posture of the hand?
TWITCHELL: Yes, what you see here is a fragment of the avoiding reaction producing the wide extension and abduction of the fingers as the hand reaches towards an object. This is seen especially during the early stages of development of voluntary reaching and it becomes less prominent as avoiding reactions and their antagonistic groping reactions become equilibrated. I would also add, however, that during the latter part of the first year of life, some opening of the hand is certainly related to the emerging instinctive grasp reaction with its highly tuned palpatory mechanism. However, during the early years of life one continues to see some evidence of partial disequilibrium of these responses when the fingers occasionally open too widely in approach to a small object.
WHITE: I think there is probably a semantic problem here. To call something "avoidance" may be a good way of assigning a label to a particular pattern which has its own integrity, but it need not always serve a withdrawal or going-away function.
TWITCHELL: In a sense, that is true; however, I might point out that, when the fingers extend and abduct too much in approach to an object, there is indeed some partial avoidance in terms of too much dorsiflexion of the fingers in relation to the object.
BRUNER: May I just get this clear? In a sense what you can say is that a particular pattern, or whatever we choose to call it, has become detached from its original function and is now being slipped into new functions, in a way serving reaching rather than avoiding. It seems a curious way to look at things.

TWITCHELL: I agree that there may be a semantic problem here; however, it is not a problem of "either" "or". I do not imply that the avoiding response is actually serving a reaching function. It is contaminating reaching. What we are concerned with here is only a fragment of the complete avoiding reaction. One might call it distal avoiding. You see, there are various degrees of exaggeration of the response. When the avoiding reaction is very exaggerated in patients with brain disease, it may be impossible for the patient to project the limb towards an object at all and any attempt only causes the limb to remain or to fly into increased flexion. When the reaction is less exaggerated, however, some extra dorsiflexion of the fingers alone as the hand nears the object may appear as the only evidence for abnormal enhancement of the response. I think this is the case with the young infant as he develops prehension. As his hand approaches the object, his fingers are dorsiflexed too much, their posture in relation to the object is one of physiological withdrawal-avoidance. Incidentally, in children and adults who have an exaggerated form of the reaction because of cerebral disease, there is also slowness in projecting the hand towards an object. We don't know whether this might also be the case in early infancy.

INGRAM: I find great difficulty in eliciting the avoiding reaction. Obviously I have been using the wrong stimuli or perhaps the wrong baby. What I get again and again are flexion responses even from the ulnar border of the hand. Are you going to call this an avoiding response? I thought the avoidance response would involve the whole limb, elbow and shoulder.

TWITCHELL: The problem may be in your stimulus. Elicitation of an avoiding reaction requires a very light distally moving contact stimulus particularly to the ulnar part of the hand, and as I have been trying to point out here, one need not produce flexion withdrawl of the whole limb. One may elicit only slight withdrawal of the fingers and this may constitute a fragmentary distal avoiding reaction.

INGRAM: Are you prepared to call extension of the wrist avoiding?

TWITCHELL: There may be a problem here in the different ways in which the anatomist and the physiologist use the terms flexion and extension. Extension or dorsiflexion of the wrist is physiological flexion and may constitute an avoiding response if it tends to withdraw the distal part of the hand from the stimulus.

The Reflex Substrata of Voluntary Activity

GENERAL DISCUSSION

Reflexes of the Hand

CONNOLLY: There are I believe certain differences between the interpretations which Prechtl places on various reflexes of the hand (whether they are specific to the hand or whether they are part of a more generalized response system) and those which Twitchell makes. I wonder if you would care to comment on this.

PRECHTL: The palmar grasp response in the newborn infant is elicited by tactile stimulation of the infant's palm. We elicit this response by putting the index finger into the infant's hand from the ulnar side and then pressing gently against the palmar surface. No traction is applied. The response is considered to be positive if the infant's fingers flex around the examiner's index finger. The response is only positive when the baby is awake and quiet. While the response is negative in sleeping infants it is exaggerated during sucking (Lenard, von Bernuth, Prechtl, 1968, *Acta Paediat. Scand.* **57**, 177). Besides this state dependency there is also an effect of head position on the intensity of the response. When the response is elicited simultaneously bilaterally (Fig. 1) the head must be centred in the midline otherwise the grasp response is increased on the side to which the face is turned. This may be due to the hand-mouth co-ordination. It is also important not to stimulate the dorsum of the hand when the response is elicited. Stimulation of the dorsum alone leads to an extension of the fingers (Fig. 2). There is a certain individual inconsistency throughout the first 9 days, as shown by Beintema (1968, *A neurological study of newborn infants*, S.I.M.P., London). As an overall tendency there is an increase in intensity from the first to the ninth day.

If passive traction is applied on the arms the situation becomes somewhat complicated. When for instance the Moro response is elicited by the head-drop method (Fig. 3) the arms are extended and abducted and the fingers spread. The electromyographic picture of this response on the left hand is illustrated in Fig. 4. If, however, the examiner pulls on the infant's arms at the wrists and the head-drop is then elicited the extensor and abductor activity is converted into the generalized flexion of the arms and the fingers. This can be clearly seen in Fig. 4 at the right hand. It should be stressed, however, that an

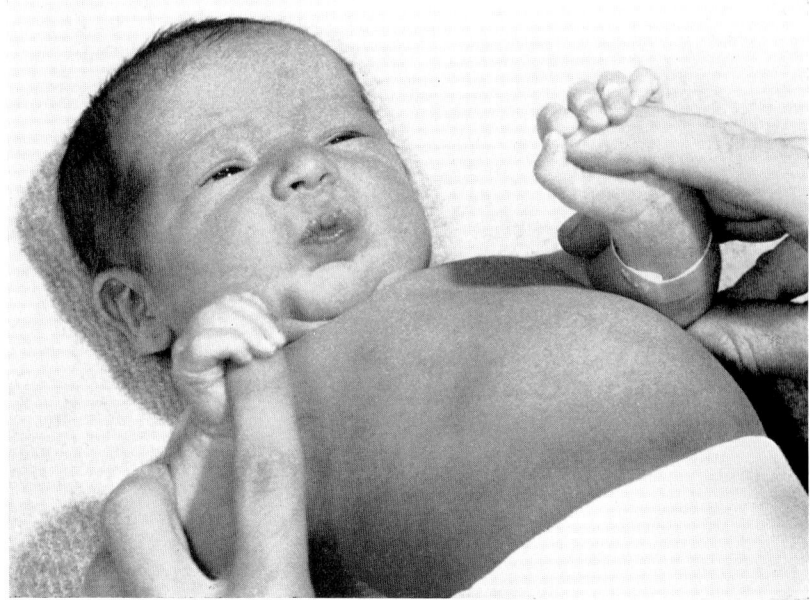

FIG. 1. Bilateral palmar grasp response elicited by tactile stimulation of the palms. Note that no traction on the hands or forearms is applied. The infant is quiet awake, age 5 days (from Prechtl and Beintema, 1964. *The neurological examination of the full-term newborn infant*. S.I.M.P. and Heinemann, London).

elicitation of the grasp response is not necessary to elicit the flexion pattern, but a pull on both wrists is sufficient (Prechtl, 1965, in *Advances in the study of behaviour*, Academic Press, London, Vol. 1, 75).

INGRAM: I think it is quite difficult to elicit the grasp reflex in many newborn babies during the first or second week of life.

WHITE: I agree entirely. It is much easier if the arm is stretched.

TWITCHELL: I took this up in some detail 3 years ago, I think the problem is first of all one of definition. When I wrote my paper on this (1965, *Neuropsychologia*, **3**, 247) there was not a consistent definition of the grasp reflex in the paediatric literature, it was elicited in a number

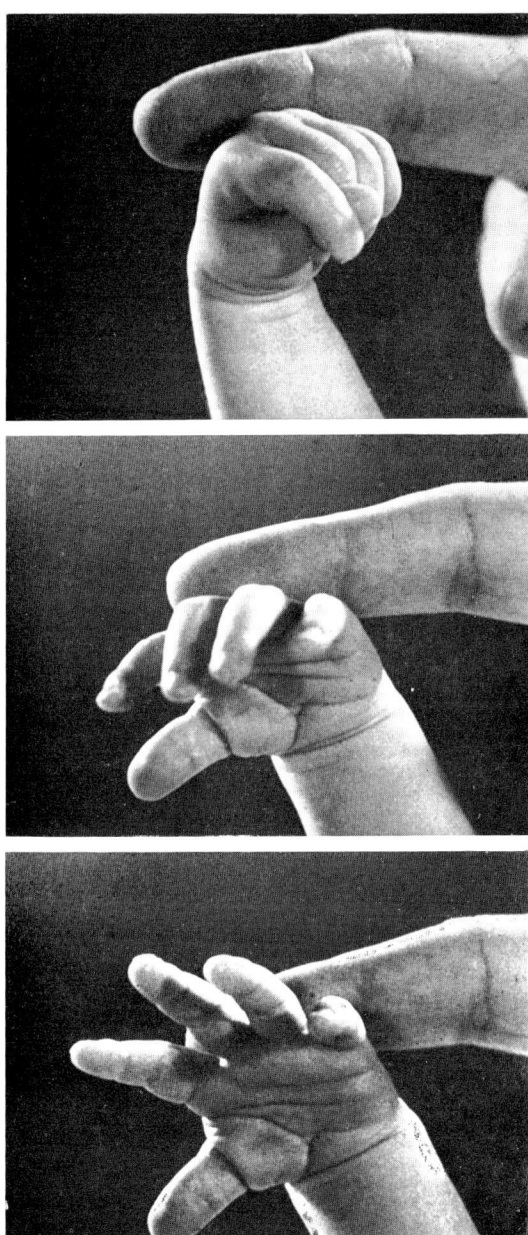

FIG. 2. Tactile stimulation of the dorsum of the hand elicits opening of the hand. Newborn, 8 days, frames from cine-film.

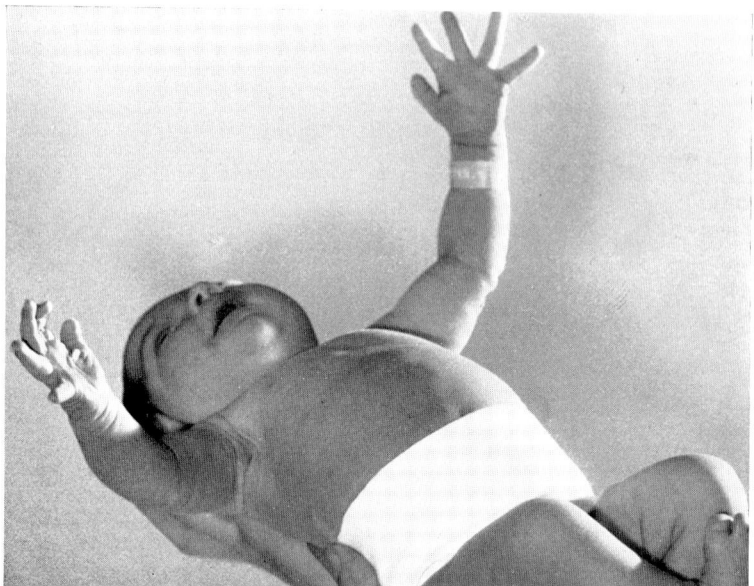

FIG. 3. Moro response elicited by head drop (from Prechtl and Beintema, 1964, *The neurological examination of the full-term newborn infant*. S.I.M.P. and Heinemann, London).

of different ways. I am sure you will agree, Prechtl, that the vast majority of paediatricians do not elicit the grasp reflex in the same way that you do. The grasp reflex as we define it is not influenced at all by the position of the head in relation to the body. This suggests to me that we have two quite different responses. I take your point that what you are calling the grasp reflex is a purely local response to contact stimulation. I have been wary of this because it seems to me extremely difficult in the infant's hand to limit the stimulus to a purely contactual one. If the stimulus to the palm is a very light one, the only response is adduction, and dorsiflexion of the fingers. I suspect that most people attempting to elicit this response also apply a good deal of proprioceptive stimulation, therefore eliciting what we call the traction response.

INGRAM: May I reiterate that during the first 2 weeks of life I find it difficult to elicit a true grasp reflex, whereas in prematures one can nearly always get it.

TWITCHELL: In prematures you can not obtain grasp reflexes as I have described them. The grasp reflex is not just the closure of fingers but rather the dual reaction—it is the snap of the fingers (closing phase), and then the proprioceptive hold. I do not think you get this,

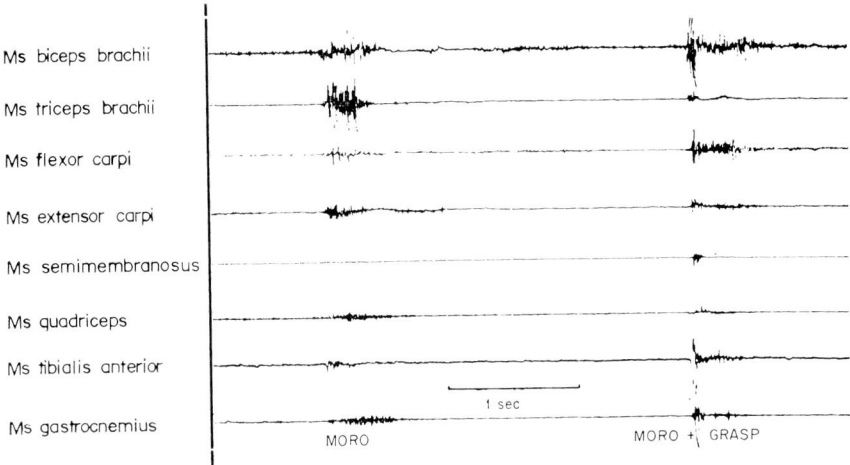

FIG. 4. Electromyogram of arm and leg muscles. At "Moro" on the left side of the recording, a head drop was carried out with the baby's arms free. At "Moro+grasp", a head drop was applied when the baby grasped the examiner's fingers and mild traction was applied in upward direction. The recording shows the shift in activity from extensor muscles (left) to flexor muscles (right). Age 6 days (from Prechtl, 1965. Problems of behavioral studies in the newborn infant. In *Advances in the Study of Behavior*, Vol. 1, Academic Press, London).

certainly I have never seen it in prematures. You can however, get a traction response in the premature.

INGRAM: I agree with you, though I would say that you get closure of the fingers in prematures.

BRUNER: Prechtl, do you have any interpretation which differs from that of Twitchell on the issue of the fractionation of responses? How do you see the fractionation pattern with the middle finger? Can you take the story a little further?

PRECHTL: I think our type of grasp response is very similar to what Vlach, V. (1968, In *Studies in infancy*, R. MacKeith and M. Bax (Eds.), S.I.M.P., London) described as a group of tonic exteroceptive reflexes which can be elicited over many joints.

BRUNER: Can you get some fine grain responses that come at that level from exteroceptive stimuli?

PRECHTL: Yes, certainly.

TWITCHELL: I am intrigued by these local responses of Vlach. When do they disappear and when is it difficult to elicit them?

PRECHTL: They disappear after several weeks, but there are obviously great individual differences. To my knowledge no systematic studies have been carried out on this topic so far.

Reflex to Voluntary Control

BRUNER: I want to come back to the general topic. We started out by talking about the reflex substrata of voluntary behaviour in general and we got down to the level of the property of individual responses Now the question is, how do they come under control so that they may be described as voluntary behaviour?

WHITE: In the case of voluntary reaching is it not clear that self-stimulation is involved, aside that is from the visual input, and that the general effect is such as to override these discrete and delicate kinds of stimulation.

BRUNER: That is an interesting hypothesis certainly, but self-stimulation means what?

WHITE: Considering voluntary reaching in the early stages, is it not the case that there is so much more affecting what happens to the child's fingers than the highly specialized individuated stimuli which emerged during the course of a neurological examination?

PRECHTL: This is certainly the impression I had. In the early weeks when voluntary, guided movements begin to appear it is very difficult to elicit the other smaller components.

BRUNER: Well suppose we exaggerate the position which you are putting forward; let us call it a question of the amount of stimulation which comes from the action itself. It becomes a question of feedback. The other suggestion is that there is a more centrally organized conception, that there is something like a kind of Bernstein (1967, *The co-ordination and regulation of movement*, Pergamon Press, London) overt reafference pattern which hinders some central segment; this then is involved in bringing the response under control. These two suggestions are not mutually exclusive.

INGRAM: Are we not trying to define different levels?

CONNOLLY: I do not think that we should jump too quickly to talking of levels, the trouble with that approach is that we do not know what goes on at each level. So far we have two alternatives. One is that under conditions of voluntary action there is suppression of more discrete movements because of the feedback from the action itself and the second is Bruner's suggestion of a central segment. I wonder if this central segment might in fact develop from the sensory feedback?

PRECHTL: Am I right in thinking that during the first 2 weeks one cannot elicit flexion of the fingers? I am not talking about the grasp reflex, but flexion of the fingers if they are touched near the tips when the hand is open. Now, at 3 to 4 months when the baby is reaching for an object we see a movement which is quite smooth until certain corrections begin to appear when the hand is close to the object. Usually the fingers semi-flex and when there is contact with the object the grasp is elicited. The reaching movement is therefore visually guided and is under voluntary control because we can see the corrections being applied as the movement approaches the terminal point but the actual grasp itself is still tactually triggered. It is in fact still a little like the reflex.

BRUNER: It is very object oriented in the sense that there are correction movements.

PRECHTL: My point is that we can break down this response into quite different components; the visually guided reaching response and the grasp component. The latter is probably a reflex component because of the tactually elicited flexion of the fingers.

BRUNER: A pattern seems to come bursting out and then be subject to correction. So that what starts off to be purposive or object oriented, and what shapes the response subsequently represent two aspects of the problem. Somehow everything, including the original response, seems to be shaped by the environment.

WHITE: At about the $2\frac{1}{2}$ month stage you very commonly see, in response either to mid-line, or right, or left presentation of an attractive object, both hands going up and staying up. This bilateral hand raising is very much like the visually elicited response that Hein and Held (1967, *Science*, **158,** 390) talked about in the cat. There are many forms of this and Prechtl described an interesting one; when the hands are thrown out, there is no anticipatory grasping but once the tips of the fingers touch then a tactually triggered grasp occurs.

BRUNER: One thing which I am struck by is that occasionally, on contact and when the baby is not looking at the object, there is something which looks like Twitchell's groping response embedded in the sequence.

WHITE: Yes, absolutely.

INGRAM: It seems to me that what you are talking about, whether you like the word or not, are certain levels or neurological hierarchies.

CONNOLLY: What are neurological hierarchies?

INGRAM: Patterns which are progressively precise in their aim and purpose.

CONNOLLY: I am afraid that I do not understand.

INGRAM: The child becomes more and more able to subordinate his original reflex behaviour and his voluntary movement improves progressively with this ability to subordinate the reflex activity. I think that what you are describing in these various stages of reaching amounts to this, and for the purposes of description I think we have to think in terms of levels.

PRECHTL: I am averse to all these levels. Let me take a rather oversimplified model of the system. If we think of it as a network, then the network of the young infant is far less complex because there are fewer connections. Now, as the complexity of the network is increased the output becomes more stable. In the early stages there is an imperative character about the response, when the stimulus occurs there is immediately an output, later when the system has become stable the output may not follow. There is the possibility to grasp or not to grasp, because we have got an increase in the degrees of freedom, so to speak. This is perhaps simply due to the increase in stability which follows from increasing complexity.

Anticipatory Grasping and Visual Guidance

CONNOLLY: I think Prechtl's formulation makes more sense since to talk of levels is nothing more than description. I wonder if we can relate these points back to Lefford's paper? What is finally described as "reach and grasp" is visually guided but there is no anticipatory grasp, as soon as the fingers are touched then the grasp appears. If we look a little later we can see an anticipatory grasp.
WHITE: I have an objection to this, the business of raising the hand up does not seem to be visually guided, it appears to be visually elicited. The visual guidance comes in when a child notes his hand near the object, I do not think the initial steps are visually guided.
CONNOLLY: What we have not yet done is to make a shift from the tactile elicitation of the grasp to the presumably visual elicitation which must be occurring when an anticipatory grasp is observed. The problem is to know what triggers the anticipatory grasp, precisely that is. Can we begin to think about the mechanisms here in terms of certain transforms being established? From a cybernetic standpoint we could talk about the increasing complexity of networks, but what Lefford was talking about, the integration of different sensory modalities, has also got something to do with this and it might provide a useful approach to the problem.
WHITE: May I throw something else in rather quickly. At a considerably earlier point the child does show a visually guided approach—the swipe response, it is very common and often very accurate.
BRUNER: This is puzzling because it is often much more accurate than it ought to be according to anyone's theory of the formation of spatial schemata.
WHITE: Yes. You get a rather peculiar system if you concentrate on

this two step prehension response. It is here that the visual input tends to assume a guiding role and an initiating role for the actual prehension. The swiping response does not occur all over the place, it occurs most commonly with a fist and the tonic-neck-reflex is involved.

CONNOLLY: Why the tonic-neck-reflex?

WHITE: Because this is the posture which the child is lying in. The child is lying with his head oriented usually about 60° to the right or left. The point I am making is that there is an interesting correlation of all these things.

BRUNER: The genesis of the swiping response may take several forms. As you know we work with children in the upright position and therefore the child has to raise his limbs. Usually before a swiping response occurs there is a general elevation of body tonus, a sort of "pumping up", and immediately following this, out comes a swipe.

WHITE: How is the stimulus presented?

BRUNER: In the mid-line position.

PRECHTL: I think a very important issue is coming in here, namely that of body posture. Cortico-spinal motor activity only makes sense if it is superimposed on a preceding body posture. You have brought your babies into a much more suitable condition by tilting them just a little. I think this means that you are dealing with much more aroused babies because of their vestibular and proprioceptive feedback, which keeps them awake.

BRUNER: But note the fact that babies in both conditions seem able to mount this visually guided swipe. Don't press me too hard on what I mean by "visually guided" here because it is not visually guided in the fine sense. However, I do not think we should lose the point that Prechtl is making, namely that the tonic framework in which this response occurs is very important.

PRECHTL: Does the vertical position facilitate the swiping? Vestibular input may be important.

BRUNER: I am afraid that I cannot answer that but certainly the eye movement patterns which we get differ depending upon whether the baby is propped up or lying down.

CONNOLLY: May I ask for more information? It has been said that the grasp at one stage is triggered by tactile stimulation and then at a later point that the child will anticipate this. Can you tell us more about how this transition is made?

WHITE: How it is made?

CONNOLLY: Yes, I mean behaviourally, I am not asking you what is going on physiologically.

WHITE: I can tell you something else which may intrigue you. You do not have to have the tactually triggered reaching before the voluntary, smooth, mature form comes in. Babies reared under our enrichment programme skipped this step.

CONNOLLY: Which step?

WHITE: The step where the hand comes up first followed by an approach with no change in the finger position of any consequence, until there is contact. This as opposed to the more mature grasp. Presumably the babies have accelerated the process markedly and therefore this step does not occur.

CONNOLLY: Can you say it does not occur or is it that you have not yet looked for it in sufficient detail?

WHITE: We have looked.

BRUNER: It may come in the form of some other activity which somehow practices this by transfer.

WHITE: I can give you some summary data. The term we use for this is a "Piaget type reach", because Piaget described it clearly. The time of onset of this with our control babies was approximately 125 days, the onset of the "top level reach", was about 145 days, approximately 3 weeks later. In the case of the babies from both enrichment groups the onset for the two behaviour patterns was reversed. The central tendency for the emergence of the mature reach response occurred in the final enrichment sample, at about 87 or 89 days. In the same sample the "Piaget type reach" occurred in only eight out of 13 babies. It indicates to me that this is not an essential step in the process.

CONNOLLY: I do not want to say that it is an essential step, just that it is a usual step.

WHITE: Yes, but that word "usual" worries me.

CONNOLLY: Well, that it is a frequently observed step, if you like; I am not implying anything by choosing that word.

WHITE: It is quite common.

CONNOLLY: I would still like to know something about the transition from the tactually elicited grasp to the anticipatory one. Your data has shown already that it did not come in that sequence but it can. What brings about the change?

LEFFORD: There appears to be a body of responses which are somehow evoked when there is stimulation of the body surface or the inner ear. In the case of the anticipatory grasp you started to describe a different kind of response where a different receptor evokes the action. It is not immediately clear just what the action is, and whether it is directly related to the source of stimulation. However, sooner or later it appears to become related to that source of stimulation.

WHITE: These reactions are all very rapid upon presentation of the stimulus, there is no lag of any kind.

LEFFORD: No, I mean in terms of the spatial directions for the arm.

WHITE: Yes, I see.

LEFFORD: So there do seem to be two sets of responses here, but I remain puzzled as to which would lead. As far as I can see it is vision that will lead even if there is kinaesthetic feedback.

TWITCHELL: How much of this early behaviour, White, is stimulus driven? Does the visual target produce it, is it in fact a visually elicited response?

WHITE: Yes, certainly.

HINDE: In a visually guided response there is a continuous feedback loop which guides the particular response on to the target. If you are learning to play darts you have an open system and each response is corrected only in terms of the previous one.

BRUNER: I agree that the question of error signals is an important one; indeed I think it is central and critical to the behaviour which we speak of as voluntary.

The Neurological Substrate

PRECHTL: There is certainly something happening at a certain point in the movement, in the contralateral motor cortex, that is. It is a great puzzle, what is firing those motor cortex neurones?

TWITCHELL: This, of course, brings up the problem of what the motor cortex does. If you ablate frontal, parietal and temporal cortex leaving only the sensory motor area then the monkey's ability is profoundly affected. The strange thing is that if you ablate the motor cortex he recovers a remarkable repertoire of movement. The animal appears very dexterous in the cage, and he is particularly dexterous if you are after him with a net. He jumps around and climbs hand over hand. However, in other ways he is not dexterous and small, delicate adjusting movements are lacking. The interesting thing is that if you take out the frontal, parietal and temporal cortex and leave the sensory motor area he cannot perform these delicate adjustments either.

If we are trying to trace down voluntary movement perhaps I could describe another curious little phenomenon. If you knock out the hemisphere, say on the left side, down to the superior colliculus then a profound spastic hemiparesis of the opposite side results (Fig. 5). The grasp reflex is abolished, instinctive grasping is abolished and

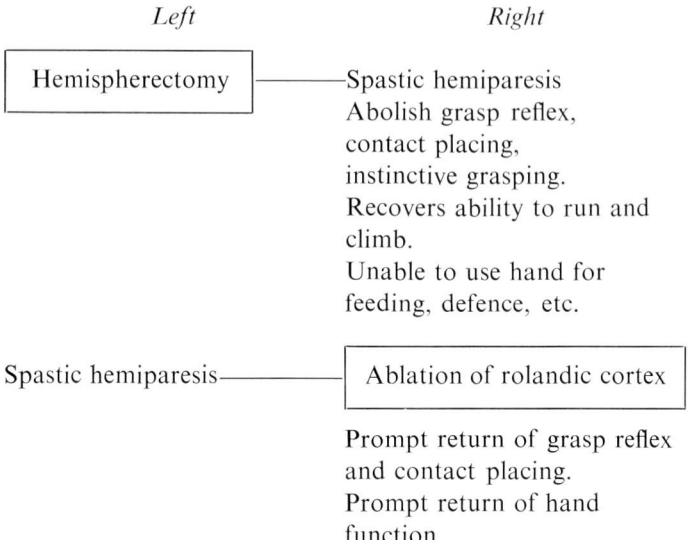

FIG. 5. Effect of hemispherectomy on hand function of a monkey.

contact placing is abolished. However, the animal recovers a remarkable ability, he can run, and climb hand over hand but he is unable to use that hand alone. If his "good hand", so called, is restrained then it is not possible to get the animal to reach out with the hemiparetic hand. Whenever he reaches out it is part of an associated movement of the other side. Now, if the motor cortex is ablated from the intact hemisphere there is an immediate return of the grasp reflex, and of contact placing on the side opposite the hemispherectomy, as well as a return of dexterous hand function, so that he will now use that hand for feeding, grooming, defence, etc.

CONNOLLY: Did you ablate the whole left hemisphere leaving only the midbrain?
TWITCHELL: Yes.
CONNOLLY: And then the whole motor cortex of the other hemisphere?
TWITCHELL: Yes.
CONNOLLY: And the responses come back entirely?
TWITCHELL: Yes they all come back. Interestingly enough some of the things that come back are what physiologists have called for a long time cortical. For years they have talked about placing reactions as a test of the integrity of the sensory motor cortex and we have not attempted to chase these things down any further. Many of the deficits

that we see have been related to what was removed but clearly we should think also of what is left in, there is certainly a balancing up between many reactions. I think it is the upset and imbalance within the hemisphere and between hemispheres that contribute to many of the deficits which we see. One of the things which this suggests to me is that in the course of the development of the infant and the young child the balance existing between a number of mechanisms may be of crucial importance. The emergence of new responses may reflect changes in this balance.

Problems of Explanation

LEFFORD: I am impressed with the actions and the way in which the arm is drawn to a visual stimulus. Would it be entirely out of the question to consider this visually elicited behaviour as an instinctive response?

WHITE: What are we prepared to consider as an explanation when we talk about innate connections between these centres?

HINDE: There is a difficulty with this sort of argument which is that usually one is just pushing the explanation back a stage. Unless there is an independent means of confirmation then it is not very useful.

CONNOLLY: In many higher organisms it seems frequently to be the case that environmental factors are necessary to make certain "pre-wired" patterns function. A certain amount of neural programming, probably specified genetically, exists and stimulation from the environment serves to bring it into operation.

KAY: I have listened with great interest to this discussion and I feel that we are back on the problem which Bruner raised in his paper; namely, that here is one piece of behaviour which a few months later has become an entirely different kind of behaviour. Now why is this later behaviour so different from the other? How did this stage of development come about? What has impressed me, listening to the descriptions, is the extensive repertoire of responses that a baby has. These responses are activated again and again, and as I see it the variability seems to increase as they are practised. I am aware that it is curious to use the term practice in the context of a reflex response but at the moment I cannot think of a better term. You have demonstrated very clearly the initial reflexes and shown us some of the variable voluntary responses which take place a few months later. Our problem is that of fitting the two of them together. But we are none too clear about our units of behaviour.

Infancy: the Emergence of Skill

The Growth and Structure of Skill

JEROME S. BRUNER

Center for Cognitive Studies, Harvard University

I. INTRODUCTION

I SHOULD LIKE to explore in this paper what it is that may be species-specific about human sensorimotor skill. My eventual hope is to understand how human skill eventuates in human tool use. Lest the discussion become too abstruse, I should like to concentrate upon a few manifestations of skill which develop during the first 18 months of life, all of them studied or in the process of being studied in our laboratory at Harvard. You will forgive me this geocentrism, for it is necessary in this case. There is simply no adequate literature on skill development in infancy, and such as there is tends in the main to be concerned with the achievement of norms rather than with the close description of behaviour, whether a norm is achieved or not.[1]

The skills in question are all pathetically simple, and in all but one case they involve the use of the hand or hands under visual guidance. The exception deals with skill in following an object with the head-eye system as it appears in a regular sequence in one or another of two windows directly before the infant. The hand skills are these:

1. Taking possession of several objects handed successively at the midline: *control of multiple objects*.
2. Raising a weighted sliding transparent lid and removing a desirable toy: *complementary use of the hands*.
3. Reaching for an object that has been placed behind a barrier screen: *detour reaching*.
4. Holding a gross object so that a fine object attached to it can be taken: *differentiation of power and precision grips*.

[1] I am greatly indebted for assistance and advice in this work on skill to Kenneth Kaye, Karlen Lyons, Lucy Lyons, Scott Present, Judy Simenson, and Derry Watkins. My former colleague, Dr. Colwyn Trevarthen, helped me enormously in the general formulation, though we rarely agreed on details.

I shall, in passing, contrast these clumsily achieved skills with a quite different skill that makes its appearance much earlier and in a highly organized form—*visual scanning*. We have only begun to study scanning and search and the manner in which they are adapted to the changing requirements of manipulation. But though this work is still far from completion, it can suggest hypotheses.[2]

In spite of the early promise of learning theory, we know very little about systems of skilled action that acquire their organization slowly, in contrast to those that have much of it built in from the start. The hands of man are a slow growing system, and it is many years before humans can exhibit the kind of manual intelligence that has distinguished our species from others—the using and making of tools. Indeed, until quite recently, the hands were regarded even by students of primate evolution as of no particular interest. Wood Jones (1917) would have us believe that there was little morphological difference between the monkey hand and that of man, but that the difference was in the function to which they were put by the central nervous system. Yet, as Clark (1959) and Napier (1962) have pointed out, it is the evolutionary direction of morphological change in the hand, from tree shrews through tarsiers through New World monkeys through Old World monkeys to man, that should reveal how the function of the hand has changed and, with it, the nature of the implementation of human intelligence. That change has been steadily in the direction of a very special form of despecialization. The hand is freed from its locomotor function, from its brachiating function, and from such specialized requirements as were answered by claws and by exotic forms of finger pads. Becoming more despecialized in function means becoming more varied in the functions that can be fulfilled. Without losing its capacity for phalangeal divergence needed for weight bearing, convergence for cupping food, prehensility for holding and climbing, or opposability—all part of an early primate heritage—the hand in later primate evolution achieves several new functional capacities while undergoing appropriate morphological change as well. A combined capacity for power and precision grip is added. The flexibility of palm and thumb increases through changes in the hamate and trapezium bones and their articulation. The thumb lengthens and its resting angle to the hand increases. The terminal phalanges broaden and strengthen, particularly the thumb. Napier may exaggerate when he says (1962, p. 62), "The present evidence suggests that the stone implements of early man were as good

---

[2] This work is being conducted in one context by Dr. Alastair Mundy-Castle and Mr. Jeremy Anglin, and in another by Drs. Eric Aronson and Edward Tronick.

(or as bad) as the hands that made them." For surely, initially stupid hands become clever when employed in a clever programme devised by the culture. But the issue becomes interesting when we inquire how the virtuoso morphology achieved by man's hands comes to be employed by clever programmes of action and, indeed, makes such clever programmes possible. Vygotsky (1962) was fond of an epigram from Bacon: "*Nec manus, nisi intellectus, sibi permissus, multum valent*"—Neither hand nor intellect left each to itself is worth much.

In the same spirit, my interest is not in the hands by themselves, but in how they both shape and express human instrumental intelligence. For it is my conviction, to state the issue prematurely, that the manner in which the hands are "mastered" by skill, how they achieve their full adaptive application, can tell us much about the nature of human problem solving and thought. I believe that the programmatic nature of human problem solving reflects the basic fact of primate evolution: that primates, increasingly, were able to use their hands as instruments of intelligence, that selection favoured those that could, and that evolution favoured in a variety of ways those organisms with a close link between hand and mind (cf. Washburn and Howells, 1960).

In rough outline, the theory of skill and its development towards which our observations lead is as follows. Skilled activity is a programme specifying an objective or terminal state to be achieved, and requiring the serial ordering of a set of constituent, modular sub-routines. Functionally equivalent variations in serial order and substitution rules for constituent sub-routines both are features of skilled activity and render skill productive in the sense that language is productive. Variations in serial order assure flexibility or productivity by making possible appropriate changes in the order with which constituent sub-routines are used. The more a skill is linked in real time with such physical requirements as gravitation, constraining velocities, etc., the fewer the functionally equivalent variations in order that will be possible: the order of steps involved in batting a ball thrown at high speed or juggling two balls is highly constrained. Where the real time constraints are reduced—as in tying a rope splice or fastening a complex lashing—there will be a variety of functionally adequate serial orders that lead to the objective. A developed skill has "rules" that include appropriate variant orders and exclude inappropriate ones.

With respect to substitution rules, they constitute one of the most intriguing features of any skilled behaviour. We have all seen the equivalent of the outfielder, thrown off balance by his effort to catch a fly ball, yet able, not only to hold on to it, but to throw it to an appropriate base while still crazily off balance. My stepson who, I assure you, is not so stylish a squash player as I am but a cleverer one, has beaten me all too regularly by such feats as hitting a return beneath a raised leg when caught facing the rear wall of the court! When humans can do this type of substitution in real time, we say they are good athletes; there are situations not so constrained by timing where we would be more likely to say that the performer who showed a flair for appropriate substitutions was "clever" rather than a good athlete.

These sources of productivity in skilled activity are crucial. To quote Professor Bartlett (1958, p. 14), ". . . skilled performance must all the time submit to receptor control, and be initiated and directed by the signals which the performer must pick up from his environment, in combination with the other signals, internal to his own body, which tell him something about his own movements as he makes them. These are the main reasons why all forms of skill, expertly carried out, possess an outstanding character of rapid adaptation. For the items in the series have, within wide limits, a fluid order of occurrence and varying qualities. So what is called the same operation is done now in one way and now in another, but each way is, as we say, 'fitted to the occasion'."

Another quotation from Professor Bartlett serves to underline the modular quality of skill. He is, of course, referring to real-time rapid skills; but that is not so crucial, as we shall see shortly. "By far the most important characteristic of expert bodily skill is 'timing' (which) . . . has nothing to do with the absolute speed at which any component response in the skill sequence is performed. Efficiency depends, more than anything else, upon the regulation of the flow from component to component in such a way that nowhere in the whole series is there any appearance of hurry, and nowhere unnecessarily prolonged delay. . . . The operator has 'all the time in the world to do what he wants' " (1958, p. 15).

All writers on skill would agree that the "secret" of such smooth flowing action is not only anticipation of what is coming next, but a sense of how what one is doing now and what one anticipates next fit into the *objective* of the serial programme in operation. There is guidance—and the parallel is quite striking—by an operation resembling analysis-by-synthesis. That is to say, each component is evaluated and corrected in terms of how well it fits into the overall performance. The components in a serially organized act of skill have not only an arrow of immediate directionality, a pointing ahead to the next component, mere chaining, but also this regulation in terms of requirements of the overall performance. Indeed, there is a point in most skilled acts (whether severely constrained by real-time requirements or not) where nothing further can be done about the act-as-a-whole, where, to use Professor Bartlett's felicitous term, the behaviour has reached a "point of no return".

Indeed, Woodworth in his last book (1958) makes much of the two-phase and polyphase sensorimotor serial patterns, with simple or complex preparatory and effective phases, the two phases being marked off by a boundary much like the point of no return. Of these components, he says, "The small but highly integrated units reveal a fundamental characteristic of organisms: their ability to integrate their behaviour into time sequences . . . They may have to learn most of these behaviour sequences, but they do not have to learn 'from scratch', for their ability and tendency to integrate their behaviour over time gives them a running start." And then he notes, "The child's developing purposiveness . . . is visible first in the little two-phase and polyphase acts, their time span being only a few seconds. Long-range purpose calls for experience and intellectual grasp" (1958, p. 39). Woodworth's emphasis upon the "context-proneness" of small units of behaviour is an attractive idea, and indeed he may be rather more conservatively an empiricist than he need be in assuming that "purpose", or what I should prefer to call the intentionality of behaviour, comes only through experience. This brings us squarely to the issue of the development of skilled behaviour, to which we turn in a moment, but only after the issue of intention has been more fully considered.

The crucial issue in the regulation of intentional action is the opportunity to compare what was intended with what in fact resulted, using the difference between the two as a basis of correction. It is immediately apparent that this is the concept of "reafference" as a source of regulation in behaviour—an idea dating from the pioneering work of von Holst and Mittelstaedt (1950), and Bernstein (1967) whose remarkable work on the physiology of action has only recently become available in English.

For Bernstein *activity* is constrasted with mere *movement*, in that the former requires the co-ordination and regulation of the latter in the *attainment of some particular objective*: a ball is to be thrown a certain distance and has a certain weight; or a screwdriver to be turned requires the application through the hand and arm of a certain torque. He says, "All systems which are self-regulating for any given parameter, constant or variable, must incorporate the following elements as minimum requirements:

"(1) *effector* (motor) activity, which is to be regulated along the given parameter; (2) *a control element*, which conveys to the system in one way or another the *required value* (S_w) of the parameter which is to be regulated; (3) *a receptor* which perceives the *factual course of the value* of the parameter (I_w) and signals it by some means to (4) *a comparator device*, which perceives the discrepancy between the *factual* and *required* values with its magnitude and sign (Δ_w); (5) *an apparatus* which encodes the data provided by the comparator device into correctional impulses which are transmitted by feedback linkages to (6) *a regulator* which controls the function of the *effector* along the given parameter" (pp. 128–129).

His diagrammatic representation of such a system is shown in Fig. 1. Quite plainly, a system of this sort requires the constant comparison of intended action (Bernstein's S_w, or *Sollwert*) with feedback from action accomplished (I_w, or *Istwert*), the two being used to generate the crucial Δ_w, or *Deltawert*, that is then converted to a necessary correction. At the centre of this system is the course of programmes, the control element that signals intention, S_w.

When one observes the early behaviour of infants—say at the onset of visually guided reaching at about 4 months of age—one is struck by the extent to which *intentionality precedes skill*. Arousal of intention, I would urge, is the initial reaction to an "appropriate" stimulus. We shall postpone until later how one may determine what constitutes appropriateness. Often, in response to an appropriate stimulus, there are evoked preparatory activities that later will make possible the performance of an adaptive act towards an object. Before the infant can reach, the presentation of an object with sharp contours and good binocular and movement parallax will induce antigravitational activity in the arms, opening and closing of the hands, and even working of the mouth. The last is particularly interesting, since it is to the mouth that the first object grasped under visual guidance will be taken.[3]

It is under the control of an object-directed intention that the modular acts of a skill are serially organized. It is this persistent intention that precedes, directs, and provides a criterion for terminating an act. In this sense, the serial structure of skilled action is, in Lashley's (1951) celebrated term, *atemporal*. Recall that Lashley was particularly concerned to dismiss the idea of *chaining* as a basis for the organization of serial skilled action, and his general proposal was that it had the properties of syntactically controlled language. "Syntax is not inherent

---

[3] I regret that an experiment now in progress under the direction of Dr. Roger Webb in our laboratory is not yet completed, but there is little question that gross action of this kind is indeed present presaging later instrumental action in support of an intention.

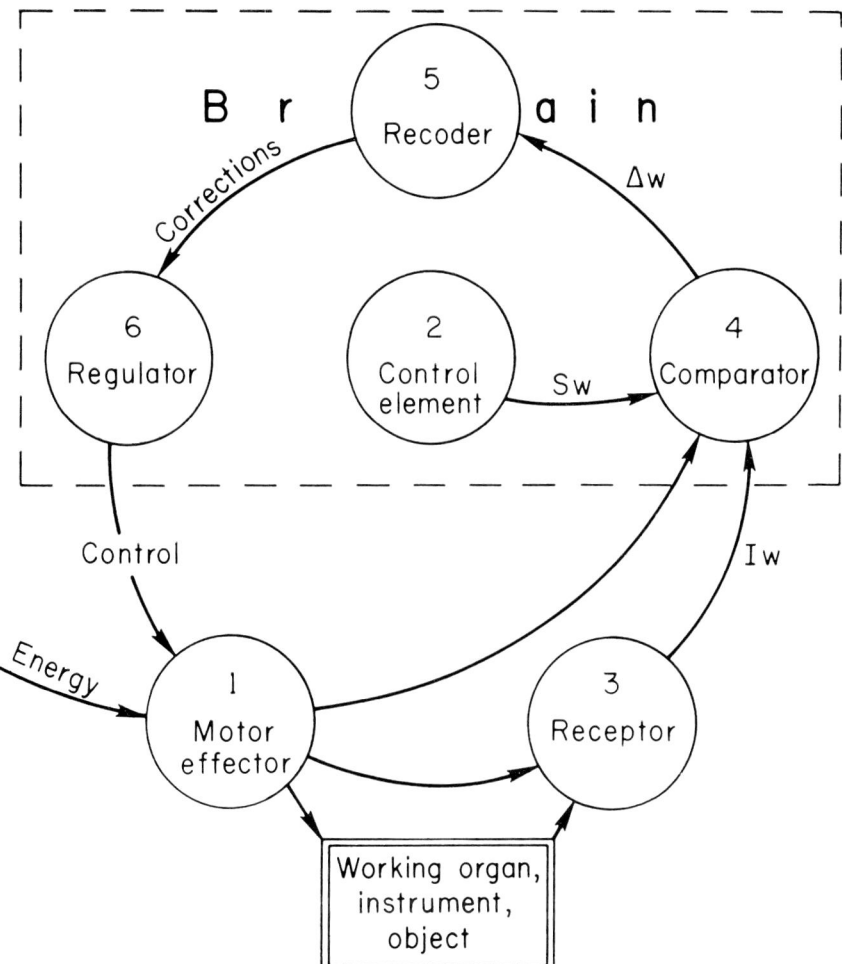

FIG. 1. Bernstein's model for a system capable of voluntary activity directed towards objects or states of the environment (modified after Bernstein, 1967, with permission of Pergamon Press, London).

in the words employed or in the idea to be expressed. It is a generalized pattern imposed upon the specific acts as they occur" (1951, p. 119). For Lashley, this is one of the three sets of events to be accounted for: "First, the activation of the expressive elements (the individual words or adaptive acts) which do not contain the temporal relations. Second, the determining tendency, the set, or idea. This masquerades under many names in contemporary psychology, but is, in every case, an inference from the restriction of behaviour within definite limits. Third, the syntax of the act . . ." (p. 122). It is the second of Lashley's trio, the determining tendency, that we have been considering under the label, intention. The issues of activation of component acts and the syntax of skill remain to be considered.

The constituents of skilled action, the component acts that are contained in the larger pattern, appear to come in their earliest development from two sources: a third source (discussed below) is completely ruled out. One source is the innate repertoire of action patterns that are evoked by appropriate interaction with the environment: the shifting of an object from one hand to another, the use of index finger to touch and explore small inhomogeneities, etc., etc. These acts appear in full but awkward completeness, gradually are shaped in a fashion described below, and are then incorporated into longer sequences. A second source of constituents is the differentiation of initially gross acts into component elements, the infant adapting these gross acts by segmentation, to the spatio-temporal structure of new tasks. The segments then achieve independence from their original context and become available for inclusion in new sequences (Bruner, 1969, 1970).

The one source from which component acts in early skilled behaviour do *not* come is from the repertory of hand-arm reflexes. The skilled behaviour we are describing is *not* effected by the beautifully precise set of reflexes described so carefully by Twitchell (1965)—traction grasping, touch-evoked grasp reflex, touch-evoked avoidance-withdrawal, non-visual groping, and tonic-neck reflex. One can observe the dissolution of these reflex patterns, I believe, in the diffuse, athetoid motion of the infant's arms and hands as an object enters his manipulatory space, motions that are pointed in the general direction of the object, as is the gaze. The beginning of manual skill is this diffusely directional awkwardness, minimally constrained. It is from this early pattern that specific patterns emerge, sometimes as specific bits of behaviour, sometimes in more orderly and predictable forms of differentiation.

For Bernstein (1967) the achievement of control always involves a reduction of or "mastery" over degrees of freedom in the action system being regulated. There are joints and tendons in fingers, wrists, elbows, shoulders, and trunk that can operate independently of each other. A tool can slip this way or that. We shall shortly see instances in which mastery in a given task requires the reduction of such freedom. Within this reduced range, with its characteristic awkwardness, there is a gradual consolidation and mastery. This is the process of modularization, whereby an act is made more automatic, less variable, and achieves a predictable spatio-temporal patterning. Bruner, Bruner and Kahneman (in preparation) find, for example, that as the child progresses in his reaching for objects, the time required for different kinds of reaches becomes uniform—whether one-handed or two, near reach or far, large object or small. This is the modularization through which innate or differentiated action patterns go.

It is when modularization is achieved and the act becomes smoothly organized, that it then goes through a process of being incorporated into new, more inclusive, and more complex serial patterns. It becomes awkward in its new context. (It is, by the way, hard to escape the conclusion that infant ungainliness or awkwardness is a highly species-specific pattern in human beings as well as the adult response of being "touched" by a display of such awkwardness.) Why is modularization so essential a preliminary to the inclusion of an act in a more inclusive, more extended routine? I believe it is a matter of attentional capacity. Prior to modularization, an act simply takes up all available attention, as we shall see from time data. We note almost on a week-to-week basis how differently infants behave in a task requiring skilled control of behaviour. One week a task such as holding a plastic plaque in one hand while capturing a pearl attached to its centre consumes an extraordinary amount of concentrated energy for as long as 30 seconds, even when it leads to failure (the infant handing the plaque from the power grip of one hand to that of the other, unable to form a precision grip or a probe with forefinger); a fortnight later the infant can bring the whole feat off effortlessly in a few seconds.

Once attention is freed, then a new pattern emerges. The new pattern appears in general to take one of three forms. It may be in the form of a more inclusive, rather grossly regulated repetitive sequence of which the previously perfected sub-routine is a part. Instead of taking possession of *one* object with a single hand while the other remains inactive, now the infant takes one and then another object, first with one hand, then with the other. It is a striking change towards inclusion of the single element in a syntactically organized sequence: the objective changes from singular concentration on "getting an object" to "getting both objects". Usually at the outset, the single component acts are more clumsily performed, principally because attention appears to be distributed over a longer sequence and "too little" is available for the single act.[4]

[4] The exception seems to be when a new repetitive pattern becomes organized rhythmically—as with banging, where a single bang on the table is followed by a rhythmic series of bangs. Under these circumstances, the behaviour appears to be better controlled. But I would not include this rhythmic patterning in the phenomenon here described.

More typically, a larger act with a more remote goal takes control of the newly modularized acts. Again, we shall see examples, one of the most interesting being the emergence of "deposit-and-storage" techniques in taking possession of objects, where the taking of an object is not for possession, but for possession within a sphere of control.

Finally, the process of inclusion consists of a virtual decomposition and recomposition of the modular act. It consists, in effect, of the initial breaking-up of an organized act into more restricted components with pauses between, and then a regrouping of these components into a modified pattern. A striking example is the transformation of initial cup use from a one-step transport of cup edge to mouth, with neither pauses nor readjustments of the cup *en route*. This is altered to include several pause points for readjusting the surface of the cup to a position parallel to sea level, so to speak, with subsequent moving of the head to meet the cup, etc. By the time the act has been perfected, it has gone to the point where adjustment of cup to water level and head requirement is continuously monitored and has no pause points at all.

Wherever we have seen the three modes of reorganization—by repetition, by integration, by differentiated elaboration—we have been struck by the complete, if gross, nature of the new form upon its first observed appearance. I find myself deeply impressed again, rereading after a thirty-year interval, the account that Coghill (1929) gives of the emergence of behaviour patterns in growth. In the third lecture of his *Anatomy and the problem of behaviour*, he writes: ". . . a nervous mechanism is established in *Amblystoma* for some time before the animal responds to stimulation, that this mechanism is such as to conduct impulses to the muscles from the head tailward, and that this order of conduction to the muscles gives the resulting movement locomotor value and thereby becomes the basic principle of both aquatic and terrestrial locomotion. The general pattern of the primary mechanism of walking is, therefore, laid down before the animal can in the least respond to its environment. . . . Accordingly, the normal experience of the animal with respect to the outside world appears to have nothing specifically to do with the determination of the form into which the behaviour of the animal is cast. On the other hand, experience has much to do with determining when and to what extent the potentiality of behaviour shall rise into action" (pp. 86–87).

Indeed, the new patterns appear in a preadapted form, a form whose dimensions are laid down in evolutionary history by the selective processes that brought primate evolution to the point of producing

Homo sapiens. It is for this reason that we must examine early behaviour, not only from the point of view of its neurophysiology and its underlying logic, but also from the point of view of its evolutionary function.

Consider now the close detail of some skilled behaviour first appearing.

II. TAKING POSSESSION OF OBJECTS

This experiment had as its objective the discovery of the manner in which infants progressed from the first appearance of visually guided reaching for an object at 4 months to the sophisticated control of several objects simultaneously a year later. Forty-nine normal infants served as our subjects, about equally divided in five age groups: 4–5 months, 6–8, 9–11, 12–14, and 15–17.

The procedure was a simple handling task, similar to an item of the Cattell Infant Intelligence Test. A small toy was handed to the right or left hand. When it was taken, a second toy was immediately presented on the side of the full hand. If not taken after 15 or 20 seconds, the second toy was shifted to the midline. A third and then a fourth object was presented at the midline if the child had taken and retained preceding objects handed to him. When, at any point in the four presentations, the child indicated clearly that he would not take the next object, the trial was ended. Each infant at each age had his four trials divided so that half would be done with the left hand initially and half with the right.

The 4- to 5-month-olds were just crossing the threshold from rather diffuse reaching accompanied by swiping, to effective, visually directed reaching. Two of the subjects in this group, though intensely attracted by the toy and visibly activated by its presence, were never able to achieve an adequately co-ordinated reach-grasp to get the toy. Others could direct their reaches precisely enough to get the object, but could not hold it for more than a brief moment. Children of this age were, for the most part, unable to deal with more than one object at a time. A second toy would either by ignored or, more probably, would so preempt attention that the child would drop the toy already in hand as he fastened visually on the new one being presented. The loss of grasp seemed inadvertent, appearing to take place when the child's attention went to the new object. The original object was retained most often when it had begun a journey to the mouth. On two-thirds of the presentations, where capture occurred, the infant took the toy to his mouth and often the mouth was open during reaching or retrieving.

The role of the mouth is nicely illustrated in Fig. 2 which attests to the sharp decline during the year in the times the mouth is used as destination—a decline from two-thirds at four and a half months to less than 5 per cent at 16 months.

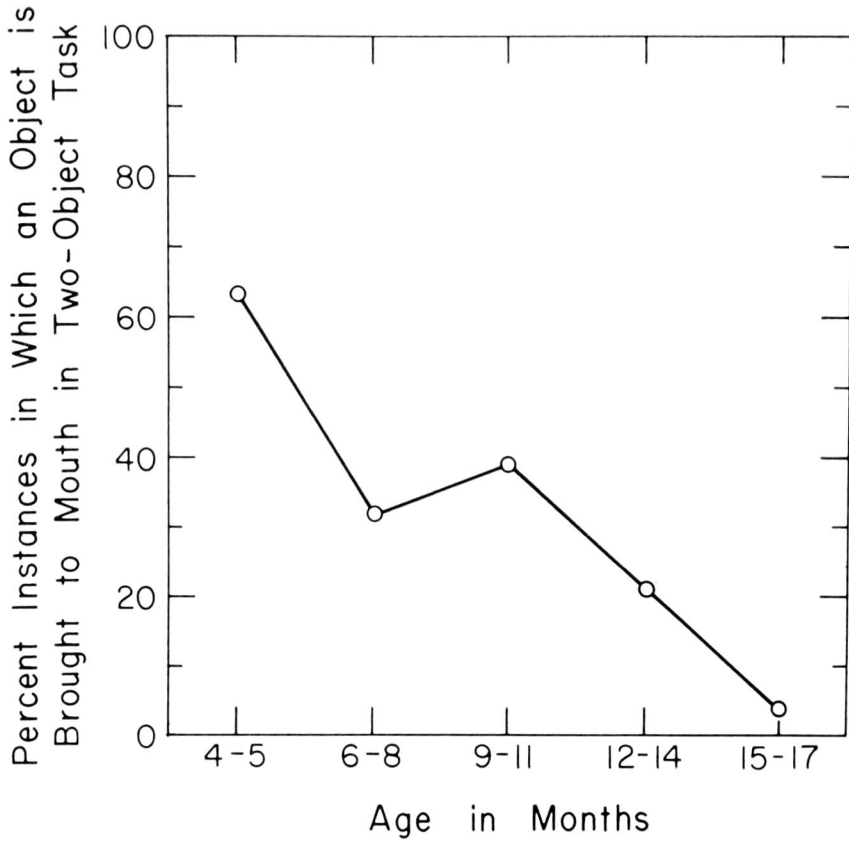

FIG. 2. Incidence of transferring a toy to the mouth as a function of age.

Six- to 8-month-olds present a sharp contrast to the younger children. All of them had clear command of simple reaching and grasping in their initial performance and were not only able to take and hold a *single* object but were able to maintain control of that first object while taking and holding a second as well. The simple reach and grasp could now be embedded in several modes of approaching the toy. They could, for one, transfer an object to the empty hand in order to free the full hand for another reach. This would most often occur after the new object had been presented several times on the side of the initially full hand. Hand-to-hand transfer had a precursor: the child would take a first object to the midline, holding it with both hands. When a second was presented, he would reach for it with the nearest hand. Gradually, this would often differentiate into anticipatory hand-over. Infants also took the second object by reaching across with the empty opposite hand, either traversing the midline slightly or reorienting it. But while all the children were able to deal eventually with two objects on at least two of their four trials, only one of them was ever able to deal with three objects successfully and then only on one of the four trials. If the barrier for the youngest subject was in going beyond one object, the barrier for our 6- to 8-month-olds was in going beyond two objects.

But note that the old programme of coping with objects has *not* been "stamped out". It is very much there. On a third of the presentations of a second object, the infant drops the one he is holding. Yet, a new programme has emerged, and its rules are strikingly powerful by comparison with the old one. It includes features for holding an object in one hand while reaching with the other, handing an object off from one hand to the other, etc. But for all its productivity in dealing with objects placed now on one side of the midline, now on the other, it is limited to a very small store of constituents, involving two hands and one mouth.

With 9- to 11-month-olds, it is immediately apparent that something new has been acquired. While a majority is not able to take up a third object initially, a significant minority is eventually able to push through to success in taking a third and even a fourth object into possession. In about one in five trials the initial response to a third or fourth object is to deposit one object from the hand either into the lap or on to one of the armrest shelves of the chair. Let it be noted, however, that this response of putting an object in reserve is sporadic and that the length of the storage is not very long. Indeed, half of the deposited toys were retrieved immediately after being deposited. For the use of storage involves at the outset several conflicting elements that are amenable to inclusion in one of two continuing programmes. As part of the deposit-and-store routine, the object must be put down. But the "put down" object then evokes a visually guided reach, particularly since it is adjacent to the hand that has deposited it. The factor that finally resolves the conflict is, of course, capacity to delay. Before a deposited object can be stored, there must be capacity to delay responding to it and a carry-over of the intention to take an object that had been presented elsewhere and that must be re-engaged now. It is much like the phenomenon of embedding in sentence formation, where an embedded clause is uttered, and then the embedded sentence resumed. It is not surprising then that only a third of the 9- to 11-month-olds dealt successfully through storage with more than two objects.

By 12 months storage is far better developed and has become so well established that it serves (as the mouth did earlier) as a terminus of expectations. Not only do we find year-old infants handing off the toy to the hand on the other side of the midline, but doing so before a second object is presented, in preparation for its appearance on a predicted side. These children, moreover, place an object in storage *before* the third or the fourth object is handed to them.

Note in Fig. 3 that not only does the incidence of deposit increase with age, but that the proportion of objects deposited that remain stored to the end of the task similarly increases until finally more than

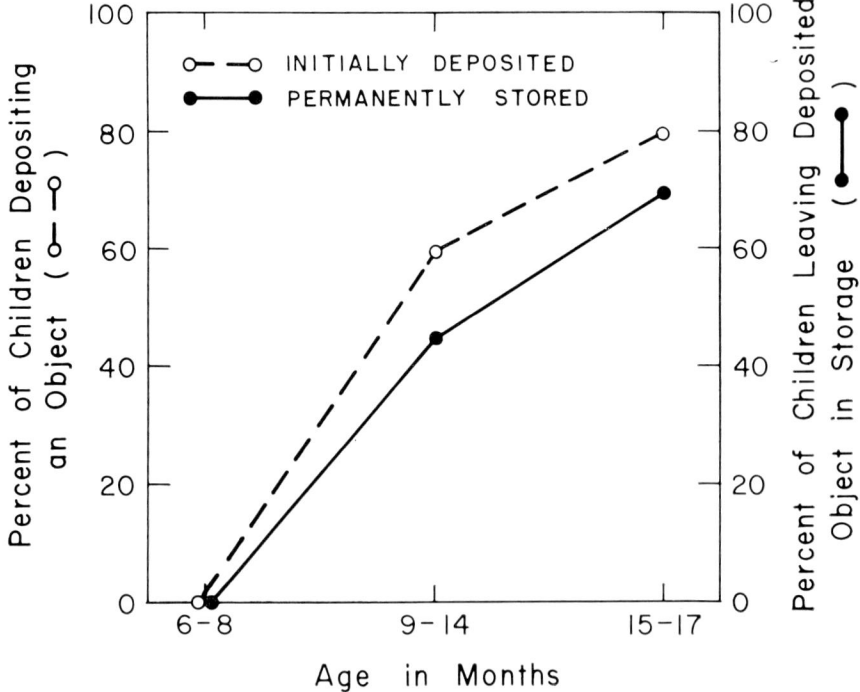

FIG. 3. Number of objects initially deposited and permanently stored by children of different ages.

three-quarters are left. Yet, the year-olds still have their old routines and, given the "wrong" circumstances, they still can slip back into an earlier programme.

But there are some real differences between the two oldest groups. The 15- to 17-month-olds are much more consistently successful than the immediately younger subjects. The 12- to 14-month-olds handle a mean of 3·0 objects successfully while the oldest subjects handle 3·7 objects. That much is not surprising; another change is less obvious and more interesting. It is a change in mode of storage. The oldest subjects not only store consistently from trial to trial but store in *one way* consistently, unlike the 12- to 14-month-olds who use any mode at any time.

One additional feature of the programme is added with the two oldest groups: more general substitution rules for deposit and storage that can now include another human being. Of objects stored by the 9- to 12-month-olds, 94 per cent are deposited in the lap or on the arm of a chair. This figure drops sharply to one quarter for the children 12- to 14-months-old; with them, over three-quarters of objects stored are handed for safe keeping either to the experimenter or to the mother. The same preference is found in the oldest group, some of whom have gone back to using a chair arm, possibly now finding agents less of a novelty.

By the time the child reaches $1\frac{1}{2}$ years, the behaviour in the task we used has the appearance of great skill, even aplomb. In fact, it has gone through a long process of transformation, involving a series of constituent acts embedded in a programme that governs their serial order. Much in this progress is the result of learning, particularly the anticipatory elements; but much involves the appearance of routines that clearly could not have been "learned" in any conventional sense, though they needed to be shaped (as with anticipation) or integrated (as with leaving an object in storage rather than retrieving it immediately).

But before we become too deeply involved in interpreting these data, let us consider another set in which the picture is much less one of *integration* of constituent acts, and much more of the order of *differentiation of constituents*, followed by their *reintegration*.

III. ACQUISITION OF COMPLEMENTARY TWO-HANDEDNESS

The skill we examine now is one that is both convenient experimentally and of interest in its own right from a biological and evolutionary

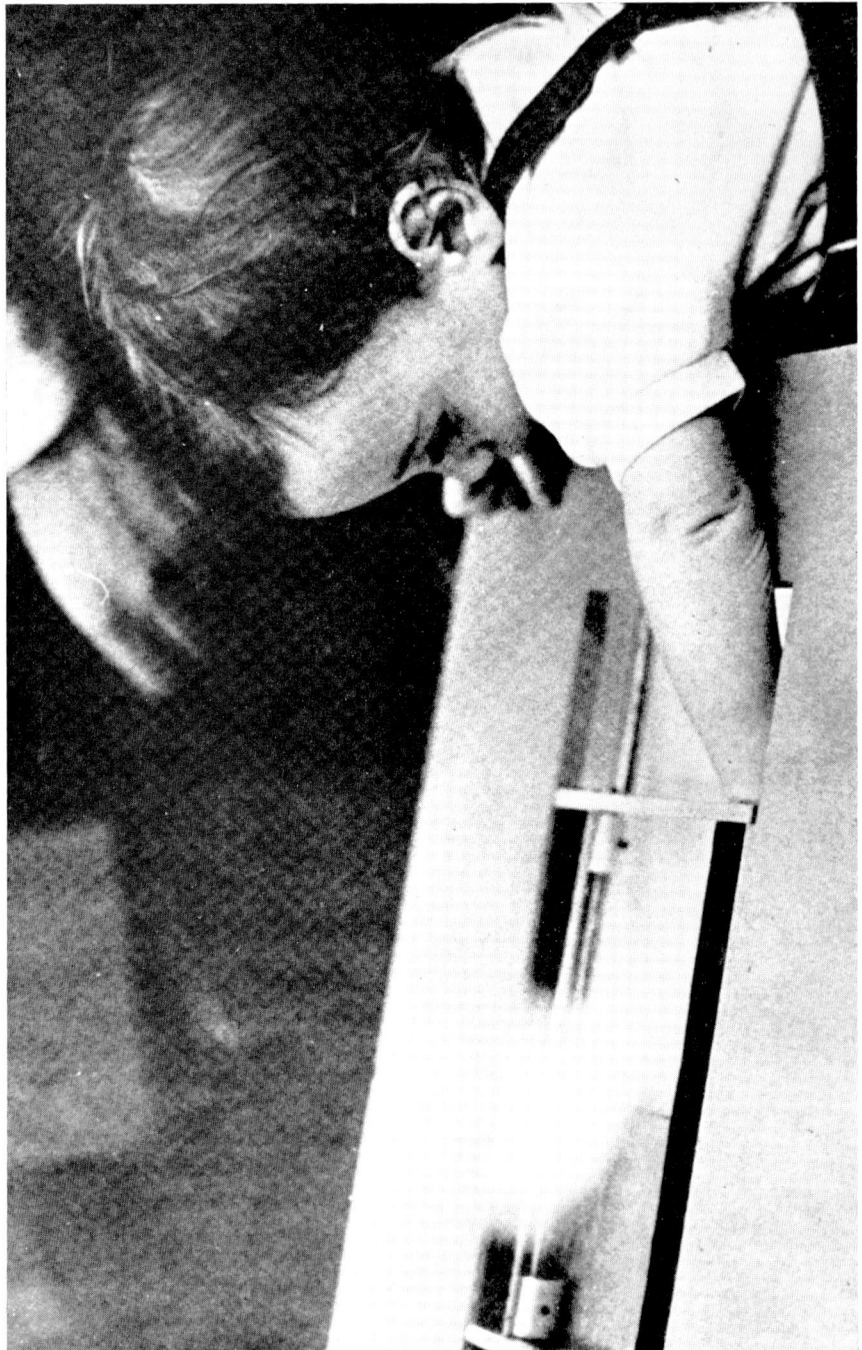

FIG. 4. Two-handed obstacle box for studying the complimentary role of right and left hand. Dimensions of the box: length, 22–25 inches; width, 16 inches; maximum height, 5 inches; minimum height, 1·25 inches. Dimensions of the sliding lid, 8·5 × 6 inches.

point of view. It is the infant's acquisition of the complementary use of his two hands with a division of labour between them. In our experiment the child is presented with a box having a transparent lid that reveals a toy inside it. The lid is mounted on sliding ball bushings so that, in order to remove the toy, the child must slide the lid up its track (which is tilted 30° from horizontal) and hold it open. The interior of the box is well illuminated by a concealed cove light. The box is pictured in Fig. 4. The most expedient way for the child to get the toy is to slide the lid up and hold it with one hand and to reach inside for the toy with the other. Thus, the skilful child uses one hand as the "holder", the other as "retriever", the work of the two being sequenced with all constituents in order.

The same subjects studied before (with the exception of the 4- to 5-month-olds) were used again. Each infant came into the laboratory with his mother and was seated in her lap before the apparatus. A small toy was visible inside the box. The temptation invariably succeeded: the infant attempted as best he could to get the toy. If the infant got the toy from the box, he was permitted to play with it for 15 to 30 seconds, after which it was gently taken from him and replaced in the box. If retrieval was again successful, four further trials were given, for a total of six. The same toy was used throughout—a brightly coloured plastic shape. No limit of time was placed on the trials, and they might last as long as 3 minutes. Six trials were given to each child.

It will come as no surprise that success increased with age, from less than a fifth of the trials ending well in the youngest subjects, to somewhat better than half in the next group, to close to nine in ten in the two oldest groups. But much more interesting than the changing frequency of success is the morphology of failure at different points in skill development. For it is in the altered nature of failure that one sees most vividly the differentiation of a gross act into a set of recombinable constituents.

The first approach to the object in the box is direct, a generalized approach behaviour that takes little account of the manipulable features of the barrier. It consisted in clawing and banging at the barrier, on a direct line to the object—a matter to be discussed at greater length in a later section. Eloquent testimony to the decline in such behaviour is contained in Fig. 5, where episodes of barrier banging are plotted for different age groups. Note that barrier banging among the young may become autonomous—a new end in itself. So often our youngest subject, presented with a task, will deal with failure by redefining the nature of the task, varying the end objective rather than holding it constant while

4

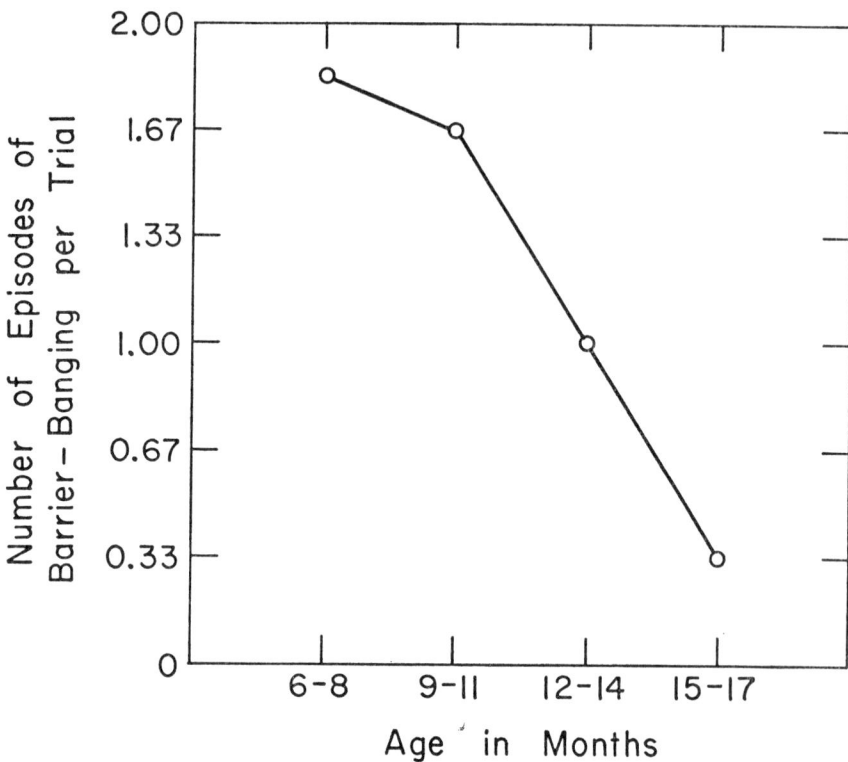

FIG. 5. Changes in frequency of barrier banging as a function of age.

varying the means. I believe this to be the heart of play, and its function is to explore means-end relationships without undue commitment. But that is a matter beyond the scope of this paper.

A second form of failure consisted in opening and closing the sliding lid without reaching for the object: each opening and return to the closed position of the sliding lid with no intervening reach counted as an incident. The average number of such incidents is shown in Table I. We believe this opening and closing also becomes autonomous since the child is diverted from the goal.

Note that autonomous opening was most frequent in the second youngest group of subjects—some four episodes per trial. There were two children in this group who never succeeded in retrieving the toy from beneath the sliding barrier; and it is an interesting fact that the same two showed *no* autonomous opening of the box. If we take the children in this group who were *most* successful on the task, they too

TABLE I. MEAN NUMBER OF INCIDENTS OF AUTONOMOUS OPENING PER CHILD AS A FUNCTION OF AGE

Age in months	Average number of incidents of autonomous opening per child per trial
6–8	2·7
9–11	4·1
12–14	1·7
15–17	1·9

showed relatively little autonomous opening (an average of 16 instances over the six trials). It was the five *middlingly* successful children in this group who were most prone to autonomous opening (an average of 26 instances per child).

The significance of this autonomous activity is in the extent to which it "breaks away" from the original intention of object capture. Requiring much concentrated attention as it does, it seems in process to achieve its own end. It is not, as with banging at the barrier, a response in failure—but rather an isolation of a step towards success.

Perhaps the simplest or most primitive successful approach to the task is one that, in effect, involves only a single hand, the other remaining inactive. The lid is slid up and the toy captured by the same hand. The hand which raised the lid must be inserted in the opening before the lid falls. This is usually accomplished with a kind of worming action rather than a darting one, extricating the toy against the wedging action of the free-sliding lid. The frequency of such one-handed attempts is shown in Table II. Note that the highest frequency is seen in the second group.

TABLE II. MEAN NUMBER OF ONE-HANDED REACHES PER CHILD PER TRIAL AS A FUNCTION OF AGE

Age in months	Average number of one-handed reaches per child per trial
6–8	0·27
9–11	0·95
12–14	0·48
15–17	0·42

But as is so often the case, in spite of the fact that the two oldest groups *can* use many more proficient techniques (as we shall see), they still occasionally use the one-handed worming technique: it is still very much part of their repertoire, although we have little idea of what conditions evoke it.

The least adept of the two-handed strategies appears in several variants. In effect, the general approach involves raising the lid with one or two hands, then going for the toy inside the box with one or two hands, but not holding the lid in the open position long enough to get in and out of the box efficiently. Both hands are involved, but with an inadequate sequencing of component acts. The incidence is not great —a little over one in six reaches in the 12- to 14-month range—but it is interesting as a case where the constituents are present, but the sequence of their execution is either confused or badly timed. It is, in a word, slightly apraxic.

TABLE III. MEAN NUMBER OF PARTIALLY COMPLEMENTARY TWO-HANDED REACHES PER CHILD PER TRIAL AS A FUNCTION OF AGE

Age in months	Average number of partially complementary two-handed reaches per child per trial
6–8	0·06
9–11	0·15
12–14	0·20
15–17	0·37

Complementary two-handed reaching is much more prevalent where virtually all the necessary constituents have become differentiated and reintegrated into an effective performance. It involves the joint use of both hands to slide the lid, retaining it in an open position with one hand, while the toy is retrieved from the box with the other. The incidence of this partially complementary two-handed reach is seen in Table III. The sequence is well organized, but the differentiation is not yet complete. Differentiation is achieved when the infant raises the lid with one hand and holds it open while the other hand retrieves the object. Not surprisingly, it shows a sharp rise in incidence after the first birthday.

From here on, the improvement that occurs with age is not one of strategy, but one of consolidating the complementary two-handed strategy, rendering it less effortful and quicker by the increasing use of the tips of the fingers and hands with an attendant decrease in the involvement of arms and trunk for lifting. In effect, by a year and a half, the act we have studied is well-structured, and differentiated, if not yet well-mastered: it still exhibits striking variability in time required. Because it still requires a considerable concentration of effort, it probably is not readily embedded into a more complex act of which it might become a component.

For the most part, the children do not *gradually* improve their approach, but rather increase the skill with which they perform old routines. Learning over the six trials seems to take the form of consolidating or perfecting constituent acts over which the child already has some mastery at the start. Two-handed efforts made their appearance abruptly rather than by some gradual route and seemed to be "ready" for triggering. It is only after a new response appears that it goes through consolidation and shaping by the opportunities provided by practice. Its initial emergence on the scene as an organized response—in any of the forms of strategy we have reported—seems independent of the practice of that organization. Some of the components, indeed, have been practised, but not the new pattern. It is in this respect, we believe, that the long evolutionary history of complementary bimanual skill provides a set of preadaptive patterns that emerge, *not* by trial and error, but in response to appropriate environmental events. These events are not so much releasers as operative requirements that are finally appreciated. Given the intention of capturing an object, it is not until a certain level of skill has been attained that the requirement of two hands is apprehended. Two-handedness then occurs in organized form, if somewhat crudely. Perhaps this is the only way so much skill can be achieved so soon with effector organs (like the hands) marked by so many degrees of freedom of movement and challenged by such a wide range of tasks.

IV. DETOUR REACHING

An infant sits in an adult's lap before a table, with a screen extending halfway across the field to approximately the infant's midline. A toy is presented to the infant in the open space and then put behind the screen, where its jingling identifies its position if the screen is not transparent. This simple outline of our experiment we varied in many ways to check a number of hypotheses about detour reaching. (These concern us here only incidentally.) As a result, 120 infants were needed as subjects, equally divided into three groups: young with median age of 34 weeks, middle with a median of 51 weeks, and oldest with a median of 69 weeks.

Several evident changes occur with growth. One is, of course, that the older the child the greater the likelihood of direct success—reaching in behind the barrier with the hand on the open side of the screen and getting the toy. The difference between ages is modulated by the depth of the object behind the screen: in general, the middle positions distinguish the different ages the most sharply, since objects in the open are easy for all, and deeply embedded objects rather more difficult for all. Figure 6 demonstrates this point.

Again we learn more about the acquisition of skill from clumsiness *en route* to perfection. The first locus of clumsiness is in activation; Fig. 7 indicates a source of difficulty that comes precisely from the

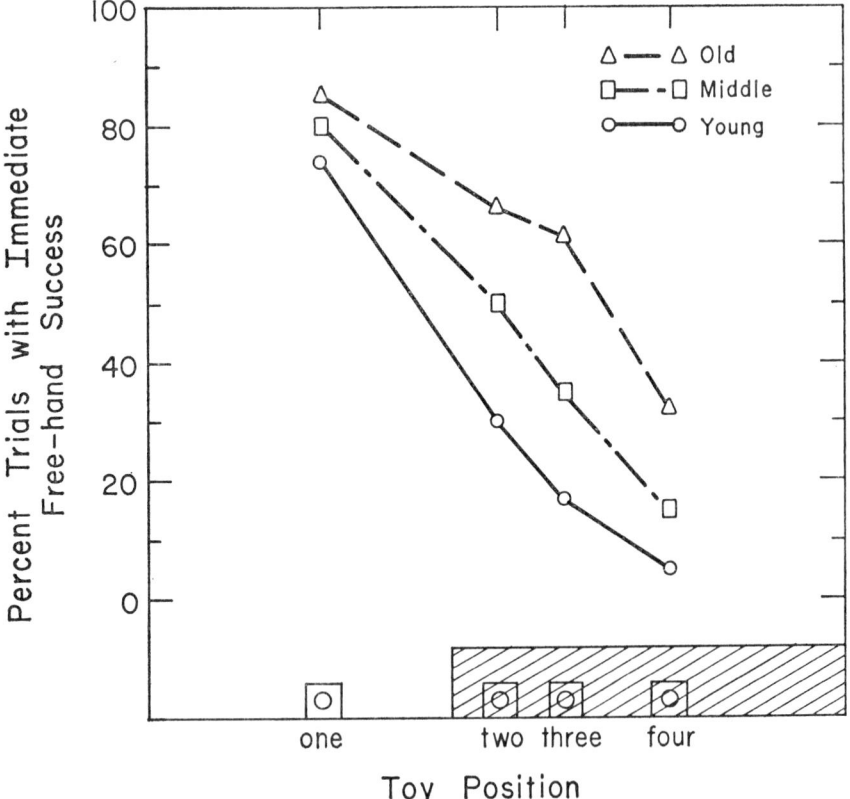

FIG. 6. Success on detour reaching problem as a function of toy position and age.

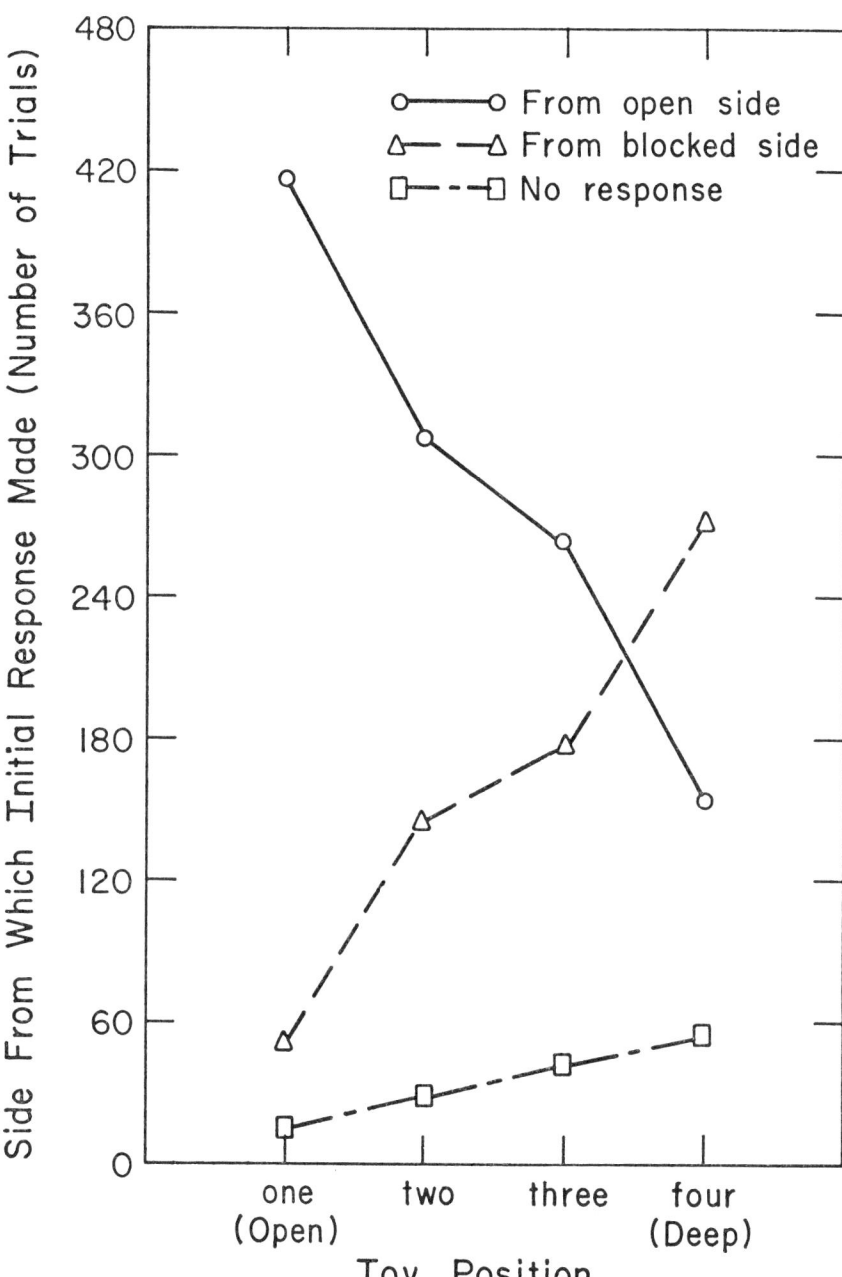

FIG. 7. Frequency of approach from open and blocked side of detour as a function of toy position.

nature of activation in this task. It shows that initial activation in the task comes on the side where the toy has been placed—either heard jingling or seen through the transparent screen.

What the activated hand is trying to do is to get directly at the objective—and in the great majority of cases when the object is well off to one side of the midline, regardless of the age of the child. Again, reaction differs at each age, depending upon the width of the detour. The young start by going straight forward at the toy half the time even when it is at the edge of the screen: and they do so with the screen-side hand. That figure is halved in the oldest children. These reactions are summarized in Fig. 8 for the transparent screen.

But the better to understand what the pattern of response is like, a closer description is needed of the way in which infants proceed on this

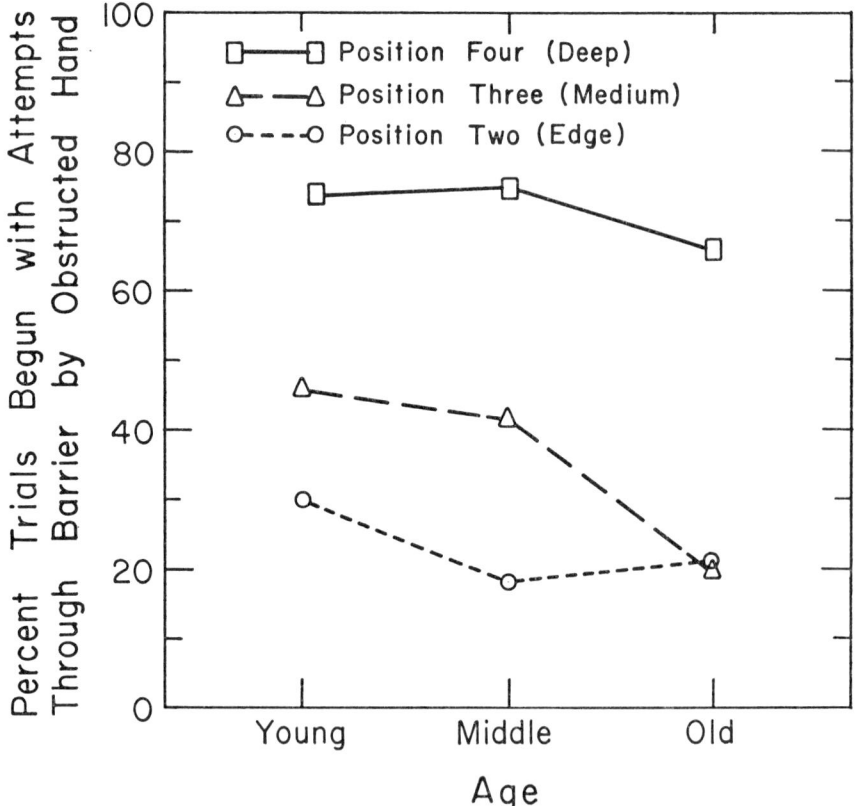

FIG. 8. Trials begun with direct approach to toy, by screen side hand as a function of age.

task. The typical initial response, most frequently found among the 8-month-olds, is a direct reaching towards the object with the screen-side hand, followed by initial scratching or banging at the barrier, followed by quitting. The contralateral hand may even be brought in to help in scrabbling against the barrier, though it could easily pass behind the barrier and take the object. Sometimes the screen-side ipsilateral hand will move to the edge of the screen, go around it in a clumsy backhand and capture the object while the contralateral hand sits idly by. In the next stage, there is initial activation again of the hand ipsilateral to the toy, a move at the barrier, and then recruitment of

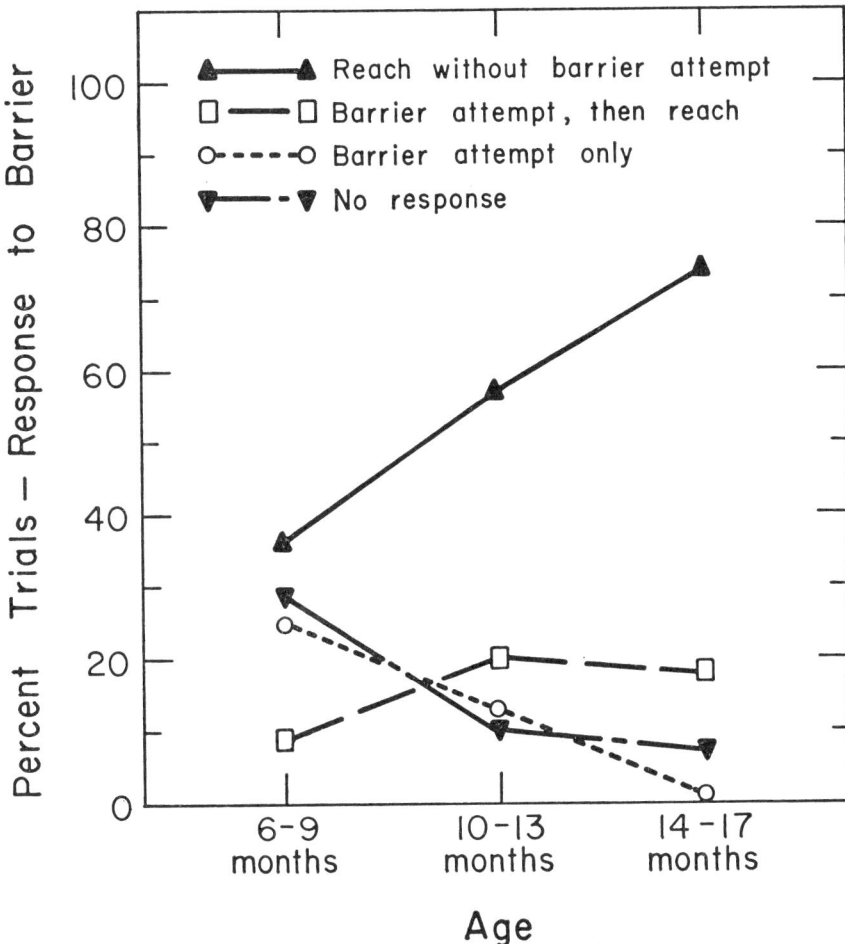

FIG. 9. Types of reach pattern in relation to age.

the contralateral hand that moves behind the screen to take the toy. About a third of the trials of the 1-year-olds are of this pattern and a quarter of the 17-monthers. There is a decreasing lag in time between ipsilateral activation and contralateral execution of the intention to capture. Finally, there is a pattern of direct reaching for the object with the hand on the open side of the screen, by far the majority response among the oldest infants. The three response patterns are summed up in Fig. 9.

Plainly, then, the acquisition of detour reaching begins from a baseline of *visual straight-line reaching* with the hand nearest the object sought. Three factors work against the replacement of this initial reaching rule. One is the continued power of ipsilateral activation which, when combined with a second rule, crowds out a contralateral approach. The second rule is to keep in operation the programme that has been started—hence the awkward backhand reaching as well as the recruitment of the contralateral hand for attacking the boundary. Thirdly, there is conflict (particularly with the transparent screen) from the tendency to be guided by visual criteria rather than by instrumental ones. In this case, the visual display (including one's hands) counteracts the tendency to use the instrumentally relevant hand.

It is important to note that there are two programmes operating, both fairly open to adaptation—the direct visual ipsilateral programme and the operational contralateral one. Each uses, in effect, the same set of constituent sub-routines of reaching, grasping, etc. We have no basis for believing that learning in any conventional sense of the word leads to a shift from one strategic programme to the other. We have counter-balanced our design in such a way that some 24 infants served to randomize out screen-type used, order of screen position, age, etc. Each child in the experiment received 16 trials. There is no indication whatsoever of any learning curve for any age, any position, any screen. The data for the completely counter-balanced subgroup are continued in Fig. 10.

I am *not* proposing that learning or experience affects eventual mastery of the detour task. Rather, the effect of experience is to "mature" new response systems which at first are slow and crude so that they may be evoked by appropriate tasks. Experience also serves to shape them; but it does not *create* them. Indeed, the anomaly is this; it is at the point where the old system begins to work smoothly and achieve goals sought that it is most likely to be superseded by a new, initially more clumsy one.

Finally, let me note the point that, in the present task, strategies or

THE GROWTH AND STRUCTURE OF SKILL

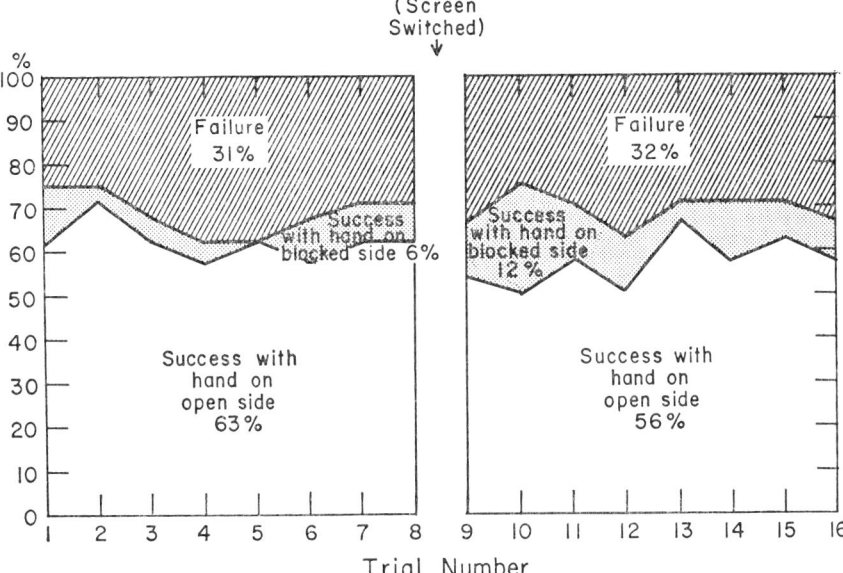

FIG. 10. Results of experiment with subgroup where age, screen-type used and screen position were randomized. The results provide no evidence of learning.

programmes continue to coexist and occasionally to get into conflict. There is one element in skill acquisition that is best called inhibition: suppressing old reaction patterns that continue to intrude. In the present instance, where two programmes (visually dominant reaching and indirect instrumental reaching) share common constituents, the requirement of such inhibition is the greater. If our task had had the requirement of real-time operation in the millisecond range, performance would have been doomed by the conflict that existed even in successful performance.

V. THE TRACKING OF EVENTS

At the outset, we remarked upon the difference in precocity between head-eye tracking and the visually guided manipulation, noting the early evident preadaptation in the former case (cf. Salapatek, 1968; Kessen, 1967; Fantz, 1961). Yet, though there is a difference in precocity, there are certain likenesses in programme that are of some interest.

The following experiment makes this clearer. It is in progress in our laboratory, a joint effort of Mundy-Castle and Anglin.

A baby—ranging in age from 10 days to 5 months—is comfortably seated in a so-called "Harvard chair", 20° reclining from upright and well supported by breech-and-belly cloth. Before him at eye level and 12 inches away are two windows side by side, each subtending about 30° of visual arc with 10° between. In these windows a beautifully jewelled ball makes successive appearances—6 seconds in one window, then after a disappearance of $3\frac{1}{2}$ seconds, 6 seconds in the other window. Record is kept of where the infant is looking, as well as of some measures such as heart rate, breathing, and gross movement.

Between 10 days and 3 months, three separate patterns emerge. The first is one in which the baby simply looks more at the windows than elsewhere in the room, but with the discernible correlation between where he is looking and where the jewelled ball is appearing. The second pattern is one in which initially the infant's gaze is directed to where the ball is until, finally, the gaze anticipates where the ball will be. During this phase there is a "stuck" quality—the baby shifts to the other window and stays there waiting if ahead of the ball. There the gaze remains until the ball disappears, when he shifts again. Finally there emerges a pattern in which the baby is plainly monitoring *both* windows. When no ball is in sight, he may spend the $3\frac{1}{2}$-second period looking back and forth between the windows; and even when looking at a ball in one window, he may glance over to the other momentarily as if to check up.

Now, let me urge that this development is comparable to one we have observed in the multiple-object manual task. At the outset the infants in this looking study have an intention to orient, but at first this expresses itself by the glance staying in the vicinity of the recurring stimulus. It is comparable to orienting to an object, arms raised and working, but with no capability of effecting a specific reach. In the second strategy, they are dealing with one stimulus at a time, "stuck" on it, to use Mundy-Castle and Anglin's phrase. In the third strategy, they are dealing with two alternative loci and objects at those loci simultaneously.

To be sure, the parallelism is not complete, for indeed we have some indication that looking and manipulating have some interesting discontinuities. But the formal similarities, I believe, are not accidents. I would urge, as Bernstein (1967) has, that all action systems have access to a common stock of programmes, programmes related to resolving spatial, temporal, relational and identity problems. Many of these programmes are, in Coghill's phrase, preadapted. And as *Amblystoma*'s neural "solution" of locomotion in water turns out to be formally identical to the solution of locomotion on land, so the solution of the problem of multiplicity has formal identities whether it is the eye-head tracking system or the hand system that is in operation.

As noted at the start, then, the management of skill may be considered as the first realization or embodiment of programmes that will be used throughout the life of the organisms not only for mastery of skilled tasks, but also for problem-solving of a kind not usually thought of as skill in the bodily sense. Indeed, the proof of the matter is that, from the infant's perspective, it is difficult to say whether the tasks reported in these pages were instances of "skill" or of "problem-solving". Perhaps we would do well in the future to explore wherein they are identical, and what makes them separate. I cannot believe that it suffices to argue simply that thought is "action internalized" or rendered into symbolic form. The task, rather, is to explore the range of development from the attainment of skill in action to the attainment of acumen: in problem-solving to explore in detail the kinship between them and the discontinuities as well. I believe that the skill of the hand, given its place in evolutionary history, may provide the ideal vehicle for such a voyage of exploration.

REFERENCES

BARTLETT, F. C. 1958. *Thinking*. Basic Books, New York.
BERNSTEIN, N. A. 1967. *The coordination and regulation of movement*. Pergamon Press, London.
BRUNER, J. S. 1969. *Processes of cognitive growth: infancy*. Vol. III. Heinz Werner Lecture Series. Clark University Press, Worcester, Mass.
BRUNER, J. S. 1970. Origins of problem solving strategies in skill acquisition. *Cognitive Psychology*, in press.
BRUNER, J. S. and BRUNER, B. M. 1968. On voluntary action and its hierarchical structure. *International Journal of Psychology*, **3**, 239–255.
BRUNER, J. S., BRUNER, B. M. and KAHNEMAN, I. The growth of manual intelligence. IV. The psychophysics of cup use. Unpublished study, Center for Cognitive Studies, Harvard University. In preparation.
CLARK, W. E. LEGROS. 1959. *The antecedents of man*. Edinburgh University Press.
COGHILL, G. E. 1929. *Anatomy and the problem of behaviour*. Cambridge University Press.
FANTZ, R. L. 1961. The origin of form perception. *Scientific American*, **204**, 66–72.
HOLST, VON E. and MITTELSTAEDT, H. 1950. Das Reafferenzprinzip. *Naturwissenschaften*. **37**, 464–476.
JONES, F. W. 1917. *Arboreal man*. Hafner, New York.

KESSEN, W. 1967. Sucking and looking: Two organized congenital patterns of behavior in the human newborn. In H. W. Stevenson, E. H. Hess and H. L. Rheingold (Eds.), *Early behavior: Comparative and developmental approaches.* Wiley, New York. Pp. 147–179.

LASHLEY, K. S. 1951. The problem of serial order in behavior. In L. A. Jeffress (Ed.), *Cerebral mechanisms in behavior: The Hixon Symposium.* Wiley, New York. Pp. 112–146.

NAPIER, J. R. 1962. The evolution of the hand. *Scientific American,* **207,** 56–62.

SALAPATEK, P. 1968. Visual scanning of geometric figures by the human newborn. *J. comp. physiol. Psychol.* **66,** 247–258.

TWITCHELL, T. E. 1965. The automatic grasping responses of infants. *Neuropsychologia,* **3,** 247–259.

VYGOTSKY, L. S. 1962. *Thought and language.* Wiley and MIT Press, New York.

WASHBURN, S. L. and HOWELLS, F. C. 1960. Human evolution and culture. In S. Tax (Ed.), *The evolution of man.* Vol. 2. University of Chicago Press.

WOODWORTH, R. S. 1958. *Dynamics of behavior.* Holt, New York.

Discussion

HEFFERLINE: I am reminded vividly of Kohler's ape, Zoltan, fitting together two sticks in order to rake a banana into his cage. Having got the banana Zoltan did not stop to eat it but continued to use the stick to rake in the rubbish that was outside the cage. He had changed his objective and the stick had become a toy as much as a tool. There is something reminiscent of insight in your use of the term *intentionality*. I think one could hypothesize that when Zoltan slotted the sticks together he was using sub-routines which were available from his previous learning history.

KAY: I too am interested in the problem of defining the objective which the child is trying to achieve in attempting to get the toy out of the box. Suppose you used a different type of apparatus where the lid is released electronically when a button, mounted let us say on the box, is depressed. Now is the child sufficiently clear at this point to suppress the groping movements of his hand and learn that he can get the toy by pressing the button?

BRUNER: There is quite an interesting thing: it is a hard thing to draw a line between an act and its arbitrary result and one we would think of as a "natural" result. If you set the child to do an arbitrary task, he can do it quite readily if he has a response system for it, and it does indeed take on some of the properties of instrumental conditioning. One of my students, Mrs. Ilze Kalnins, is in the process of writing an experiment in which infants suck as a means of bringing displays into focus. The picture is drawn into focus when the infant sucks at or above a rate of 1·5 per second. If he sucks below that rate, or stops sucking, the picture drifts out of focus. In a control condition, if the infant sucks at the criterion rate, it drives the picture out of focus. If he does not suck it comes into focus. Now under these circumstances children as young as 30 days of age do indeed learn how to handle this task very handsomely, sucking for focus and desisting to avoid blur. Now what is interesting about arbitrary links between response and consequence is the ritualization of response of the type we saw in Guthrie and Horton's study where the cats pushed a striped pole with their rear end to cause a door to open and let them escape. They finally developed a kind of ritual minimal act of banging to open the door. Under these circumstances they do develop a skill. But what is the difference?

We have been doing studies of the eye–head system to find out in the saccade of tracking how much it is the head and how much it is the eye that moves in tracking an object. The apparatus is very simple in principle, requiring summating of two matched inputs from eye and from head. The infant wears a "velcro" cap to which is attached an adhering crown with a stalk that turns easily in a potentiometer to register rotary motion. The whole system is gimballed and counterbalanced so that it is virtually weightless and the child can move his head in any direction. As soon as he moves it around the axis, it turns the stalk in the potentiometer and registers. We also have output from the eyes coming from a couple of d.c. electrodes on the external canthi. We turn the infant's head while he holds his eyes on an object so that we can calibrate the head and eye systems and thus know where the line of sight is.

If you tell an adult subject to watch what you are doing as you move objects in the field, the eyes will lead the head in moving and will move more than the head. If the subject himself is now asked to move the objects over comparable distances, the head will lead and will move more. We are just now starting comparable work with infants. But obviously there is *some* kind of skill even in this arbitrary task—skill as in the experiment of Wickens where the subject, having learned to remove his finger from threatened shock by the use of his adductors, is able to shift immediately to his abductors when his hand is turned upside down. One learns *place*. But the arbitrary response patterns simply are not of the same order as the subtle, synergistically organized systems like, say, head-eye-hand. If the infant has to take the initiative in scanning (in contrast merely to tracking an event) again the hand leads. Passive action produces again a priority of the eye system.

I want to argue that, as Kay said this morning, skill involves a series of acts like identifying an appropriate object, estimating the space in which it operates, organizing the motor platform on which action is to be carried out, estimating conditions of time, space, etc., that may alter in order to have transformations for coping with displacements in space or time, etc. I would argue that under the arbitrary conditions where the cat moves that stick in the Horton and Guthrie experiment, there is virtually no skill acquired in Kay's sense. Because *specific* responses have been learned, there is no longer full appropriate correction to go with the response.

Experience and the Development of Motor Mechanisms in Infancy[1]

BURTON L. WHITE

Harvard University

I. THE AIM OF THE INQUIRY

THE SUBJECT OF this paper is related to some long-standing research in which I have been specially interested, namely the role of experience in the development of man's adaptive abilities. In the narrower field of human infancy my work began with a study of the development of visual-motor capacities and in particular with the acquisition of visually directed reaching. In order to pursue this, facilities were required for prolonged observation of infants during the period leading up to its emergence. At this time one can look for early forms and precursors of the behaviour and examine variables of a subjective or environmental nature such as postural factors, grasp developments and the influence of targets for visual and tactual exploration. Fortunately the ideal situation was offered at a local institution for illegitimate children where physically normal infants could be studied in relatively invariant environmental conditions. The material circumstances making up the "world" of these infants from 3 weeks to approximately 4 months is shown in Fig. 1. Routine care consisted in bottle-feeding and diaper-

[1] At various stages, extending over the last 6 years, this research has received support from Grant M-3657 from the National Institute of Mental Health; Grant 61-234 from the Foundation's Fund for Research in Psychiatry; Grants HD-00761 and HD-02054 from the National Institute of Health, the Optometric Extension Program; Grant NSG-496 from the National Aeronautics and Space Administration; Grant AF-AFOSR354-63 from the Office of Scientific Research, United States Air Force; the Rockefeller Foundation; and contract number OE5-10-239 from the Office of Education. The research was conducted at the Tewksbury Hospital, Tewksbury, Massachusetts. I am very grateful for the assistance of Dr. Richard Held, Mr. Peter Castle, Mrs. Kitty Clark, Mr. Richard Light and Mrs. Cherry Collins, and for the consideration and aid given by Drs. John Lu, Solomon J. Fleischman, Peter Wolff, and Lois Crowell and head nurses Helen Efstathiou, Frances Craig, and Virginia Donovan.

changing every 4 hours, with a 5-minute bath each morning. Apart from this the infants were left alone and usually supine.

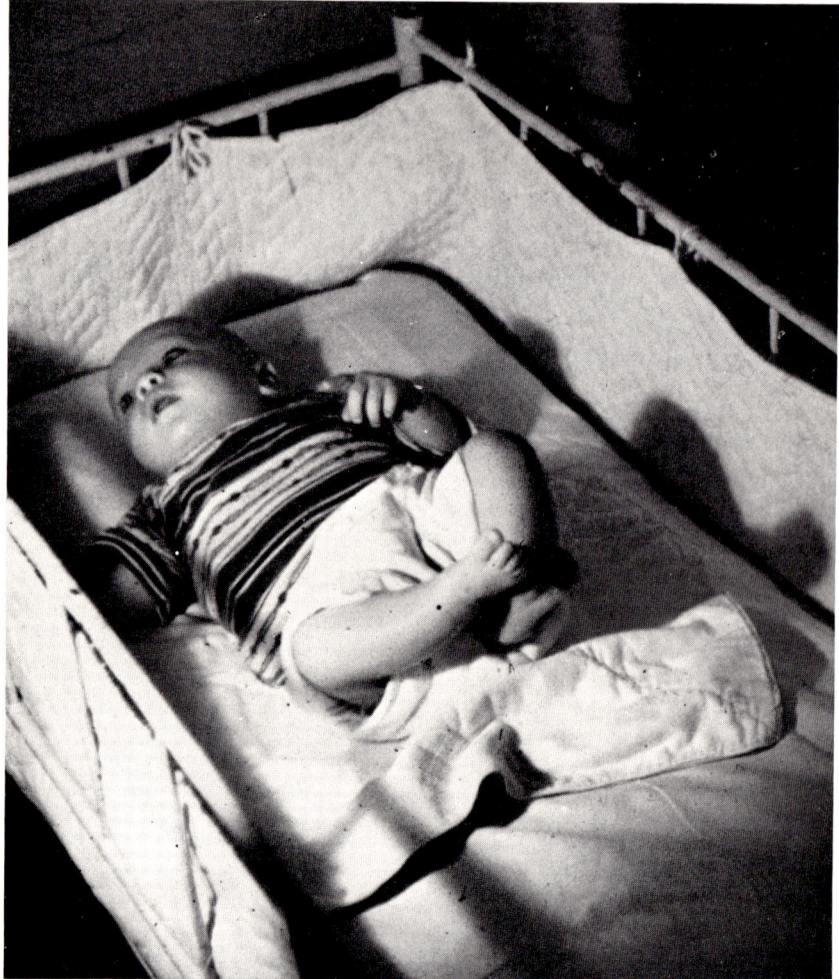

FIG. 1. The typical nursery ward facility for control infants 1-4 months of age (from White and Held, 1965. Copyright by Allyn and Bacon, Boston).

II. THE COURSE OF DEVELOPMENT

Detection of Salient Behaviours and Experiences

The early studies were concerned with a thorough understanding of what the infant was like in that world, and with the identification of

EXPERIENCE AND THE DEVELOPMENT OF MOTOR MECHANISMS   97

developments and experiences worthy of quantitative assessment. Fairly early in the programme visual exploration, hand regard, visual pursuit and visual convergence were selected for study, in addition, visually directed reaching. Later the prerequisite function of visual accommodation and the diagnostically interesting blink response to an approaching target were added. A wide variety of other behaviours,

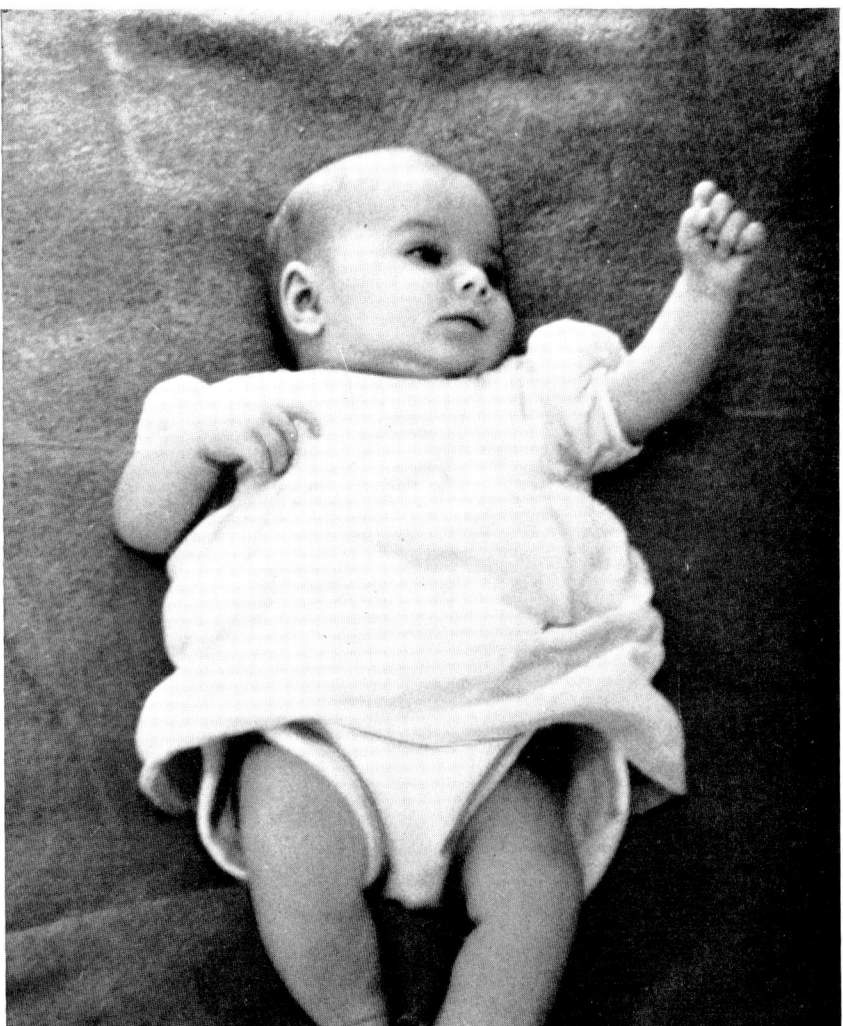

FIG. 2. Hand regard (from White *et al.*, 1964. Reprinted with permission by the Society for Research in Child Development, Chicago).

such as postural developments, were dealt with by regular administration of the Gesell scales (Gesell and Amatruda, 1941). Among our experiences several facts stood out with great clarity:

(a) The first month of life is a poor time to study visual-motor function, at least under routine conditions (our subjects were only visually alert above five per cent of the time during daylight hours);
(b) hand regard is a surprisingly frequent activity at which most infants spend dozens of hours, especially during the third month of life (Fig. 2);
(c) tactual exploration with the hands is minimal until the third month of life probably because the modal position of the fingers up to that time is flexion, and also because the influence of the tonic-neck-reflex virtually precludes mutual explorations by the hands (Fig. 3);
(d) most infants are visually alert and easily pleased during the third and fourth months of life;
(e) young infants are considerably less oral than psychoanalytic theory would lead one to believe.

The Problem of Quantitative Techniques

This field of study, as we found, is far from being well equipped with good tests or techniques for assessment purposes. The best non-specific instruments available to us appeared to be the Griffiths scale and the Northwestern infant intelligence scale devised by Griuland. However, by force of circumstances we were prevented from using these and accordingly the Gesell schedules, in spite of their weaknesses, were substituted; along with the Rosenblith modification of the Graham scale for screening newborns. The latter test was dropped after 200 babies had been tested without a single defective one, which was not manifest to the naked eye, being detected by it.

For behaviours such as visual accommodation and exploration there were no established techniques; we therefore devised our own. These, though effective because they were adapted for an infant's specific stage of development, were of uneven quality due to heavy reliance on subjective measurement. (No apology should be needed in this respect; one should surely measure as well as possible what is judged to merit measurement, rather than measure only when it can be done with absolute precision.)

Visual exploration or attention. To assess the sheer amount of visual

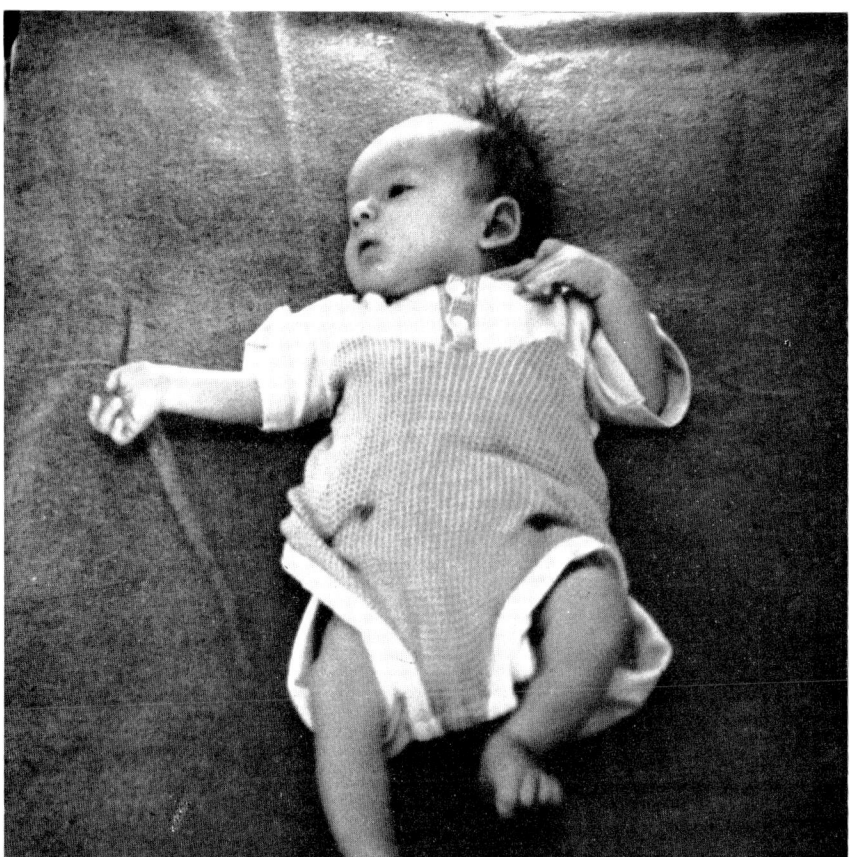

FIG. 3. The tonic neck reflex posture of the second month (from White et al., 1964. Reprinted with permission by the Society for Research in Child Development, Chicago).

exploration we used a subjective technique consisting of weekly 3-hour continuous watches of each subject. With the use of a simple definition of visual alertness—eyes more than half open, direction of gaze shifting within 30 seconds and criteria for ruling out periods of high distress— we were able to achieve inter-observer reliabilities in the region of 90 per cent agreement after brief training periods (White and Castle, 1964).

Prehension. For plotting the emergence of visually directed reaching we instituted a standardized test session on a weekly basis. This procedure also relied on the subjective assessment of behaviour, but unlike the measures on visual exploration inter-observer reliabilities were not obtained (for details see White et al., 1964). We depended on a consensus between tester and recorder which is not much better than conventional clinical testing. However, such a procedure is not devoid of scientific value; it is simply a poorer method of data collection than we should have liked. Departures were made from the Gesell procedures in certain important ways, such as the design of a more attractive stimulus object (White et al., 1964); in the presentation of the object at 45° right and left as well as at the midline; and in the use of an extension rod rather than the hand with which to offer the object.

Visual accommodation. In a paper in 1965 (Haynes et al.) we reported preliminary data on the development of focusing ability in infants, expertise in measurement being provided by Haynes whose assessment technique was an adaptation of a common procedure used in testing the vision of adults. After verification that the infant was attending to the target, the optometrist would make a subjective judgement of accommodative performance with a retinoscope and then check the judgement by using lenses of known power to standardize the appearance of the infant's response. Occasionally the results were checked but on the whole the optometrist's statement that he had confidence in his results was accepted, especially since certain other behaviours were regularly consistent with his assessment of accommodative status.

We are now completing the analysis of a replication of the earlier normative study, an inter-observer reliability study, and an attempt to enhance the development of accommodative ability. Preliminary indications are that the normative data are nicely confirmed, though the inter-observer reliabilities vary as a function of the subject's age and test distance.

The palpebral response to an approaching visible target. We managed to devise a reasonably sophisticated and objective assessment procedure for this response (Figs. 4, 5 and 6). Details of the test procedure have been published elsewhere (White and Clark, 1968). A polygraphic record of stimulus and response was obtained which was sensitive enough to allow fairly precise analysis of latency, amplitude and frequency of response (Fig. 7).

Our methods of measurement as regards the independent variable, however, were rather less sophisticated: most commonly we used duration of application of an experimental procedure. For example, in one study we administered 20 minutes of extra handling per day for 30 days; in another we placed infants in prone posture in front of interesting visible displays for 15 minutes after feeding, three times per day for 85 consecutive days. A third method was simply to change the environment in a particular way at one point in an infant's development

EXPERIENCE AND THE DEVELOPMENT OF MOTOR MECHANISMS 101

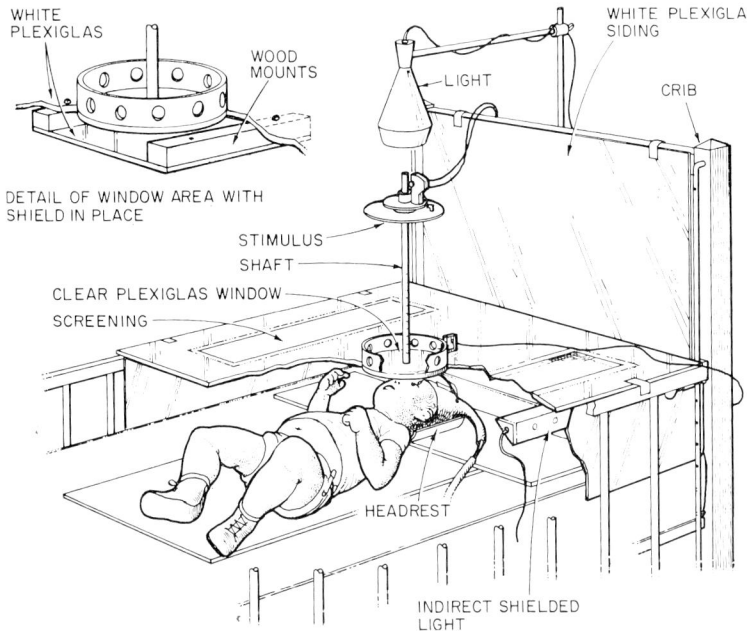

FIG. 4. Apparatus set up on conventional hospital crib, infant in test chamber (from White and Clark, 1968. Reprinted with permission of author and publisher).

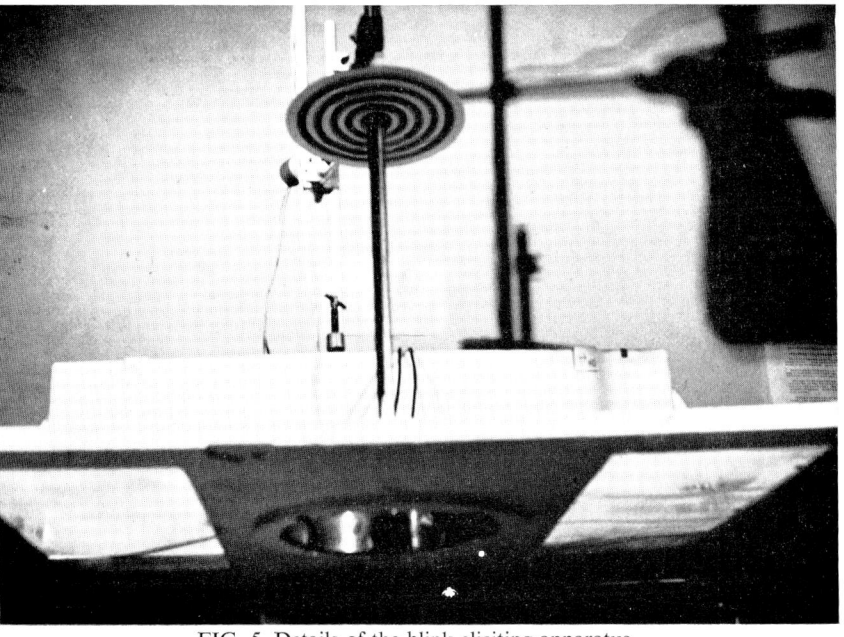

FIG. 5. Details of the blink-eliciting apparatus.

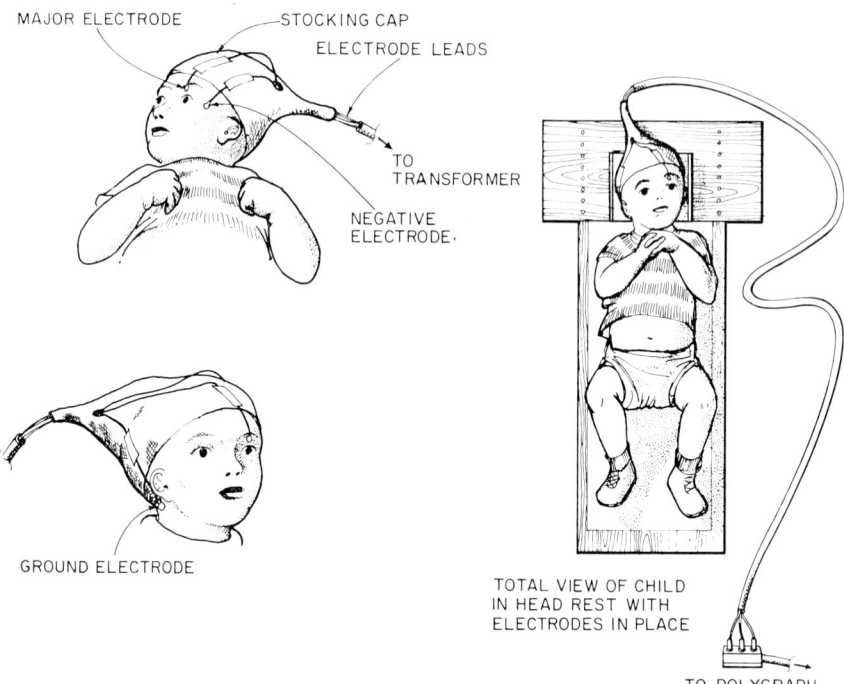

FIG. 6. Details of the electrode placement for the blink test (from White and Clark, 1968. Reprinted with permission of the author and publisher).

and let him live in that "world" for 24 hours per day, until such time as a new sensory environment was called for. In this last case there was an added measurement to be taken, because the extent to which subjects undergo different experiences as a consequence of an experimentally changed environment is quite variable. For example, in one study two-thirds of the subjects viewed and batted the experimental objects repeatedly over a 30-day period, but the other third hardly noticed them. Obviously, counts of interaction are a more accurate guide of the functional value of the experimental conditions than the crude statement of duration of exposure.

III. DATA ON VISUAL MOTOR DEVELOPMENT

Visual Attention

Figure 8 illustrates the development of this activity from birth to 4 months of age; each point represents the average of two scores taken

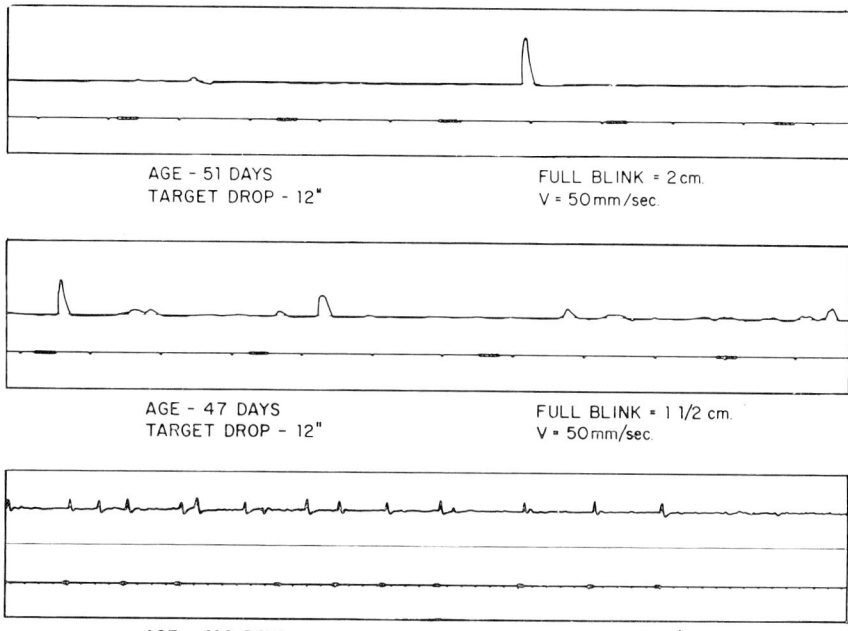

FIG. 7. Sample blink records, human infants (from White, 1969. Reprinted with permission of the Merrill-Palmer Institute).

during successive 2-week periods. It is interesting to note the correspondence between rather dramatic changes in the visible environment and the shape of this curve. For example, the sharp increase in slope between 45 and 60 days of age occurs at about the same time as the onset of sustained hand regard (approximately 49 days); for the next 6 weeks or so, the child spends much of his waking time observing his fist and finger movements. The next major change in the visible environment occurred for these infants between $3\frac{1}{2}$ and 4 months (see vertical line of Fig. 8) when they are transferred to large, open-sided cribs. About this time, the slope of the curve again shows a sharp increase, when the combination of greater trunk mobility, enabling them to turn from side to side, and the more diverse visual surroundings gave them access to a much more varied stimulus array.

Visually Directed Reaching

Figure 9 shows the results of our study: a ten-step analysis culminating in visually directed reaching just before 5 months of age (White *et al.*, 1964).

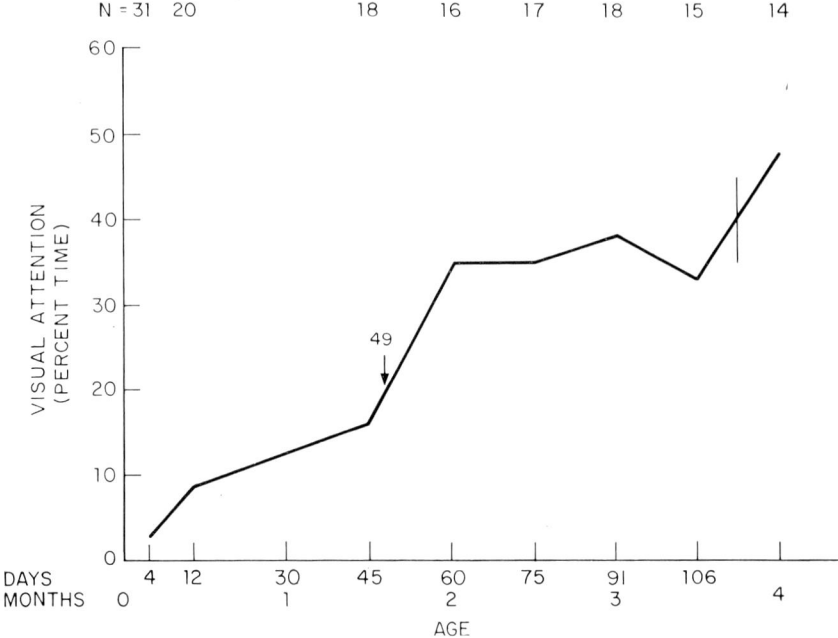

FIG. 8. Visual attention as a function of age, data for control group. The arrow at 49 days indicates the median age at which sustained hand regard appeared. The vertical bar at about 110 days indicates relocation to large open-sided cribs (from White and Held, 1966. Copyright by Allyn and Bacon, Boston).

Visual Accommodation

The development of visual accommodation during the first 4 months is shown in Fig. 10. Perfect adjustment to changing target distance would be represented by zero slope, whereas the complete absence of accommodative change would be indicated by a value of 1 (Fig. 4). Under 1 month the infant's accommodative response does not adjust to changes in target distance; the system appears to be locked at one focal distance, with a median value for the group of $7\frac{1}{2}$ inches. This is indicated by a slope of 1. Occasionally, infants of this age did not remain alert long enough to allow complete calibration of their responses; so in these few instances the magnitude of error was estimated (see legend to Fig. 10). Flexibility of the response begins about the middle of the second month, and performance comparable to that of the normal adult is attained by the fourth month, as shown by a median slope of 0·03.

In addition to these measurements 11 infants were retinoscoped while asleep in the nursery; in all 11 cases the accommodative system

Response	Observed N	Total N
Swipes at object	13	13
Unilateral hand raising	15	15
Both hands raised	16	18
Alternating glances (hand and object)	18	19
Hands to midline and clasp	15	15
One hand raised with alternating glances, other hand to midline clutching dress	11	19
Torso oriented towards object	15	18
Hands to midline and clasp and oriented towards object	14	19
Piaget-type reach	12	18
Top level reach	14	14

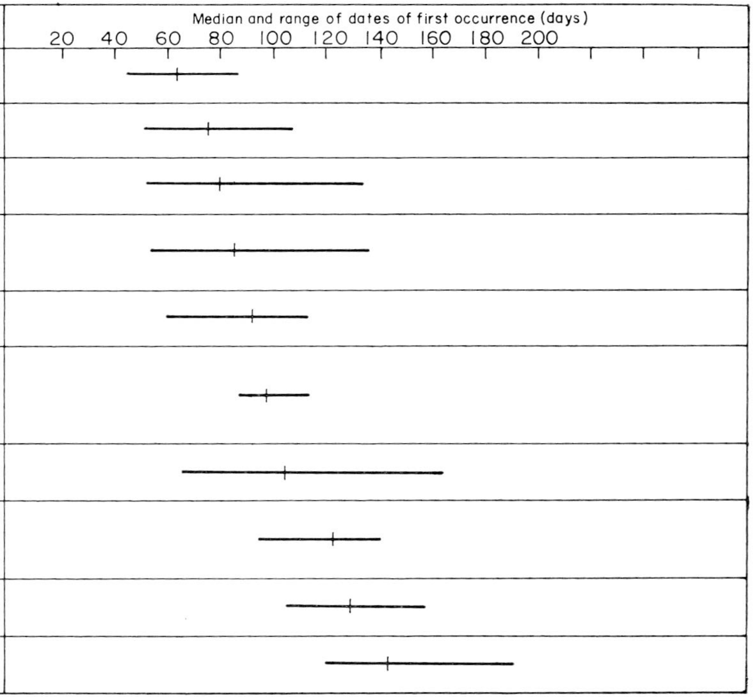
Median and range of dates of first occurrence (days)
20 40 60 80 100 120 140 160 180 200

FIG. 9. Normative data on the development of visually directed reaching. These data were compiled by combining the scores of control and handled infants (which did not differ significantly). From White *et al.*, 1964. Reprinted with permission by the Society for Research in Child Development, Chicago.

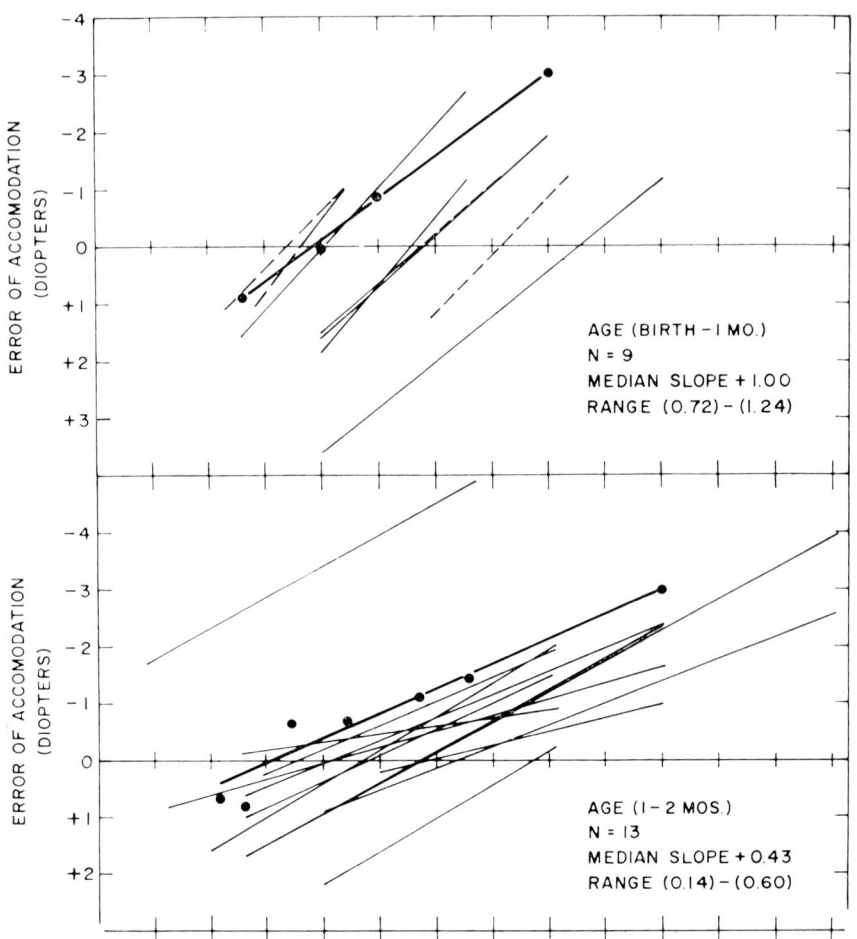

FIG. 10a. Four stages in the development of accommodation in the first 4 months of life. The heavy lines fitted to the filled circles illustrate both the progress of a typical infant and also the closeness of fit of the lines to the plotted points. During the first month, the data that were estimated are represented by dashed lines. Plus values indicate deviations in the hyperopic direction (from Haynes *et al.*, 1965. Copyright by the American Association for the Advancement of Science).

was found to be totally relaxed. Infants less than 1 week old occasionally exhibited slow changes in accommodation, but they were in no way related to the distance of the target. Older infants, when drowsy, exhibited a gradual drift of accommodation towards optical infinity, suggesting that drifting seen in the first week of life is a function of level of drowsiness.

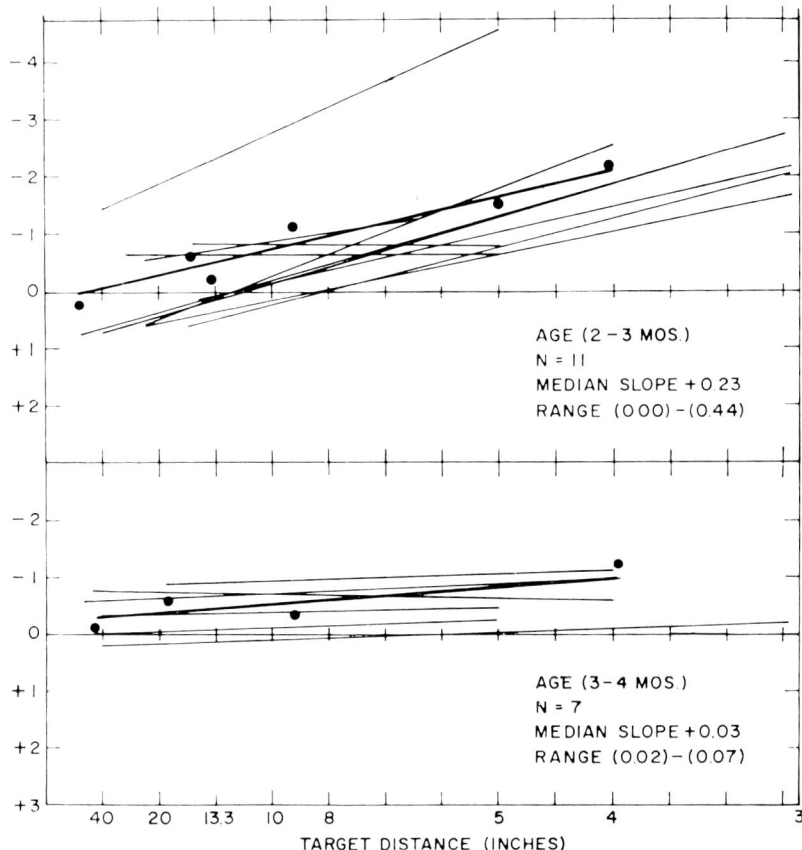

FIG. 10b. Same as 10a. Copyright 1965 by the American Association for the Advancement of Science.

The Blink Response to an Approaching Visible Target

Data on the development of this function are set out in Table I and Figs. 11–17.[2] The general conclusion to be gathered is that little stimulus-related response occurs before the middle of the second month of life. After that, development proceeds rapidly during the next 8 to 10 weeks

---

[2] Since spontaneous blinking occurs throughout the age range of this study (see Fig. 17), it is possible, especially with very young infants, that not all test-trial responses are elicited by the target action. Though data analysis is incomplete, it appears that our test trials influence the *timing* of blink responses more than their frequency. Though frequency is generally increased somewhat over time, the developmental changes are manifested most clearly by the growth of machine-like regularity of blink responses following immediately upon target action. Figures 13 and 14 indicate response latencies (measured from cessation of target action) shifting from 5–600 milliseconds at 1 month to about zero at 4 months.

TABLE I. NORMATIVE DEVELOPMENT OF THE BLINK RESPONSE

Target drop	18-32	33-47	48-62	63-77	78-92	93-104	105-119	120-134	135-149
Frequency[a]									
2 inches Ns	18	14	14	10	13	9	8	7	6
Med	0	0·75	0·5	3	3	6	5	8	9·5
Range	0-4	0-4	0-7	0-8	0-4	3-9	1-10	3-10	5-10
7 inches Ns	18	14	14	10	13	9	8	7	6
Med	1	2	2	7·5	7	9	8	10	10
Range	0-6	0-10	0-10	1-9	5-10	7·5-10	9·75	9-10	9-10
12 inches Ns	18	14	14	10	13	9	8	7	6
Med	3	3	4·5	8	7·5	10	10	10	10
Range	1-6	0-10	0-10	3-10	5-10	9-10	3-10	7-10	9-10
Overall median score across 2-7-12 inches	2	2	2	5	6	9	9	10	10
Latency									
2 inches Ns	8	8	7	8	10	9	8	7	6
Med	500	400	475	425	203	120	73	80	55
Range	340-600	-80-780	-120-760	160-1,060	90-835	60-400	40-530	40-360	-5-140
7 inches Ns	10	13	12	10	13	9	8	7	6
Med	550	650	810	200	80	40	25	0	10
Range	360-1,060	100-1,110	90-1,140	60-800	0-255	-5-120	-95-200	-30-30	-80-30
12 inches Ns	18	13	13	10	13	9	8	7	6
Med	650	600	350	35	40	40	5	-20	-15
Range	20-1,200	0-960	0-1,050	0-320	-50-880	-30-80	-120-100	-60-60	-125-0
Overall median score across 2-7-12 inches	555	640	580	250	90	60	55	30	0
Amplitude									
2 inches Ns	8	8	7	8	10	9	8	7	6
Med (%)	66	66·5	47	40	51	57	70	70	116
Range (%)	30-107	26-140	30-120	25-100	32-93	40-67	25-174	67-143	53-144
7 inches Ns	10	13	12	10	13	9	8	7	6
Med (%)	58	52	53	61	73	87	100	147	114
Range (%)	33-136	27-130	32·5-100	25-147	36-140	40-160	35-175	80-214	67-208
12 inches Ns	18	13	13	10	13	9	8	7	6
Med (%)	56	47	70	80	93	120	106	113	113
Range (%)	25-113	30-107	27-150	30-275	40-140	53-74	35-174	58-166	98-208
Overall median score across 2-7-12 inches	50	60	50	67	67	65	90	115	116

[a] There were ten randomly spaced target drops of 2, 7 and 12 inches. In all trials, the target bottomed at from 1·5-2 inches from the corneal surfaces of the infant's eyes.

EXPERIENCE AND THE DEVELOPMENT OF MOTOR MECHANISMS 109

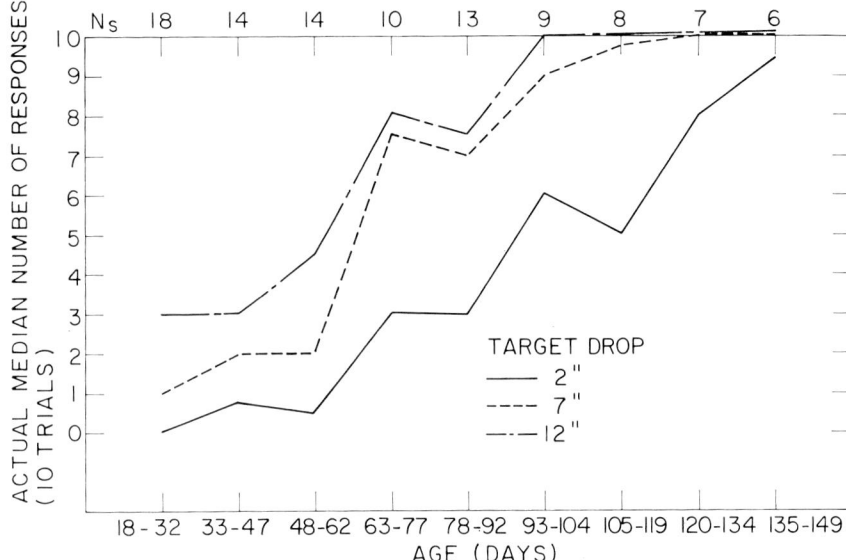

FIG. 11. Frequency of blink responses as a function of length of target drop, normative group.

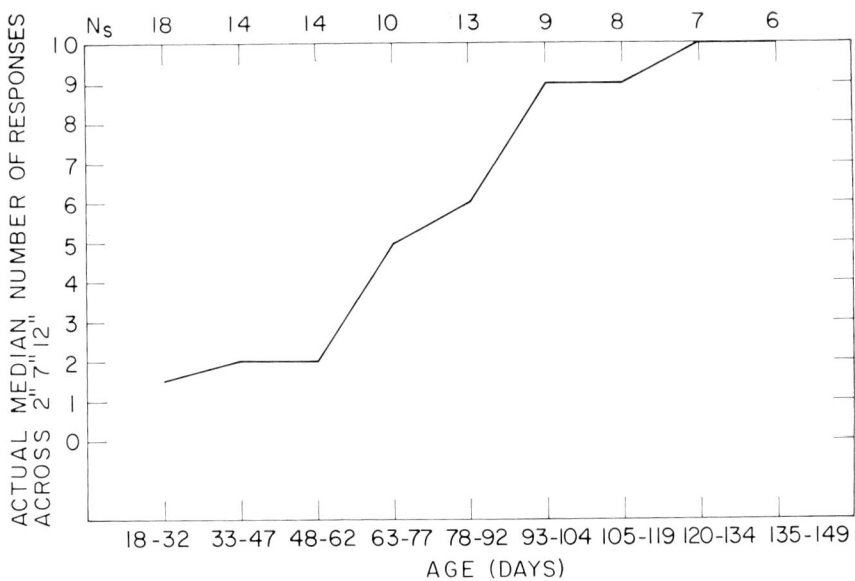

FIG. 12. Frequency of blink responses across three target distances, normative group.

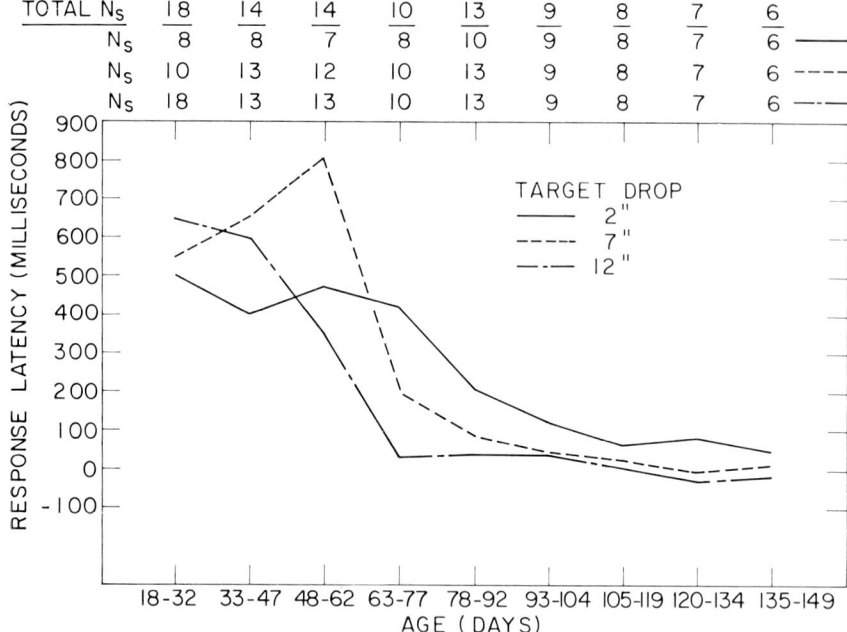

FIG. 13. Latency of blink responses as a function of length of target drop, normative group.

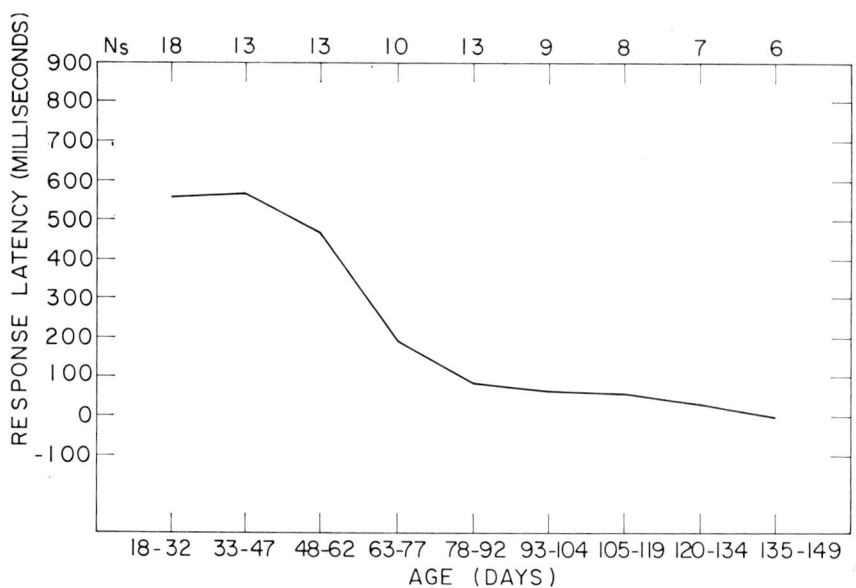

FIG. 14. Latency of blink responses across three target distances, normative group.

and seems to be complete by 4 months of age. There is a close correspondence between the development of this response and the flexibility of the accommodative system.

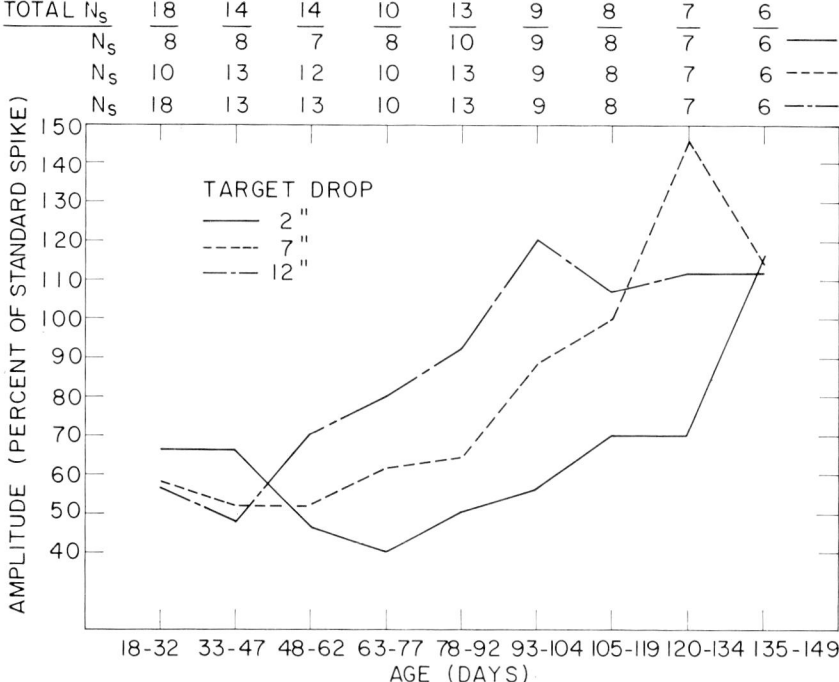

FIG. 15. Amplitude of blink responses as a function of length of target drop, normative group.

Hand Regard

The onset of sustained hand regard (more than 3 seconds of continuous viewing) occurred at 49 days of age for the first control group ($n = 16$).

Theories

Elaborate theorizing is out of place in the study of infancy at this stage, although one must acknowledge the importance of Piaget's (1952) general biological view of development as being a continuous process of adaptation, and the value of his concepts of assimilation and accommodation. His theory, however, does not deal with the

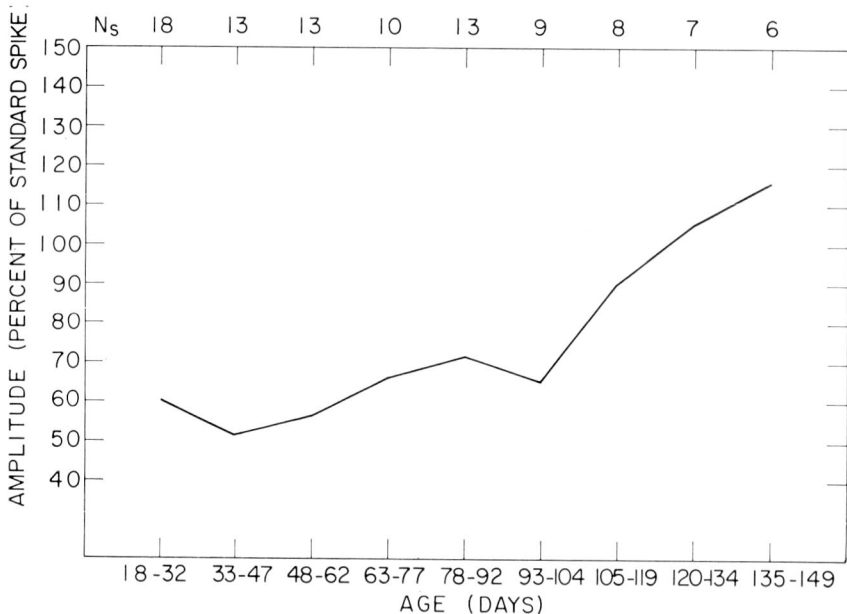

FIG. 16. Amplitude of blink responses across three target distances, normative group.

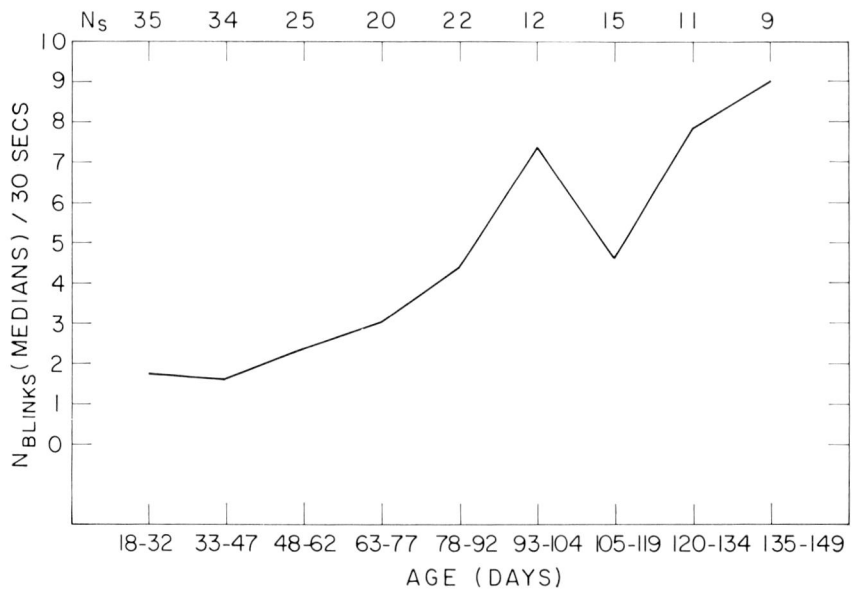

FIG. 17. Spontaneous blink rate, experimental and control groups combined performance.

mechanisms of development in the moment-to-moment experiences of the child. As regards mechanisms, Held claims that information is processed, and the infant develops, only when he performs certain motor acts within certain kinds of sensory surroundings, while Hunt argues that the infant's motor involvement is restricted to the ocular and extra-ocular muscles in the first month and that more extensive motor development only becomes necessary later. Such discussion of mechanisms addresses a very practical level of experimental investigation (in contrast to the concepts of assimilation and accommodation which belong in the realm of abstractions), and it is preferable to the theoretical notions about infancy, espoused by many leading authorities, which do not meet the facts.

IV. LONGITUDINAL EXPERIMENTAL STUDIES

First Modification of Rearing Conditions: Handling Study

We carried out one handling study because of the weight of evidence, from several sources, consistent with what we had learned about infants in the first weeks of life and on the assumption that active involvement by the infant is, in general, a prerequisite for development. I shall concentrate on that involvement. Major clues regarding the types of experience to foster come from what we discovered about the emerging abilities and interests of infants. An additional assumption, therefore, is that "feeding" newly emerging abilities holds the key to designing the optimal "match" between the infant and the environment.

Many recent studies have reported the remarkable effects of post-natal handling on the subsequent development of laboratory reared animals (Denenberg and Karas, 1959; Levine, 1957; Meier, 1961). Mice, kittens and dogs given a little extra handling grew up to be "better" animals as measured by a wide variety of tests—they were superior in many physical and adaptive respects. Surveys of maternal deprivation studies by Yarrow (1961) and Casler (1961) suggest that early handling appears necessary for adequate human development. Brody (1951) noted that infants who received moderate handling were consistently more visually attentive than those receiving minimal handling. A test was accordingly devised to discover whether extra handling of our subjects, who normally received minimal amounts, would result in accelerated visual-motor development.

From day 6 to day 36, nurses administered 20 minutes of extra handling each day to each of ten infants; thereafter measures of overall development, physical growth, general health, development of reaching,

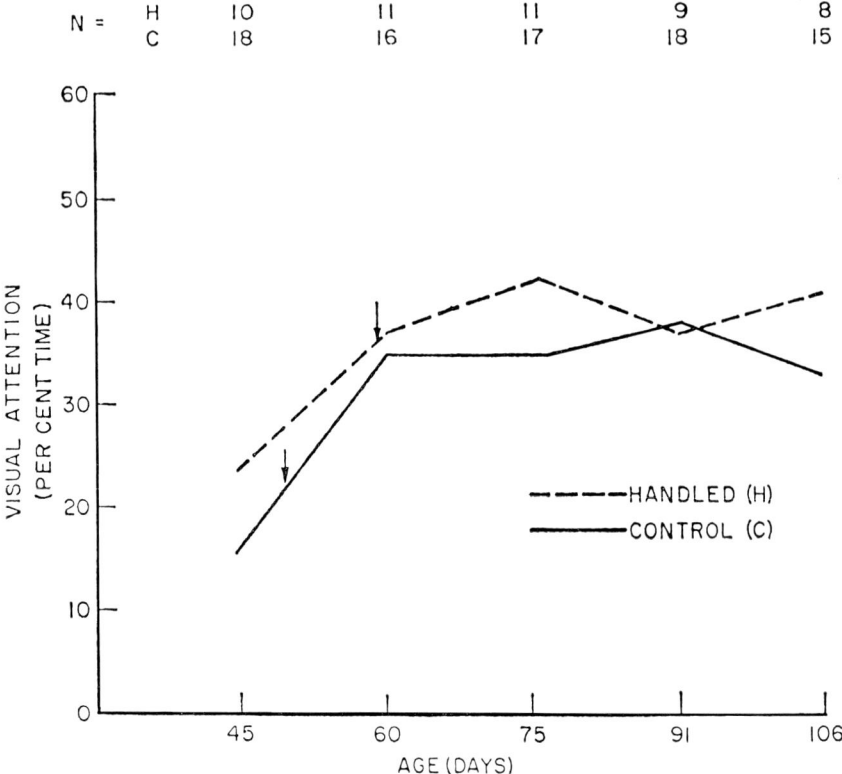

FIG. 18. Comparison of visual attention in control subjects and in those given extra handling (from White and Held, 1966. Copyright by Allyn and Bacon, Boston).

and visual attention were taken at weekly intervals between days 37 and 152 (White and Castle, 1964).

Results

No changes were found in any developmental process except the growth of visual attention; the handled group was more visually attentive than the control group.[3] Note that the shapes of the curves in Fig. 18 are quite similar. Sustained hand regard appeared somewhat later in the handled group (day 60) than in the controls (day 49). Upon transfer to large open-sided cribs the handled group, like the control

[3] In a previous report (White and Castle, 1964) we indicated that this increase in visual attention was statistically significant; in fact, the analysis used was inappropriate. Moreover, we added data from one new subject. Subsequent analyses (see Table IV) indicate a strong trend that fails to reach significance at the 5 per cent level.

group, exhibited a sharp increase in visual attentiveness (see Tables II–IV).

TABLE II. SUMMARY OF VISUAL ATTENTION DATA

From White, 1969. Reprinted with permission of the Merrill-Palmer Institute, Detroit.

Group and Period observed	N subjects[a]	N scores[a]	Mean percentage of time attending
37–112 days			
Control	45	113	32·1
Handled	11	102	36·8
Massive enrichment	13	118	32·8
Modified enrichment	14	146	40·1
Total	83	479	
37–75 days			
Control	34	59	29·9
Handled	10	58	34·2
Massive enrichment	13	68	26·3
Modified enrichment	14	78	36·7
Total	71	263	
76–112 days			
Control	16	43	33·5
Handled	8	37	41·4
Massive enrichment	9	43	46·9
Modified enrichment	13	70	42·5
Total	46	193	

[a] Number of subjects and observations varies because subjects, though overlapping, were not identical for the three periods.

This investigation suggested that innocuous environmental modifications might alter the development of important visual-motor functions such as exploratory behaviour; however, no evidence for comparable plasticity in other visual-motor developments was found following the extra handling. It is possible that further research into the effects of early handling would establish the possibility of still greater increases in visual exploratory behaviour.

Second Modification of Rearing Conditions: Massive Enrichment Study

Several studies indicate that visual-motor performance depends to a significant extent on experiences of particular kinds for its development. Riesen's (1958) work demonstrated that chimpanzees require exposure to patterned visual stimulation for normal visual-motor development. His later studies have suggested that movement within a patterned

TABLE III. SUMMARIES OF ANALYSES OF VARIANCE PERFORMED ON VISUAL ATTENTION DATA

From White, 1969. Reprinted with permission of the Merrill-Palmer Institute, Detroit.

Treatment groups in analysis[a] and period observed	Source	ss	df	ms	F	p
37–112 days old						
C, H, ME, Mod E	Between	4,696	3	1,565	3·95	<0·01
	Within[b]	188,259	475	396	—	—
	Total	192,955	478	—	—	—
C, H, ME	Between	987	2	494	1·10	NS
	Within[b]	148,084	331	447	—	—
	Total	149,071	333	—	—	—
37–75 days old						
C, H, ME, Mod E	Between	4,550	3	1,517	4·56	<0·01
	Within[b]	86,137	259	333	—	—
	Total	90,687	262	—	—	—
C, H, Mod E	Between	1,615	2	808	2·43	NS
	Within[b]	63,714	192	332	—	—
	Total	65,329	194	—	—	—
76–112 days old						
C, H, ME, Mod E	Between	3,560	3	1,187	2·87	<0·05
	Within[b]	78,011	189	413	—	—
	Total	81,571	192	—	—	—

[a] C=Control Group; H=Handled Group; ME=Massive Enrichment Group; Mod E=Modified Enrichment Group.

[b] In nested analysis of variance designs, between- and within-subject mean squares may be pooled if they do not differ significantly (Winer, 1962). In the data of this study, such was the case. Since neither between- nor within-subject variability was of interest, the variances were pooled to test for treatment differences.

environment is also required for adequate development (Riesen, 1958). Held and his collaborators (Held and Bossom, 1961; Held, 1961; Mikaelian and Held, 1964) have repeatedly demonstrated the importance of self-induced movement in dependably structured environments for adaptation to rearranged sensory inputs in human adults. Held and Hein's (1963) study of neonatal kittens showed the applicability of these findings to developmental processes, and their results indicated that movement *per se* in the presence of dependable surroundings was insufficient for normal visual-motor development. Kittens whose movements were externally produced rather than self-induced did not develop normally; self-induced movement in dependable surroundings was found to be necessary for adequate development as well as for maintenance of stable visual-motor behaviour.

TABLE IV. SIGNIFICANCE OF DIFFERENCES BETWEEN MEAN VISUAL ATTENTION SCORES FOR EXPERIMENTAL AND CONTROL GROUPS OBSERVED AT AGE 37–75 DAYS AND/OR 76–112 DAYS

From White, 1969. Reprinted with permission of the Merrill-Palmer Institute, Detroit.

Group means compared[a]	t	df	p[b]
37–112 days old			
C (32·1) vs H (36·8)	1·72	213	<0·05
C (32·1) vs ME (32·8)	—	—	NS
C (32·1) vs Mod E (40·1)	3·10	257	<0·005
H (36·8) vs ME (32·8)	—	—	NS
H (36·8) vs Mod E (40·1)	—	—	NS
ME (32·8) vs Mod E (40·1)	2·96	262	<0·005
Mod E (40·1) vs C+H+ME (33·8)	3·50	477	<0·0005
37–75 days old			
C (29·9) vs H (34·2)	—	—	NS
C (29·9) vs ME (26·3)	—	—	NS
C (29·9) vs Mod E (40·1)	3·21	135	<0·005
H (34·2) vs ME (26·3)	2·42	124	<0·01
H (34·2) vs Mod E (40·1)	1·87	134	<0·05
ME (26·3) vs Mod E (40·1)	4·56	144	<0·0005
ME (26·3) vs C+H+Mod E (33·9)	2·97	262	<0·01
76–112 days old			
C (33·5) vs H (41·4)	1·73	78	<0·05
C (33·5) vs ME (46·9)	3·06	84	<0·005
C (33·5) vs Mod E (42·5)	2·29	111	<0·025
H (41·4) vs ME (46·9)	—	—	NS
H (41·4) vs Mod E (42·5)	—	—	NS
ME (46·9) vs Mod E (42·5)	—	—	NS

[a] C = Control Group; H = Handled Group; ME = Massive Enrichment Group; Mod E = Modified Enrichment Group.

[b] Because six significance figures are being calculated in each group, a conservative position would increase the required level of significance to $10/K(K-1)$, where K = Number of Groups. In this case, K = 4, and the more stringent level required would be 0·0083 (Ferguson, 1959, p. 238).

Our subjects were usually reared under conditions which are less than optimal with respect to the kinds of experience discussed above. Mobility was hampered by soft mattresses where the infant easily sank into depressions, as well as by the supine posture in which they were placed. The visual surroundings were poorly figured. Consequently, according to our hypothesis, improved conditions for mobility and brighter surroundings would produce accelerated visual-motor development.

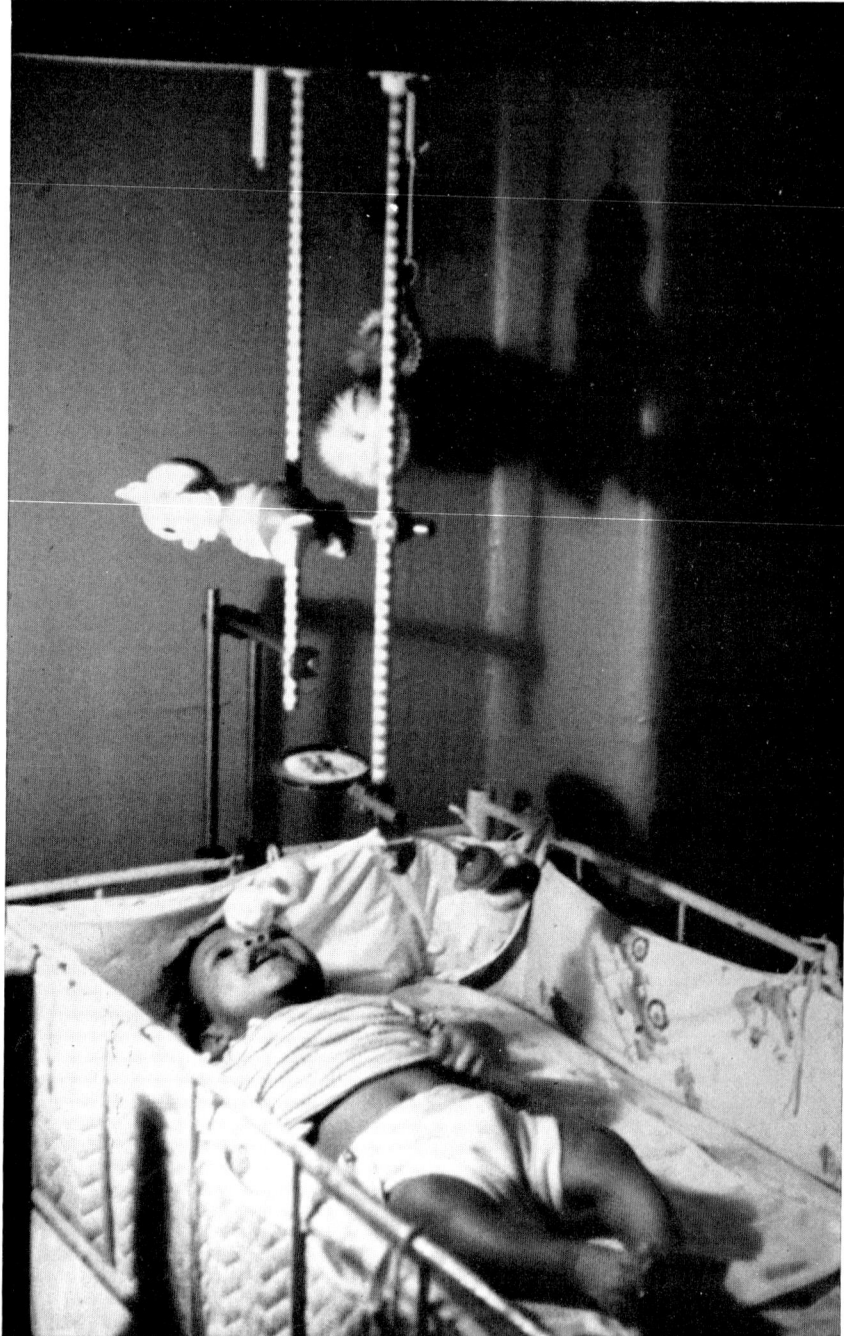

FIG. 19. The massive enrichment condition featuring many brightly coloured objects around the infant at distances of 5–36 inches (from White and Held, 1966. Copyright by Allyn and Bacon, Boston).

As a first test we enriched the environment of a group of 19 infants in as many respects as was feasible (White, 1967). First, tactual-vestibular stimulation was increased; each infant received 20 minutes of extra handling each day from day 6 to day 36. Secondly, mobility was increased; infants were placed in a prone posture for 15 minutes after the 6 a.m., 10 a.m. and 2 p.m. feedings each day from day 37 to day 124. At these times the crib liners were removed, making the ward activities visible to the child, so that movements of the head and trunk resulted from the normal tendency of infants to rear their heads in the presence of figured visual surroundings. Moreover, the crib mattresses were flattened to facilitate head, arm and trunk mobility. Thirdly, the visual surroundings were brightened; a special stabile, featuring highly contrasting colours and numerous shapes against a dull, white background, was suspended over these infants from day 37 to day 124 (see Fig. 19); and printed multi-coloured sheets and bumpers were substituted for the standard white ones. These changes were designed to heighten the visual interest and increase the hand movement because of the normal tendency of infants to swipe at visible objects nearby.

Prehensile responses and visual attention were measured weekly. The rates of development of spontaneous behaviours related to visual-motor function such as hand regard, hands touching at the midline, mutual fingering, and turning of the torso were assessed from the records of the 3-hour observation periods. Performance in the Gesell tests was recorded at bi-weekly intervals to determine general developmental progress. Records of rate of weight gain and general health were also kept.

Results

Hand regard and swiping. Hand regard, as such, was less frequently shown by this group than by the controls; instead, the hands were generally first observed as they came in contact with portions of the experimental stabile. We called this pattern "monitored stabile play" and considered it together with "monitored bumper play" as forms of hand regard. By these criteria the onset of hand regard was delayed for some 12 days in our experimental group (not significant, see Table VIII). The onset of swiping was also set back by about 5 days, which was also not significant (Mann-Whitney U Test). The responses to the test object leading to reaching is illustrated for this group in Fig. 20.

Prehension. The median age for the first appearance of top-level reaching was 98 days for the experimental group, an advance of some 45 days over the control group ($p < 0.001$; Mann-Whitney U Test).

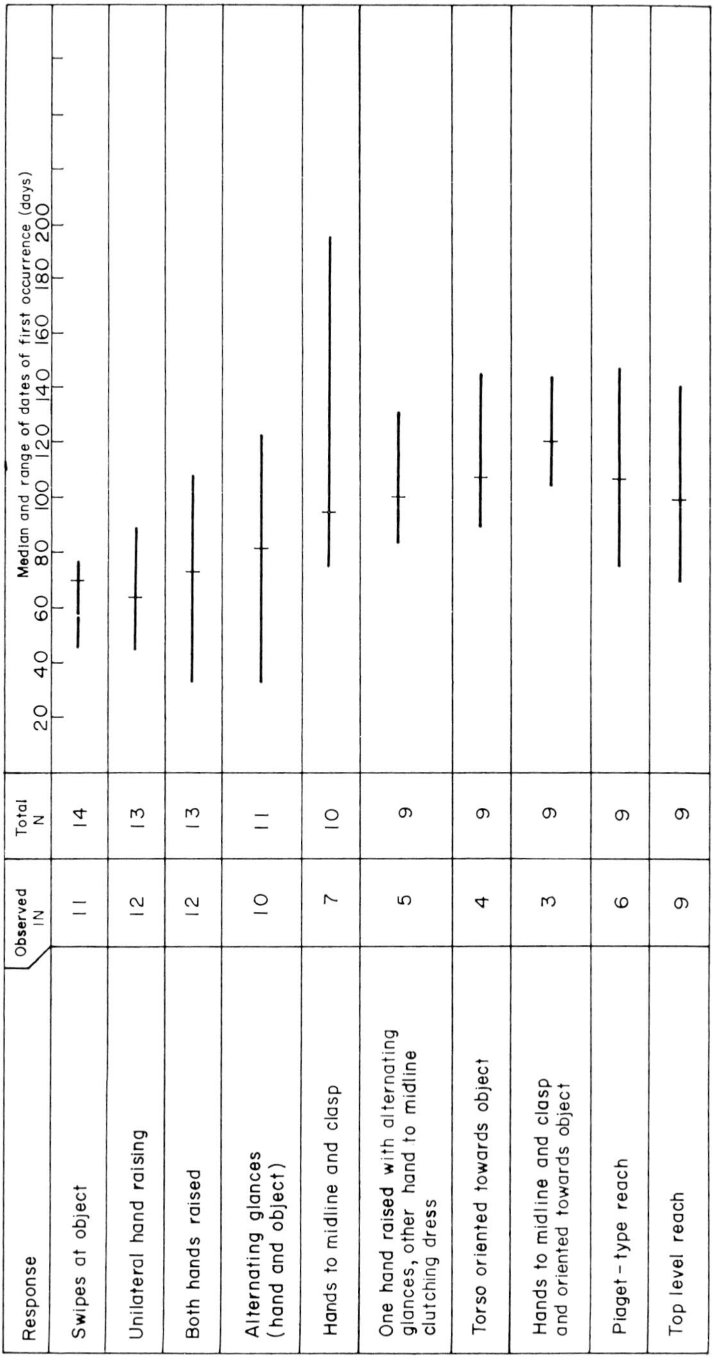

Response	Observed IN	Total N	Median and range of dates of first occurrence (days) 20 40 60 80 100 120 140 160 180 200
Swipes at object	11	14	
Unilateral hand raising	12	13	
Both hands raised	12	13	
Alternating glances (hand and object)	10	11	
Hands to midline and clasp	7	10	
One hand raised with alternating glances, other hand to midline clutching dress	5	9	
Torso oriented towards object	4	9	
Hands to midline and clasp and oriented towards object	3	9	
Piaget-type reach	6	9	
Top level reach	9	9	

FIG. 20. The development of visually-directed reaching. Study B—massive enrichment (from White and Held, 1966. Copyright by Allyn and Bacon, Boston).

Some types of preliminary responses reported to our control group did not occur before the onset of top-level reaching.

Visual attention. The course of development of visual attention was also altered dramatically in our experimental group, as illustrated by Fig. 21 and Tables II, III and IV. Whereas the delay in the onset of

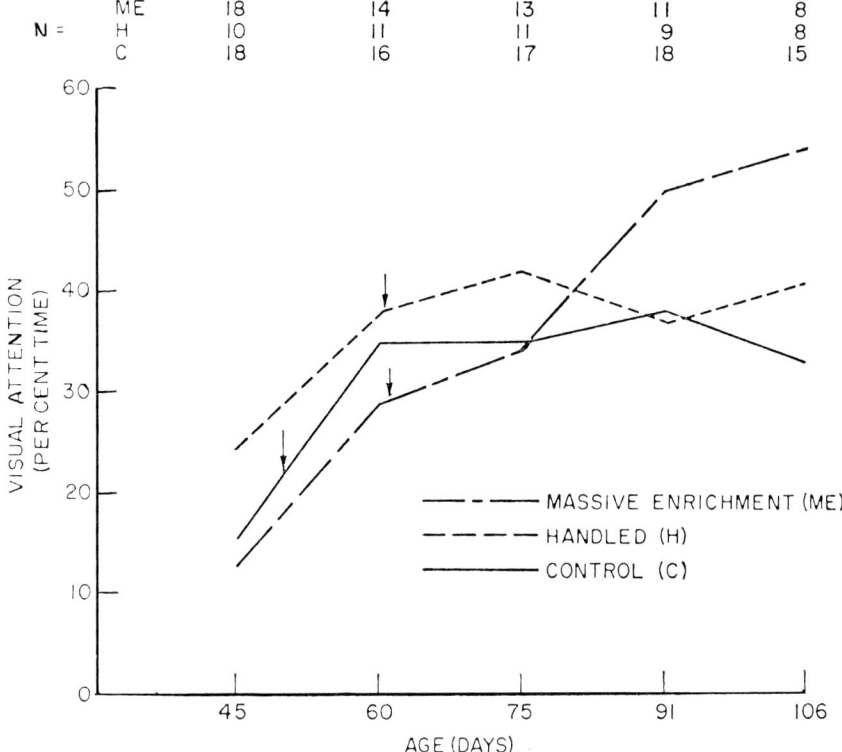

FIG. 21. Comparison of visual attention among control subjects, handled subjects, and those given handling followed by massive enrichment (from White and Held, 1966. Copyright by Allyn and Bacon, Boston).

hand regard was accompanied by a decrease in visual exploratory behaviour for the first portion of the test period, once the group began to engage in prehensile contacts with the stabile and the figured bumpers, visual attention increased sharply.

Clearly the results of this study demonstrated the plasticity of several visual-motor developments. The notion that the onset of hand regard is in part a function of environmental factors is not novel. On the Gesell scale hand regard is a behaviour for day 84. Our control infants, however, with virtually nothing else to look at, discovered their hands before 50 days of age; and Piaget (1952) noted that the onset of this behaviour varied by as much as 30 days among his own children as a function of differing environmental circumstances. Therefore, the fact that infants provided with enriched surroundings were late in discovering their hands as compared with controls was not totally unexpected.

To our surprise the group exhibited less visual attention during the first 5 weeks in the brightened surroundings; in fact, not only did they tend to ignore the stabile and bumpers but they seemed to spend much more time crying than did the control group during the same period. Then at about 72 days of age this group began to engage in a great deal of stabile play. The rattles were repeatedly swiped at, thereby producing far more monitored hand regard and arm movements than would normally have occurred. Subsequently in less than 1 month, the integration of the group with the approach movements had been completed, a transition for which control infants required almost 3 months.

Earlier it was noted that the course of development of visual exploratory behaviour seemed to reflect the availability of interesting things to look at; in the control and handled groups the slope of the curve of visual attention increased sharply when the hands were discovered and then decreased during the next 6 weeks. In this experimental group for about a month, beginning at day 37, the new attractions were actually ineffective and perhaps even upsetting. However, once positive responses to the surroundings were aroused, visual attention increased sharply, in striking contrast with the previous groups; the dip seen at $3\frac{1}{2}$ months in both previous groups was absent.

Third Modification of Rearing Conditions: Pacifiers

Until day 37 procedures for the third study were the same as in the second study; then instead of the enrichment provided by prone position, the stabile and printed sheets and bumpers, just one modification was introduced from day 37 to day 68 (White, 1967). Two pacifiers were mounted on the rails of the crib and made to stand out visually by fixing to them a red and white patterned disc against a flat, white background (Fig. 22). The objects were set 6 to 7 inches away from the corneal surfaces of the infant's eyes, in a position to elicit maximum attention from 6 to 10 week-old infants, whose eyes normally accommodate at about 8 to 10 inches. It was assumed that the pacifiers might have the effect of helping the infant to discover his hands; these objects might furthermore provide appropriate anchor points in space intermediate between the locus of spontaneous fixation and the ordinary

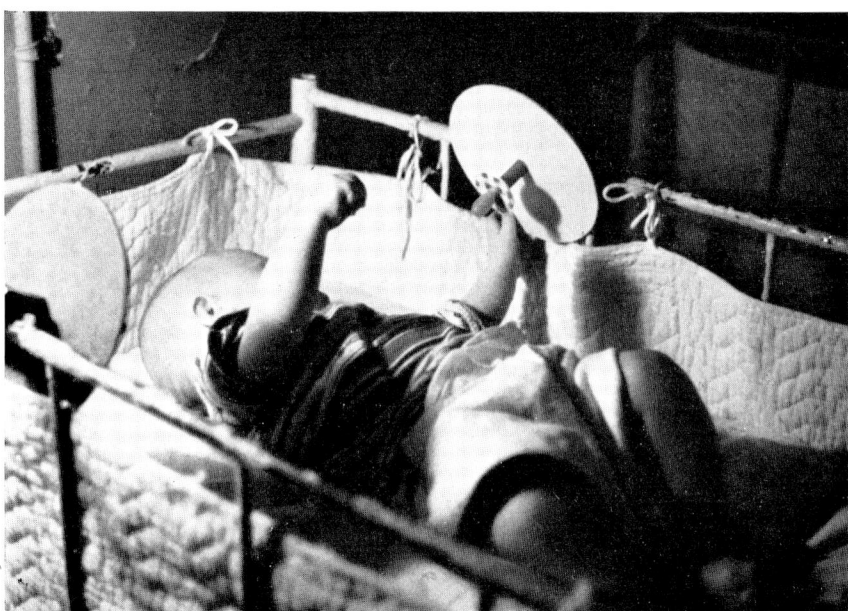

FIG. 22. The modified enrichment condition with two highlighted pacifiers placed according to postural and visual characteristics of the 4–8-week-old-infant (from White and Held, 1966. Copyright by Allyn and Bacon, Boston).

path of motion of the hand extended in the tonic-neck-reflex posture.

At 68 days, the infant was placed in a crib with a stabile similar to the one used in the previous study until he was 124 days old. According to our theory these infants ought to have been consistently precocious in the attainment of visually directed reaching, and shown consistently higher visual attention.

Results

Hand regard and swiping. In the control group the onset of sustained hand regard occurred at day 49; infants in the handling study were behind (day 60). Infants in the second study were even later in this respect (day 61), supporting the idea that the discovery of the hand is in part a function of the availability of interesting visible objects. The modified enrichment of this third study seemed more appropriate for the infant during the second month of life; and infants exhibited sustained hand regard at day 44 (see Table V). It should be noted that control infants reared in ordinary unenhanced surroundings are about as advanced in hand regard at this age. The onset of swiping responses

TABLE V. SIGNIFICANCE OF DIFFERENCES BETWEEN EXPERIMENTAL AND CONTROL GROUPS IN AGE AT ONSET OF SUSTAINED HAND REGARD[a]

From White, 1969. Reprinted with permission of the Merrill-Palmer Institute, Detroit.

Condition (N of Ss; Mdn age in days at onset)	Handled (N=10; Mdn=60)	Massive Enrichment (N=14; Mdn=61)	Modified enrichment (N=15; Mdn=44)
Control (N=16; Mdn=49)	0·1469, NS	0·0571, NS	0·1867, NS
Handled (N=10; Mdn=60)	—	0·4168, NS	0·0136
Massive enrichment (N=14; Mdn=61)	—	—	0·0016

[a] Table entries are significance levels based on Mann-Whitney U (1-tailed) tests. In order to conclude that the groups compared come from significantly different (0·05 level) parent populations, compensation must be made for the fact that a number of pairs have been sampled. In this case, six pairs are sampled, and the significance level must reach 0·008 before it can be concluded that the two groups differ. This value was derived from the following formula: $p=(1-\alpha)^n$, where $p=0.05$, $n=$ number of pairs compared, and $\alpha=$ the level of significance which must be found for any single pair in order to conclude that there is more than one parent population involved.

followed the same general pattern, with infants in this third study making an earlier start than any other group (day 58; see Fig. 23).

Prehension. Apparently the modified, or paced, enrichment of the third study was the most successful match of external circumstances to internally developing structures. This was indicated by the acquisition of top-level reaching at less than 3 months of age, namely, day 98 which is significantly earlier than the controls ($p < 0.001$, Mann-Whitney U Test).

Visual attention. Figure 24 shows the data on visual attention for the subjects from the four groups. The depression of visual interest shown by the infants in the second study from day 37 to 74 has been eliminated, and the "modified enrichment" group consistently is more attentive ($p < 0.0005$) throughout the test period (see Tables III and IV). It is curious to note that the third group was more consistently attentive than the others, the reduction of such behaviour at 3½ months appeared as it had in the control and the first groups. It seems that some uncontrolled variable is interacting with our various attempts at modifying the function.

Fourth Modification of Rearing Conditions: the Mitt Study

The three major kinds of experience that seemed appropriate for manipulation during the first three months of life were hand regard,

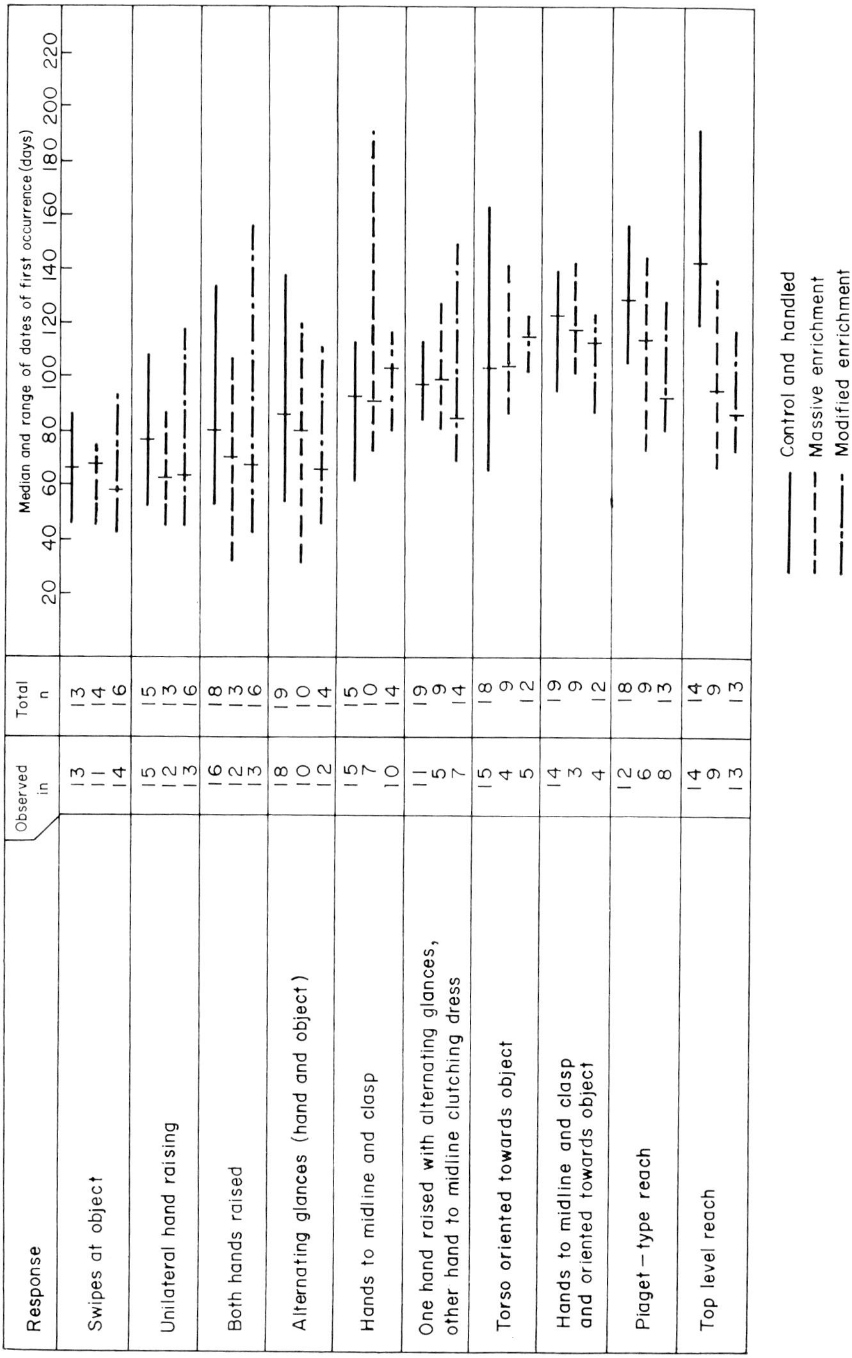

EXPERIENCE AND THE DEVELOPMENT OF MOTOR MECHANISMS 125

Response	Observed in	Total n	Median and range of dates of first occurrence (days)
Swipes at object	13 11 14	13 14 16	
Unilateral hand raising	15 12 13	15 13 16	
Both hands raised	16 12 13	18 13 16	
Alternating glances (hand and object)	18 10 12	19 10 14	
Hands to midline and clasp	15 7 10	15 10 14	
One hand raised with alternating glances, other hand to midline clutching dress	11 5 7	19 9 14	
Torso oriented towards object	15 4 5	18 9 12	
Hands to midline and clasp and oriented towards object	14 3 4	19 9 12	
Piaget-type reach	12 6 8	18 9 13	
Top level reach	14 9 13	14 9 13	

——— Control and handled
– – – Massive enrichment
–·–·– Modified enrichment

FIG. 23. Comparison of prehensory responses among all groups (from White and Held, 1966. Copyright by Allyn and Bacon, Boston).

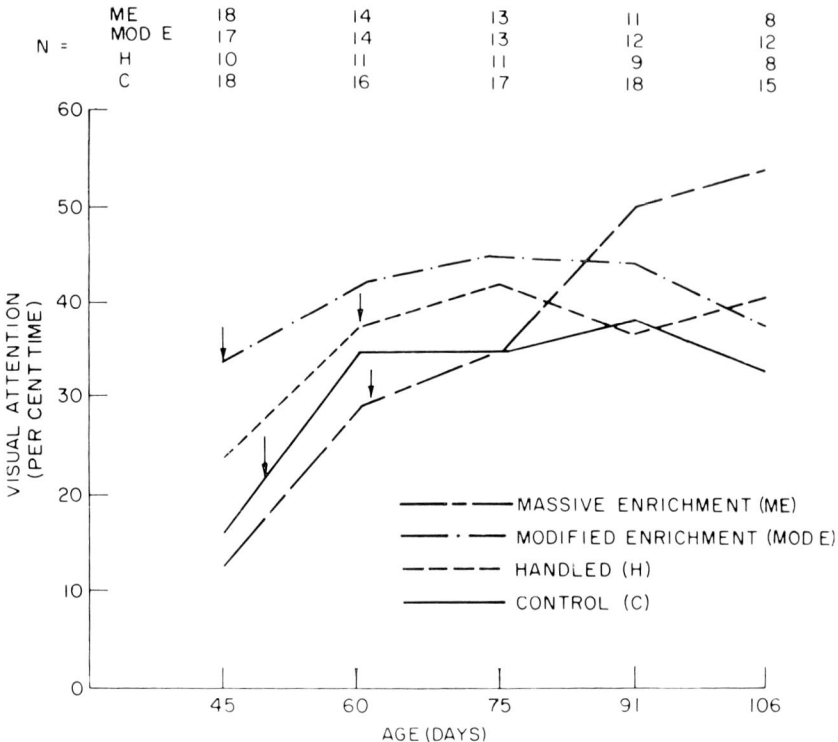

FIG. 24. Comparison of visual attention among all groups (from White and Held, 1966. Copyright by Allyn and Bacon, Boston).

non-specific visual attention while supine, and visual attention whilst prone and with head elevated. In this last study the purpose was to induce earlier requisition of flexible accommodation and whatever perceptual mechanisms underlie the blink response to approaching visible targets.

The following alterations of rearing conditions were instituted from 21 to 105 days of age. Red and white striped golfer's mitts were worn by the experimental subjects (Fig. 25); their plain white sheets and bumpers were replaced by others featuring various colours and forms; and they themselves were placed in the prone position for 15 minutes after the 6 a.m., 10 a.m., and 2 p.m. feeds. These procedures were designed to hasten the visual discovery of the hands and to provide more noticeable and stimulating surroundings. Whether passive visual scanning or scanning while moving head, torso and hands is more effective in early development, is an open question. We hoped to test the more fundamental general ideas of the plasticity of the behaviours in question by increasing both kinds of learning opportunities.

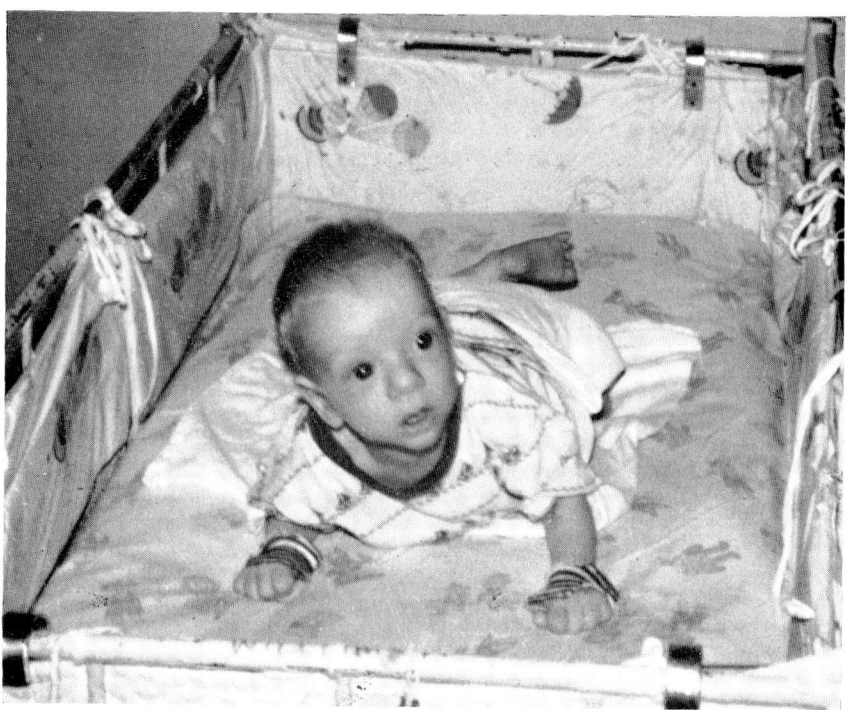

FIG. 25. Rearing conditions in the Mitt study featuring red and white mittens, brightly printed bedding and regular prone placement.

Results

Hand regard. The onset of sustained hand regard was markedly advanced, as is shown by Fig. 26.

Visual attention. The total amount of visual attention was unchanged but the distribution of attention while alert was altered considerably (Figs. 27 and 28). Hand regard occurred in the experimental group as a common activity during most of the second month of life, whereas virtually none was seen in the new control group.

Visual accommodation. There was no significant change in the development of visual accommodative ability, Table VI. A slight trend might be present, since group performance for the experimental infants was slightly behind at the outset of the study and slightly ahead at the end.

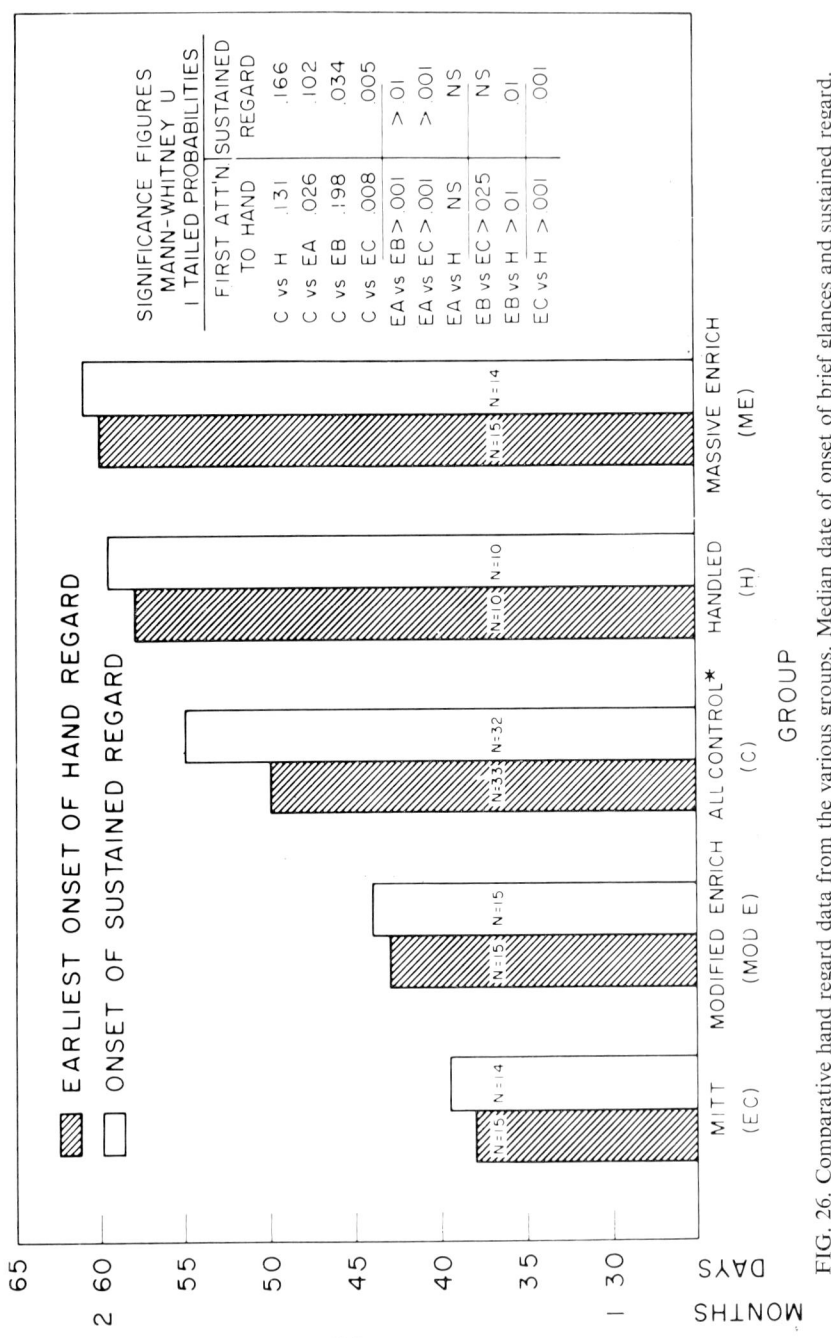

FIG. 26. Comparative hand regard data from the various groups. Median date of onset of brief glances and sustained regard. * Old and new control combined (from White, 1969. Reprinted with permission of the Merrill-Palmer Institute, Detroit).

EXPERIENCE AND THE DEVELOPMENT OF MOTOR MECHANISMS 129

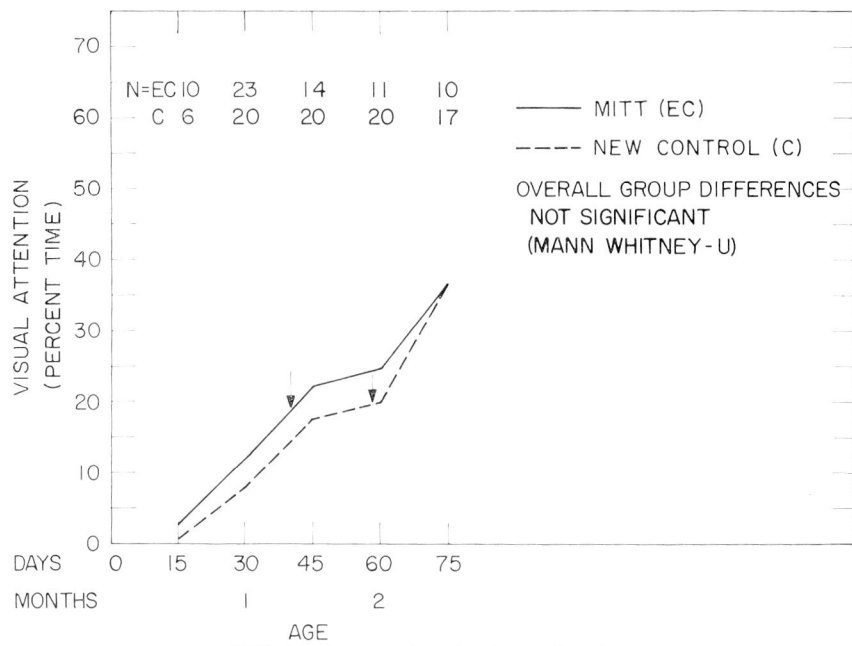
FIG. 27. Comparative visual attention data.

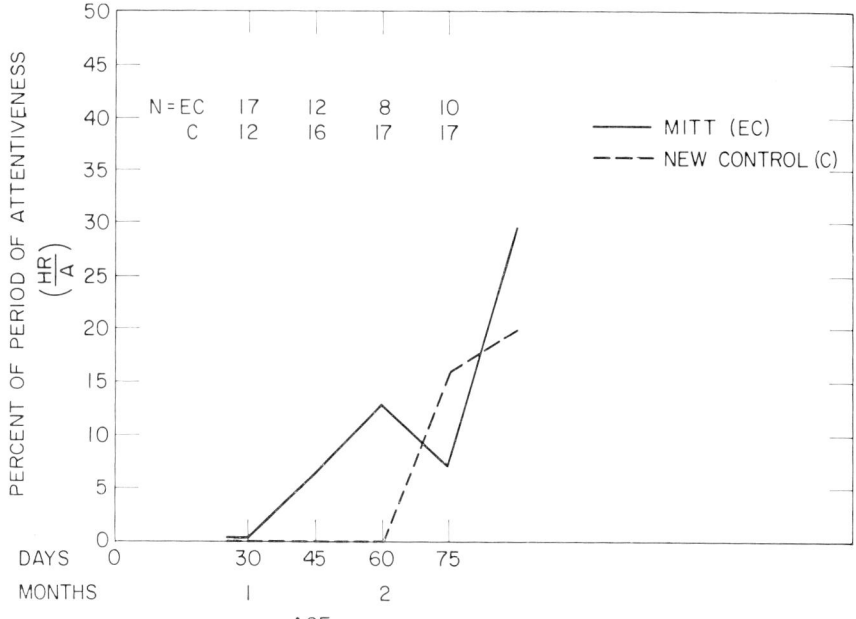
FIG. 28. Comparative hand regard data. Development of proportion of visual attention devoted to sustained hand regard (both figures from White, 1969. Reprinted with permission of the Merrill-Palmer Institute, Detroit).

TABLE VI. THE DEVELOPMENT OF VISUAL ACCOMMODATION COMPARISON OF CONTROL VS EXPERIMENTAL GROUPS

Age (days)		Subjects		Significance levels (Mann-Whitney U Test)
		Control	Experimental	
18–31	N_s	15	9	
	Median slope values	+0·40	+0·55	NS
32–80	N_s	16	26	
	Median slope values	+0·19	+0·28	NS
81–105	N_s	9	12	
	Median slope values	+0·10	+0·28	NS

The Blink Response

Table VII and Figs. 29, 30 and 31 show the comparative performances of experimental versus control subjects. It is obvious that no dramatic alteration of the course of this developmental process has been effected.

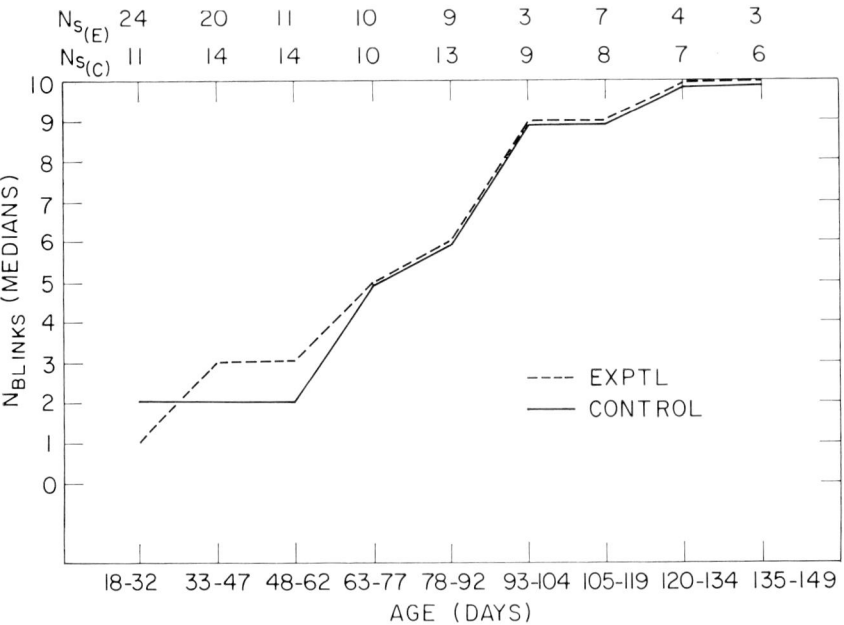

FIG. 29. Data on blink responses. Frequency of responses over ten trials, experimental vs control groups.

EXPERIENCE AND THE DEVELOPMENT OF MOTOR MECHANISMS 131

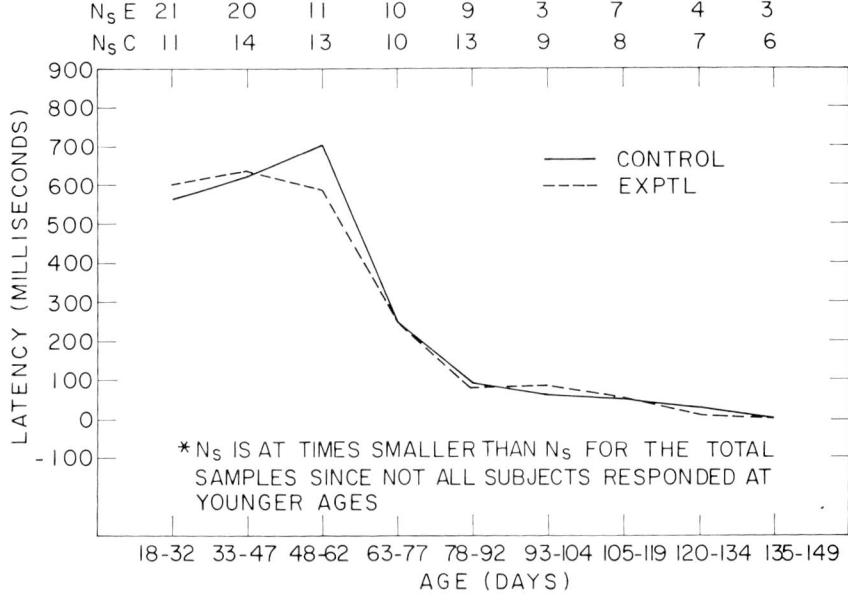

FIG. 30. Data on blink responses. Response latency, experimental vs control groups.

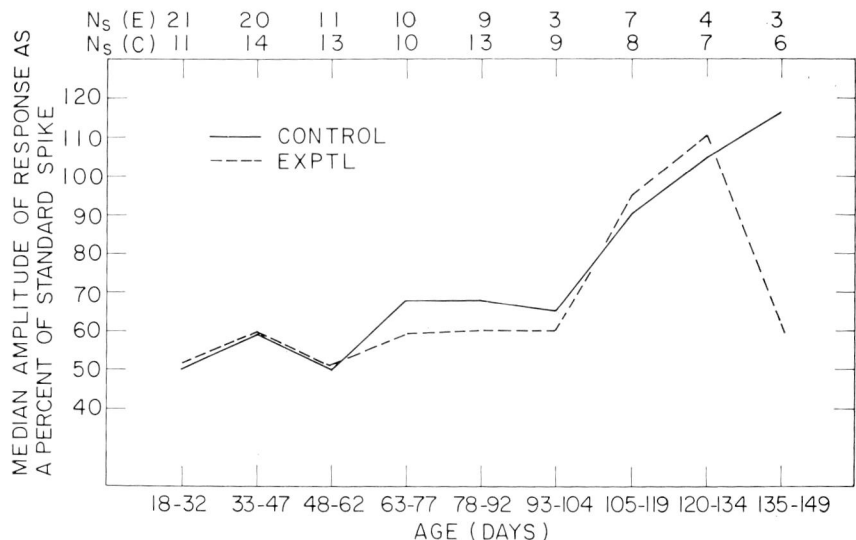

FIG. 31. Data on blink responses. Amplitudes of response, experimental vs control groups.

TABLE VII. THE DEVELOPMENT OF THE BLINK (PALPEBRAL) RESPONSE TO AN APPROACHING VISIBLE TARGET—
COMPARISON OF EXPERIMENTAL VS CONTROL GROUPS

Target drop		18–32		33–47		48–62		63–77		78–92		93–104		105–119		120–134		135–149	
		E	C	E	C	E	C	E	C	E	C	E	C	E	C	E	C	E	C
Frequency																				
2 inches	N_s	24	11	20	14	11	14	10	10	9	13	3	9	7	8	4	7	3	6
	Med	1	1	2	0.75	2	0.5	4	4	4	3	3	6	7	5	7	8	5	5
	Range	0–4	0–4	0–5	0–4	0–3	0–7	0–6	0–8	1–10	0–4	1–5	3–9	5–9	1–10	2–10	3–10	4–10	9–10
7 inches	N_s	24	11	20	14	11	14	10	10	9	13	10	9	7	8	4	7	3	6
	Med	1	3	3	2	1	2	5	8	4	7	10	9	7	10	10	10	10	10
	Range	0–6	0–6	0–8	0–10	1–7	0–10	0–9	1–9	1–10	5–10	9–10	8–10	9	5–10	4–10	9–10	9–10	9–10
12 inches	N_s	24	11	20	14	11	14	10	10	9	13	10	9	7	8	4	7	3	6
	Med	2	4	4	3	7	5	8	10	9	8	10	10	10	10	10	10	10	10
	Range	0–8	1–6	2–10	0–10	2–9	0–10	1–10	3–10	5–10	5–10	4–10	9–10	7–10	3–10	4–10	7–10	8–10	9–10
Overall median score across 2–7–12 inches		1	2	3	2	3	2	5	5	6	6	9	9	9	9	10	10	10	10
Latency																				
2 inches	N_s	15	6	17	8	9	7	8	8	9	10	3	9	7	8	4	7	3	6
	Med	430	500	430	400	500	475	562	425	150	203	180	120	100	73	130	80	70	55
	Range	310–	340–	50–	–88–	300–	–120–	110–	160–	60–	90–	0–	60–	60–	40–	10–	40–	40–	5–
		1,010	600	1,000	780	1,060	760	918	1,060	650	835	400	400	140	530	570	360	420	140
7 inches	N_s	17	7	18	13	11	12	10	10	9	8	3	9	7	9	4	7	3	6
	Med	640	460	542	650	460	810	250	200	40	80	100	40	20	25	0	0	–10–	–10
	Range	0–	360–	–120–	–100–	–30–	–90–	–60–	–60–	–60–	0–	–60–	–5–	–30–	–95–	–80–	–30–	–10–	–80–
		1,020	1,060	1,040	1,100	920	1,140	1,000	800	160	255	400	120	170	200	140	40	20	30
12 inches	N_s	19	11	20	13	11	13	10	10	9	8	3	9	7	8	4	7	3	6
	Med	440	650	775	600	800	350	10	10	50	40	40	40	0	5	–30	–20	–20	–15
	Range	–260–	20–	140–	0–	–100–	0–	–20–	35–	–60–	–50–	–20–	–30–	–20–	–720–	–60–	–60–	–50–	–125–
		1,200	1,200	1,130	960	1,030	1,050	1,200	320	400	800	80	80	100	100	160	60	0	0
Overall median scores across 2–7–12 inches		540	560	640	570	500	473	250	180	87	85	80	60	50	55	5	30	0	0
Amplitude																				
2 inches	N_s	15	6	17	8	9	7	8	8	9	10	3	9	7	8	4	7	3	6
	Med (%)	45	66	47	66.5	40	47	69	40	50	51	53	57	80	70	130	80	53	116
	Range (%)	20–	30–	27–	26–	27–	30–	31–	25–	30–	32–	50–	40–	40–	25–	10–	40–	40–	53–
		125	107	147	140	92	120	100	100	113	93	67	67	210	174	570	360	420	144
7 inches	N_s	17	7	18	13	11	12	10	10	9	13	3	9	7	8	4	7	3	6
	Med (%)	67	50	79	52	53	53	60	61	67	73	60	87	93	100	95	147	67	114
	Range (%)	30–	30–	33–	27–	26–	32.5–	27–	25–	40–	36–	40–	40–	50–	35–	25–	80–	40–	67–
		160	136	200	130	150	100	160	147	168	140	140	160	160	175	370	214	90	208
12 inches	N_s	19	11	20	13	11	13	10	10	9	8	3	9	7	8	4	7	3	6
	Med (%)	53	56	73	47	67	70	57	80	80	93	70	120	100	106	105	113	90	113
	Range (%)	30–	25–	26–	30–	40–	27–	33–	30–	40–	40–	40–	53–	80–	35–	80–	58–	53–	98–
		220	113	131	107	200	150	107	275	174	140	107	74	153	179	160	166	113	208
Overall median																				

REFERENCES

BRODY, S. 1951. *Patterns of mothering.* Internat. Universities Press, New York.

CASLER, L. 1961. Maternal deprivation: a critical review of the literature. *Monog. Soc. Res. Child Develop.* **26**, 1–64.

DENENBERG, V. H. and KARAS, G. G. 1959. Effects of differential infantile handling upon weight gain and mortality in the rat and mouse. *Science*, **130**, 629–630.

FERGUSON, G. A. 1959. *Statistical analysis in psychology and education.* McGraw-Hill, New York.

GESELL, A. and AMATRUDA, C. S. 1941. *Developmental diagnosis.* Hoeber, New York.

HAYNES, H., WHITE, B. L. and HELD, R. 1965. Visual accommodation in human infants. *Science*, **148**, 528–530.

HELD, R. 1961. Exposure-history as a factor in maintaining stability of perception and coordination. *J. nerv. ment. Dis.* **132**, 26–32.

HELD, R. and BOSSOM, J. 1961. Neonatal deprivation and adult rearrangement: complementary techniques for analysing plastic sensory-motor coordinations. *J. comp. physiol. Psychol.* **54**, 33–37.

HELD, R. and HEIN, A. 1963. Movement-produced stimulation in the development of visually-guided behavior. *J. comp. physiol. Psychol.* **56**, 872–876.

LEVINE, S. 1957. Infantile experience and resistance to physiological stress. *Science*, **126**, 405.

MEIER, G. W. 1961. Infantile handling and development in siamese kittens. *J. comp. physiol. Psychol.* **54**, 284–286.

MIKAELIAN, H. and HELD, R. M. 1964. Two types of adaptation to an optically-rotated visual field. *Am. J. Psychol.* **77**, 257–263.

PIAGET, J. 1952. *The origins of intelligence in children.* 2nd ed. Internat. Universities Press, New York.

RIESEN, A. H. 1958. Plasticity of behavior: psychological series. In H. F. Harlow and C. N. Woolsey (Eds.), *Biological and biochemical bases of behavior.* Univ. Wisconsin Press, Madison. Pp. 425–450.

WHITE, B. L. 1967. An experimental approach to the effects of experience on early human behavior. In J. P. Hill (Ed.), *Minnesota symposium on child psychology.* Univ. Minnesota Press, Minneapolis, **1**, 201–225.

WHITE, B. L. 1969. Child development research: an edifice without a foundation. In S. Irving (Ed.), *Merrill-Palmer Quarterly.* Merrill-Palmer Institute, Detroit. **15**, 47–48.

WHITE, B. L. and CASTLE, P. 1964. Visual exploratory behavior following postnatal handling of human infants. *Percept. mot. skills*, **18**, 497–502.

WHITE, B. L., CASTLE, P. and HELD, R. 1964. Observations on the development of visually-directed reaching. *Child develop.* **35**, 349–364.

WHITE, B. L. and CLARK, K. R. 1968. An apparatus for eliciting and recording the eye blink. *Percept. mot. Skills*, **27**, 959–964.

WHITE, B. L. and HELD, R. 1966. Plasticity and sensorimotor development in the human infant. In J. F. Rosenblith and W. Allinsmith (Ed.). *The causes of behavior: Readings in child development and education psychology.* Second edition. Allyn and Bacon, Boston.

WINER, B. J. 1962. *Statistical principles in experimental design.* McGraw-Hill, London.

YARROW, L. J. 1961. Maternal deprivation: toward an empirical and conceptual re-evaluation. *Psychol. Bull.* **58,** 459–490.

Discussion

TWITCHELL: In the younger infant do you get any visual pursuit when you are outside his focal range?

WHITE: Yes, in fact pursuit is usually of better quality at 15 inches.

TWITCHELL: How about at 30 inches?

WHITE: I don't think we have tested often enough at that distance to say. A problem which arises at such distances is that the necessary target size for eliciting these early pursuit responses becomes unmanageable.

BRUNER: The sharpness of the contour is also very important.

WHITE: Yes, certainly. We can usually go out to about 2 feet quite successfully; of course, the optimal distance varies between subjects.

TWITCHELL: It should be relatively easier within that narrow range of focus.

WHITE: Perhaps it should be, though such an idea pre-supposes that acuity is of central importance to the response whereas this does not appear to be the case. I am convinced that the pursuit in the first 2 weeks of life consists of a series of movement induced centralizing reflexes.

TWITCHELL: I have always been a little curious about whether an infant in the course of development shows what has been called by some, visual groping reactions and visual avoiding reactions. I have never looked carefully for it myself but I wonder if some of your findings might be considered as examples of a visual avoiding reaction. Swiping is not very accurate initially, the arm is as it were flung at the target but eventually the response does become quite accurate. Some of our own studies on infant development and on adults in various stages of dissolution of neural function lead me to believe that some tactile mechanism is particularly important here. I have another question. Are these early reaching responses purposive; is this really purposive prehension? If it isn't, when does purposiveness appear?

WHITE: Bruner, perhaps you would care to respond on the question of potential visual avoidance phenomena.

BRUNER: I wish the issue were not so clouded. We have obtained some curious data in situations rather similar to those which you have described. We (Berry Brazelton and Colwyn Trevarthen did the actual work) involve the mother in our test situation. She is positioned in front of her baby, who is strapped upright in a special (Harvard) chair. A camera is positioned behind a curtain, the lens peeping through a small aperture and focused on the baby. A mirror is placed behind the baby so that we can see the mother's face reflected in the mirror, and baby's face directly. We ask the mother to get the baby to smile, though not to touch him because this introduces a whole range of additional variables and it is so easy for the baby to bring the mother under stimulus control. The babies we studied were aged between 3 and 4 months. Now, with an inanimate object which is not reciprocating to the baby in any way, gaze aversion is rare. However, when the mother's face, which is reciprocating to the baby, is substituted for an inanimate object, the baby appears to have to avert his gaze after a while. He simply cannot look at the mother for very long without having to turn away and then come back. This may be one of the things which starts the very important inter-play between the mother and the baby. However, I am not sure that we should call gaze aversion of this kind visual avoidance. I think the gaze aversion is probably a response to an overload of interaction rather than simply a consequence of looking at an object. With an inanimate object, in our case a little 35-cent monkey, the baby continues to look directly at it and even movements on the periphery of the visual field have little effect.

I would like to say a little more about this because I want to raise the question of whether it is aversion or diversion. In the situation where a baby is looking at a configuration which reciprocates to it, such as the mother's face, then if any movements in the periphery distract it, immediately its attention is drawn to them. When the baby is looking at an object which is not reciprocating to him, the effects of peripheral distraction are barely noticeable. It seems to me that it is not so much aversion as a readiness to be lured off by another object.

TWITCHELL: There is another very common visual avoidance response which Ling (1942, *J. Genet. Psychol.* **61,** 227) pointed out in her study of the development of visual fixation. If an infant is fixating a target disc and this gets too close (by too close I mean within 4 to 6 inches), then the infant will attempt to increase the distance between the disc and himself. When he is supine about all he can do is to rear back and try to turn his head back. We have seen this response regularly in tests of visual function during the first few months of life, particularly during the second month. If the target comes too close the child will back off rather rapidly.

HOWARD: Is novelty important here at all? The mother's face is of course a very familiar stimulus, quite apart from whether she interacts with the baby.

CONNOLLY: Presumably the monkey becomes a familiar stimulus, though.

BRUNER: Yes, we only have one 35-cent monkey.

HOWARD: I see, I hadn't quite appreciated that.

BRUNER: On thing that is really important is to examine this question of posture (the baby upright and the baby supine) in situations which are as comparable as possible. I have a feeling that we shall bedevil the literature if we assume that babies behave in a typical fashion in each of these positions. When the whole tonic framework is activated, behaviour such as hand watching and the extent to which a grasped object is brought to the mouth probably differ greatly.

HINDE: May I add a comparative observation at this point, not about 35-cent monkeys but about real ones. Rhesus monkey mothers spend a great deal of time peering into their infant's face and the infant does exactly what has been described. The mother goes down and tries to get her face right in front of the baby's face; it happens quite suddenly when the baby is in the ventral position and also when it is older and sitting up on its own.

CONNOLLY: Are these laboratory reared monkeys?

HINDE: Yes, they are laboratory reared rhesus monkeys living in largish social groups.

The Experimental Analysis of Skill

Analysing Motor Skill Performance

HARRY KAY

University of Sheffield

I. INTRODUCTION

WE WITNESS so many examples of motor skills as we move around in the world that it is not surprising we ignore the common-place and turn attention to the outstanding performance of skill; the world-class competitors, the Olympic athletes. This paper is written from the standpoint that, contrary to popular opinion, the significance of human skills lies not in their uniqueness but their ubiquity. There are a vast range of motor activities which we all, or nearly all, learn to perform and these are the skills which reveal the basic functional mechanisms of the human system.

Ultimately we have to ask: "What kind of system controls human skills and in what way does it differ from other systems?" Before any satisfactory answer can be attempted we need to be able to say what exactly we are trying to understand; and the beginning lies in a precise description of the essential features of skilled performance.

Fortunately developmental psychologists and paediatricians have been well aware of the importance of describing what is taking place as a baby begins to control its movements. As a result of their work a number of stages in motor development have been identified, providing a detailed record of how a child progresses as it gains increasing control over its motor functions. It is not my intention to rehearse these well-known facts but to acknowledge the care and precision with which workers such as Bayley (1935), Gesell (1940), Halverson (1932, 1940), McGraw (1943), Illingworth (1966), Shirley (1931) have studied and presented this evidence.

Our problem now is to ask what should be the next stage in research. How should we be building on this work to increase our overall understanding of skills? How do we relate developmental studies of skilled responses to the laboratory research that has taken place on this subject in the fields of experimental and applied psychology? To date, the two fields of developmental studies and the analysis of adult skills have had curiously little influence upon each other. Each has gone a separate way, each has made a notable contribution but neither has contributed to the understanding of the other. It is the main thesis of this paper that each can in fact contribute very considerably to the other and that the time for this is ripe.

Accordingly I am taking as read the work on motor development in babies and young children which has been discussed in Connolly's[1] paper; but I do wish to state briefly some of the main features of the work of the experimental psychologist studying skilled performance. I hope this will set the stage for one side of our discussions and we may then turn to discuss how this work may throw further light upon the mechanisms of motor skill development.

II. THE EXPERIMENTAL STUDY OF SKILLS

A. *Information Flow*

The psychologist trying to analyse the motor skills of an adult is faced with a paradox which in many respects holds the secret to our understanding of skilled actions. On the one hand performance may be intermittent, with a measurable delay as an individual initiates a response to an external signal; the standard reaction time experiment typifies this delay. No matter how well prepared the subject may be to initiate a response to a signal he still takes, as Helmholtz said a long time ago, a measurable time of some 100–200 milliseconds, before he can respond. If all human performance were like the reaction time we should move around in a series of jerks punctuated by relatively long time gaps, and, of course, we do no such thing.

For the surprising paradox is that most skills are characterized by continuous, fluid movements which are flexible and astonishingly rapid. The concert pianist may make ten responses in a second. Where then is the intermittency and delay? How does it come about that this serial ordering of events is so different from the response to a discrete signal? It is apparent that we tend to regard as a skill those actions where the apparent limitations of the human system are most successfully surmounted. This is fair enough, but let us note in passing that it is something most of us achieve in our everyday actions as we move

[1] Skill development: problems and plans, this volume.

around and respond to our environment. It would follow that the monitoring of a sequence of skilled responses is of a different order from the reaction time situation where it takes so long to initiate a response. If we ask why the reaction time is so long, the answer from the psychologist used to be in terms of perceiving the signal, deciding upon and initiating the correct response and carrying it out. Today this would be described in the language of communication theory as a process in which information is being transmitted and where the time delay is predictable according to how much uncertainty (the amount of information) there is in the situation. The greater the probability of a signal, the shorter the reaction time to it. If we are responding to one signal out of two it takes longer than if we are responding to one signal alone, or again it would take longer the less predictable the time of onset of the signal. This concept of the human operator processing information allows us to examine widely differing skills and point to where the limitations in their performance lies. It was expressed most directly by Hick (1952) in his statement that, "the rate of gain of information is, on the average, constant with respect to time, within the duration of one perceptual-motor act".

We now appreciate that this is not the whole story: other variables apart from information also influence the rate of responding. Nevertheless the basic concept of the human operator as an information processing system has been helpful in contributing to our understanding of motor responses; in particular it has helped us to appreciate that what might have happened does in fact often influence a situation just as much as what did actually occur. This is especially relevant to our understanding of children's performance. If we consider a child's performance only in terms of the known world of the adult, then often its difficulties are not apparent. But when we consider it from a child's point of view where so much is unknown and literally almost anything can happen, we begin to appreciate how much more complex is the situation for a child. It is often facing possibilities which the adult has ruled out of consideration, because on the basis of his previous experience, he can say that some events, or classes of events, are most unlikely. A child who lacks this experience has to consider more eventualities, and to that extent is having to process more information.

Another long-standing problem which this approach has answered is the query about how many things a person can do at the same time. The answer is not clear because the question itself is ambiguous—it depends upon how we define our independent events. But we can state the question much more directly by asking how much information the human system can process or, in other words, what is the channel capacity of the system. When considered from this standpoint we appreciate that it may well be possible for the human system to cope with a number of simultaneous events. The actual number may not be so important as their degree of uncertainty: where many events are predictable, and therefore are carrying little information, the system is not overburdened. However, two simultaneous events, each highly improbable, may represent too high an information load.

B. *Anticipation and Internal Signals*

One other feature should be mentioned in the preliminary survey—anticipation. If the human operator can only respond with delay to a stimulus, then an obvious technique for circumventing the difficulty is to begin responding before the onset of the signal. This implies some form of learning, since anticipation is only possible where something is already known about the situation and the occurrence of signals. Such anticipation may take many forms; a person may be anticipating the next stimulus in a sequence as you may be anticipating correctly the next word which I shall speak. As we all know, listening to spoken languages is only possible because we are keenly aware of the sequential dependencies in the language structure. There is much redundancy in ordinary speech and, I wish to argue, in most other skills.

One reason for this arises from the different sources of signals. In motor responses there are obvious visual signals to which the operator attends. But often there is also an anticipation of a number of signals which are internal to the performance. We monitor our motor skills partly by reference to the extent to which the results of our actions accord with some external criteria, and also by attending to the internal signals we inevitably receive from the muscles controlling our responses. It is the hall-mark of so many practised skills that the operator is monitoring them by these internal signals; indeed, in those instances where we have a high-speed, time-stressed operation it would often be impossible to carry out the responses if they were not so monitored. The reason for this is two-fold. The internal signals often precede the external signals by a useful time gap, as when the tennis player hits the ball. The skilled player can feel the impact of the ball on the racquet and judge whether the stroke is sound, but he has to wait some time before he can see whether the ball pitches correctly. He acts on the internal signals because it would in fact be too late to begin action if he waited for the visual signal. The faster the game the more important this feature becomes.

But the second reason is equally basic to skills. The internal signals are the inevitable accompaniment of the skill itself; kinaesthetic and proprioceptive feedback originates from the limbs and muscles which are directly concerned with the motor responses. They are, literally, an integral part of the activity. To this extent the skilled player learns as much as possible about such signals and can eventually control his responses from such a source. This enables him to do two things. He learns to predict the sequence of signals which he will receive from responses. As his responses become more practised he is able to repeat his movements with some precision and this in turn implies that the feedback from his muscles is becoming less varied. This increasing predictability is all important because we are now saying that, as long as the operator makes the response as intended, the ensuing feedback signals will carry little or no information for him—they will be redundant. But as soon as the response does vary the feedback will correspondingly differ from the expected and the information content may be such as to demand the full channel capacity of the system. We now see in action the evergreen principle that the poorer the operator the harder is his task. It is indeed so, because the more random his responses the greater the uncertainty of the internal signals which he has to monitor. Hence the learner who is performing indifferently is trying to pick out a constant pattern of signals when the variability of his own responses is largely contributing to their high information content.

A further point follows from this. Because the skilled performer is faced with little or no uncertainty from the internal signals, and yet is able to monitor his performance from them, he is free to attend to other events. He therefore has time to switch his attention to, say, the overall strategy of his performance. This may be essential since so many skills depend upon a dual characteristic: the operator has to try to control his own performance in a predictable manner and at the same time he has to be prepared to initiate further action if external events demand it. For example, in walking or driving a car we make many routine responses, but at any point we must also be prepared to respond appropriately if external events, such as another car or pedestrian, or a change in road surface, require it of us.

Now it is so often a feature of the beginner's motor skill that he masters one without the other—he does the right thing at the wrong time. He runs off a set routine of responses which are, alas, not appropriate to the changing circumstances. (Politicians are rather practised at this too.) I think it is fair to say that it is this linking of the practised set of responses to accord with the external demands of time and place that signifies the true skills; this is what we mean by flexibility and timing. In the cumbersome language I wish to adopt later, it is the point where the macro-strategy has successfully linked together the micro-structure or, in other words, the overall plan of the skill has taken over the individual sequences of routine responses.

C. *A Filmed Example: Catching a Ball*[2]

It is my contention that this general view of skills provides an understanding of many of the problems in a child's motor performance, and I wish to illustrate this by commenting on the movements of three children of different ages catching a ball, and by noting the general features.

1. *At 2 years old.* The little girl, Oona, is 27 months and is not too sure what this catching game is really about. She has clearly played it before and she knows that she positions her hands together in front of her body. But for her there are many unknowns in this situation. For example, she does not know when the ball is going to be thrown; that is, she cannot appreciate from the actions of the thrower's arm and hand when he will release the ball and throw it to her. She cannot anticipate at any point in the ball's flight where it will land: knowledge of trajectories, force of throwing and speed through the air are still mysteries to her. For the most part she is doing something after it has happened, often very long after, as when she eventually turns to fetch the ball that has fallen. But the most striking example of this late timing is in the all important co-ordination of the fingers to grasp the ball, when it is clear that she knows what she has to do but does not know when to do it. The ball falls gently on to her hands, it rolls up her wrist and then off and only after this does she begin to curl up her fingers as if trying to catch the ball. Throughout, her hands are held in a static position in front of her and there is no attempt to match their position with the flight of the ball. We see that the ball passes closely by the hands but the hands are held passively until after the ball has passed and it is too late to catch it.

2. *At 5 years old.* Caroline, aged 5 years, is by contrast with the 2-year-old child familiar enough with this game. She knows where to stand, how to position her hands and she moves her hands to catch the ball—in other words she can correctly anticipate the trajectory of the ball and its flight. Certainly she can move her hands to the correct spatial position, even if her timing and co-ordination are not outstand-

[2] At this point in his presentation Kay showed a 3-minute film of children catching a ball (Ed.).

ing. She does in fact generally catch the ball but sometimes her fingers are a little slow in closing around it. We witness then an improvement in the overall strategy and a better appreciation of what she is trying to do and at the same time we have an increased motor ability to carry out the skill. The one obvious deficiency is that the whole skill is being carried out as if it were in slow-motion—it is apparent that if we speed up the operation there will be no reserve of abilities to meet the new conditions.

3. *At 15 years old.* This is effectively what we have done with the 15-year-old boy, Mark. The game is now moving much faster as the ball is thrown with more force and the trajectory is varied. The general strategy of the skill is now clearly learned, the stance is not so rigid but more ready for action and the arms and hands move freely to take the ball in its flight. The overall impression is one of smoothness and ease. The eyes are concentrated upon the ball; they do not watch the hands which are controlled entirely from the boy's own awareness of the position of his limbs. This is a typical feature of skills—the freedom of movement resulting from an ability to receive information from a variety of sources. In this example we see that visual information about the flight is matched against proprioceptive-kinaesthetic information about the movement of the hands. The two are brought together so that we now have a beautifully correlated sequence of external events and motor actions, almost as if the hand-arm actions were tied to the ball. These responses are certainly anticipatory, in that the action is begun long before the ball arrives at its final spatial position, but we should note that the response is based on information which to the skilled player is highly predictable. In other words to the skilled player the initial trajectory of the ball enables him to predict its future position with great accuracy.

The performances of these three children is summarized in Table I.

From this brief description of one example let us now consider how the psychologist's analysis of skills may contribute to our understanding of the development of motor functions, and what recommendations might follow from it.

D. *Reducing the Information Flow*

At all stages of motor skills we are trying to reduce information flow. This may be done in two ways. First, we can so manipulate a situation that the number of choices in it are reduced, or we can slow down the operation so that the number of events in unit time is curtailed; these would be examples of reducing information by changing the external

TABLE I. SUMMARY OF THE PERFORMANCE OF THREE CHILDREN CATCHING A BALL

	2-year-old	5-year-old	15-year-old
General strategy	Almost nil	Some features; say approximately 50 per cent	Complete
Hand movements	Static	Intentional, appropriate but excessive	Directed and effective Smooth
Timing and co-ordination	Almost nil	Effective but slow	Co-ordinated and unhurried
Eye gaze	On thrower	On thrower, ball and hands	On ball
Stance	Rigid	Jerky	Adaptive

events themselves. Secondly, a biological system, and some recent forms of adaptive devices made by man, may follow an alternative procedure of learning the probabilities of events by assessing their past frequencies or rates of occurrence. We have discussed how the skilled performer is prepared to predict, say, a sequence of events and can plan a series of responses on the basis of the first few events as they occur. To the unskilled onlooker this series of responses may seem remarkably quick but the exponent has in fact initiated them well ahead of the point where they were required. As Craik said (1947, 1948), the skilled performer must detect the constants in the situation and one of the most important is to appreciate how far one signal is the inevitable forerunner of another. We all appreciate that serial responses are an outstanding feature of skills but we now see why this is so necessary. If a person were continuously referring back to each incoming event as he controlled his responses, we should have the intermittency of the reaction time. The performance would become a hectic oscillation as the operator directed his attention between the incoming signals and the response he wished to make to them.

But it will be rightly pointed out that this is exactly the problem with so many skills. We often cannot control external events but our actions must be in tune with them. As we have seen, the skilled craftsman does this by working with an extended series of events. He is not initiating and monitoring single events but a series of them, thereby gaining the necessary time to switch between incoming and outgoing sequences. What in fact he does is to simplify his problem, partly by his ability to predict a sequence of future events on the basis of the first signals which are presented, and partly by his ability to trigger off a whole sequence of responses. Thus the time gaps between the different actions are lengthened. It will be readily appreciated that this feature has implications for a child in the early stages of learning motor skills.

It would seem that we need to control the speed of presentation of events if a child is to cope with a situation. We must remember that many events will not be grouped together but be treated as independent items. One of the striking results that has emerged from our experiments in Sheffield is that children may often respond as accurately as adults (Connolly, Brown and Bassett, 1968); but if put under a time stress, their performance deteriorates. They have greater difficulty than the adult in balancing the trade-off between speed and accuracy. We are now in a position to say why this must be so. We know a child, like any other performer, is limited by the amount of information he can transmit; but just because there are so many unknowns in the situation for a child the task will be all the more difficult because he will have to transmit far more information than the adult. For example, a child may be unaware of constraints that are obvious enough to an adult; he might think a ball harder, heavier, even larger than it was. An adult lives in a world where a vast number of objects are utilized and where, when he sees these objects, he implies their function. This does not hold for a child who may still be looking with wonder and few preconceptions upon his everyday surroundings.

E. *Necessity for a Preprogrammed Sequence in Children's Learning*

From our discussion there follows an essential teaching dictum. We must reduce to a minimum any intervention from external events; we must so arrange the situation that a child is insulated from environmental distractions. This begins to sound as if we are proposing a type of Skinner-box for children's motor learning. If we are, the reasons are not altogether identical with Skinner's. We are trying to ensure that a child can respond with the minimum reference to external conditions and attend only to those signals which are essential to this task. To this extent the Skinner-box analogy holds. But we are primarily interested in a child making not one response but putting a series of motor responses together to form a skilled sequence. We think that he may learn to do this more efficiently by attending to his own responses and programming them against the constraints of external events. Of course the time will come when a child has to carry out the full skill where environmental demands dictate the pace and onset of responses but before facing a child with these conditions we should ensure that his repertoire of responses is adequately practised to meet the requirements.

F. *Compatibility of Stimulus-Response*

If we now turn to the situation where we actually confront children with responding to the environment, we can simplify the task considerably by ensuring that the responses are compatible with the stimuli. One of the striking results that emerged from reaction time work was the speed with which subjects could respond to multi-choice situations when the stimuli and responses were highly compatible, as in Leonard's (1959) situation. His subjects had to press with the finger which received tactile stimulation and they found this choice remarkably easy; indeed, there was no difference between two- and four-choice reaction times. On the other hand, it required a lot of practice to achieve a similar equality between reaction times for different numbers of choices when the compatibility between signal and response was less, as in the Mowbray and Rhoades (1959) experiment.

There is good reason for thinking we may save practice if we use compatible responses as far as possible when teaching young children. Adult motor responses are often so over-learned that we fail to appreciate how even simple translation processes, such as a symbolic transformation of a number to a key position, have all to be laboriously learned and will increase the difficulty for a child.

G. *The Need for Redundancy: the Joy of Repetition*

Fortunately nature seems to be on our side at this point. If children are to learn complex serial motor responses they need to carry them out again and again, and there are many examples which illustrate how much enjoyment a child does in fact get from repeating a response. This a is necessary feature of children's learning at all levels. A child faces novelty everywhere. There may be Wordsworth's "freshness of a dream", lending an air of unreality to the child's world, but biologically a child is struggling to come to grips with a strange environment where it is only possible to survive by knowing the contingencies of events. In his strange world a child comes to love repeatable happenings; by repetition he begins to control the world around him. Eventually he will acquire such control that he will seek out the spice of life—variety— but for the present he has too much of it and so he pleads for the familiar story with its known ending, or the practised game which he has mastered and where he can demonstrate his proficiency.

We may consider this feature in terms of redundancy. How much information is a child having to process in a given situation, and of the signals which are being presented how many are expected by a child and to that extent redundant? We find that at so many levels of a child's relatively unpractised skills—his ability to stand, to walk, or to listen to a language—they all entail maximum attention being given to them. There seems little or no redundancy at this stage of learning. It is not surprising therefore that where so much is unknown a child creates its own redundancy by its love of repetition. We have to build on practised units of behaviour.

H. *Planning the Macro-Strategy*

Our analysis so far has highlighted the fact that in most skills an operator has to strike a balance between maintaining his own responses and observing the changing environment. The skill is to match a planned motor sequence against a continuously changing input: this we shall call the macro-strategy. It is never easy for any system to achieve such a balance, and it must be harder for a child than an adult, for at each point a child will inevitably be so much more uncertain of events, whether they originate from his own more varied responses or the novelty of the external world. In such circumstances he will inevitably have difficulty in controlling this key feature in skills—how to divide attention between input and output.

This points to the need for a child to acquire control over a sequence of responses. Until he can run off a sub-routine of responses, as if in a pre-programmed sequence, he will never be able to turn his attention to meet the external requirements because the channel capacity of the system will be overloaded. It would seem that by repeatedly carrying out a series of motor responses the *micro-structure* of a skill is established. But the crucial stage is reached when this motor sequence is phased with changing external events. At some stages of development a child has to learn to continue making a response, or responses, whilst perceiving and initiating action to new stimuli, and in these circumstances it is only too easy for one element to become predominant and for the other to be neglected.

The macro-strategy, then, demands an interaction between input and output monitoring which matches the varying demands of the two streams of information. It will be easier to achieve where the units of identification are as large as possible, thereby permitting the minimum amount of switching compatible with efficiency. We can think of such examples as the first few notes which indicate a whole tune, or a few words of a sentence, or the beginning of an arm movement which foretells a complete gesture. Almost inevitably the units for a child will not be large or varied and to this extent the macro-strategy will be built up slowly as the micro-structure of the skill is practised.

In terms of the whole system controlling human skills, we may conclude that is easily overloaded and that learning is very much a strategy of identifying events so that the organism can operate in larger units, and to this extent be free from the immediate constraints of time and place. It is a laborious process and yet another demonstration of why human development takes so long.

III. SUMMARY

A general framework of analysing motor skills was discussed and emphasis was placed upon the limitations of a human operator transmitting information. A skilled performer was viewed as a communication channel, receiving signals from both the external and internal environment. The internal signals arising from a performer's own limbs are all important to skills and are difficult to learn when motor performance is irregular. The need to overcome the inevitable intermittencies in the system by anticipating signals and co-ordinating responses into larger serial units was stressed. A child has to learn these sequences of signals and as he learns he increases the redundancy in the skill.

A simple example of catching a ball was recorded on cine film and the marked difference in the behaviour of a 2-, 5- and a 15-year-old child were analysed. The examples support the view that with practice the units of responses were enlarged so that eventually whole subroutines may be triggered off. It is useful to distinguish between the macro-strategy where the effort is to match a planned motor sequence with a continuously changing environment, and the micro-structure of a skill, where a child is learning to enlarge the single responses of behaviour into co-ordinated units. One of the difficulties experienced by a child arises because his units of behaviour are so small and require a frequent oscillation of attention between input and output.

REFERENCES

BAYLEY, N. 1935. Development of motor abilities during the first three years. *Monog. Soc. Res. Child Develop.* No. 1.

CONNOLLY, K., BROWN, K. and BASSETT, E. 1968. Developmental changes in some components of a motor skill. *Brit. J. Psychol.* **59**, 305–314.

CRAIK, K. J. W. 1947. Theory of the human operator in control systems. I. The operator as an engineering system. *Brit. J. Psychol.* **38**, 56–61.

CRAIK, K. J. W. 1948. Theory of the human operator in control systems. II. Man as an element in a control system. *Brit. J. Psychol.* **38**, 142–148.
GESELL, A. 1940. (Ed.) *The first five years of life.* Harper, New York.
HALVERSON, H. M. 1932. An experimental study of prehension in infants by means of systematic cinema records. *Genet. Psychol. Monogr.* **10**, 107–286.
HALVERSON, H. M. 1940. Motor development. Chapter VI. In A. Gesell (Ed.), *The first five years of life.* Harper, New York.
HICK, W. E. 1952. On the rate of gain of information. *Quart. J. exp. Psychol.* **4**, 11–16.
ILLINGWORTH, R. S. 1966. *The development of the infant and the young child.* Livingstone, Edinburgh.
KAY, H. 1969. The development of motor skills from birth to adolescence. In E. A. Bilodeau (Ed.), *Principles of skill acquisition.* Academic Press, New York.
LEONARD, A. J. 1959. Tactual choice reactions: 1. *Quart. J. exp. Psychol.* **11**, 76–83.
MCGRAW, M. B. 1943. *The neuromuscular maturation of the human infant.* Columbia University Press, New York.
MOWBRAY, G. H. and RHOADES, M. V. 1959. On the reduction of choice reaction times with practice. *Quart. J. exp. Psychol.* **11**, 16–23.
SHIRLEY, M. M. 1931. *The first two years: a study of twenty-five babies.* Vol. 1. Postural and Locomotor developmental. University of Minnesota Press, Minneapolis.

Discussion

BRUNER: I was struck, looking at your film and by your comments, that there may be another way of describing the strategy of an unskilled operator. When a skill is initially being brought under control, one of the first things a child does is to decrease the number of degrees of freedom deployed within the situation. This is a point Bernstein (1967, *The co-ordination and regulation of movements.* Pergamon Press, London) makes a good deal of in his study of controlled movements. Perhaps I can give you an example from an analogous type of situation; the early reaching behaviour of the young child is done with a hand spread wide, with no anticipatory grasping at all. When he contacts the object this leads to grasping. It is essentially a sequential organization, one that minimizes degrees of freedom controlled per unit time. In the case of the little girl attempting to catch the ball, by holding her hands out and converging in a bilaterally symmetrical way she is in fact reducing degrees of freedom. You would probably find that under conditions where a certain amount of predictability was possible there would be an anticipatory movement in the direction of, or to the side of, the ball. I should be extremely interested to see the way in which additional components come into the behaviour, and the way in which segmentation and anticipation develop.

You commented on the fact that when a skill is being learned, the learner, be he infant or be he an inept adult, is learning probabilities within the situation. I have had grave doubt that what in fact is going on is the learning of probabilities. The child could not possibly master so many probabilities without learning a supporting structure of rules of a highly generic kind. Superimposed upon such rules is an appreciation of the invariability. The kind of thing I have in mind here are rules concerned with such things as trajectories, rules having to do with the intersection between a movement in one direction and a movement towards you. This kind of rule learning consists of going from instances in the environment, general if crude notions, some of them probably species specific versions of the structure of space and movement. Further experience with the environment then leads to shaping in terms of the probability which exists within the application of the rule. I think that in talking about the learning of probabilities pure and simple we are making assumptions about learning capacity and how much learning can occur that exceeds the limits of information processing capacity.

A further problem which stems from the probabilistic approach relates to the question of transfer. Motor transfer could not be so good if the child were only learning probabilities. Nor could we learn probabilistically how to reduce degrees of freedom appropriately. Nor could there be fail safe strategies. So I would wish to argue that on the response side we have preadapted response patterns that are generated by the stimulus-processing side which has ways of converting encounters with the environment into rules for processing information and for signalling the requirements of a response.

KAY: I should like to think a lot more about that; I am sure you are discussing one of the basic issues. I was pondering about the relationship between the macro-strategy and the sub-routines. How do they get built up? It seems to me that the child has practised over and over again in certain situations and I was impressed by the fact that he got satisfaction from this. It seemed to me that at each point a child was not necessarily analysing what was happening but was making a repetitive response and from this getting a repetitive feedback, the situation such as throwing a ball against a wall is a suitable example. This would lead to the child being able to predict what would happen in such a situation. Now, if you contrast the 2-year-old and the 5-year-old children, the 2-year-old would be quite unable to say at what speed the ball will come. She does not seem to be able to make any analysis from the trajectory of the ball, or the way in which you throw it. She does not seem to know where it will go. Do you remember when I hit her on the chest deliberately, I was not being nasty; I was trying to show her that this was what happened.

BRUNER: It was perfectly plain that no learning would occur if you had gone on doing this all day.

KAY: No, I wouldn't like to say that; I think there may well have been some learning. I think what one had to do in a case like this was to try to get the child to see what was going to happen, to prepare her for it. And then you saw certain little sub-routines did in fact come in. If you threw the ball very carefully so that it would roll up on her hand, then she had time to cup her hands and it would stay, she caught the ball. If one threw the ball deliberately to hit her fingers then it would drop off, there would be no cupping. It seems to me that this little sub-routine was being learnt in this way. With practice this became increasingly co-ordinated. Now with the 5-year-old girl this of course has been learned. She has got what I think you are calling the rules; that there is someone standing in front of her, that he is going to throw the ball towards her, that the ball is going to come at a certain sort of speed etc., and that she must have her hands ready to catch it. Is there really so much difference here between what you and I are saying? I am saying that she knows the probabilities and you are saying, I think, that she knows the rules—she knows what is going to happen in terms of velocity, gravity, trajectory, etc.

BRUNER: I would say that both of these children are using rules, but they are using somewhat different rules. This is one of the reasons why I would be prepared to bet that there are certain aspects of behaviour of the 2-year-old which would not change even though you threw the ball time and time again.

KAY: As to your point that the little girl would not have learned had I gone on throwing the ball all day, she is a bright little child and I think in fact she would have learned.

BRUNER: What I would say is that, if you had continued to throw the ball she would learn to catch like a 2-year-old and not to catch in the way the 15-year-old or the 5-year-old caught the ball. This to me is the crucial thing; all that practice does is to shape the response pattern which comes out crudely at the outset. It is a response pattern which has certain strategic features in it and one question to which we need the answer is: what happens upon the perfection of that behaviour, in what way can we describe this behaviour as following the rule? However much practice you give the little girl she is not going to wind up like an American short-stop or a British cricketer, at least not for a very long time.

LEFFORD: In looking at the film I was particularly impressed with the differences in eye movement among the three children. The boy's eyes seemed to search for information almost becoming a prehensile organ which seeks information and data. Another feature which impressed me greatly in the film was the adaptive function of the body and the hands as a whole. I think this indicates that other sources of information are coming into play—kinaesthetic and proprioceptive information. I suspect that there is an interchange and co-ordination of information from within the body with information obtained from the distance receptors (information about the object in space). This is where I put my money; skill comes from an integration or inter-relationship between the different sensory processes. I doubt if there are any pre-programmed plans. I think the programme is created as the information comes in from the eyes and from the body.

HINDE: May I take up this question of eye-movements which was one of the most striking things about the film for me. It seemed to me that in the case of the little 2-year-old the experimenter was having to catch her eye so that she focused on the ball first. What was so clear about the 15-year-old was that he was not focusing on the ball as it came towards him but using his peripheral vision. This reminds me of work done during the early development of the Comet, which was the first jet airliner, British of course. In the course of high-speed taxiing trials, down the middle of the runway at London Airport, it was found that the pilot's swing was much smaller if he used peripheral vision. This was in contrast to the situation where he focused on a light in front of him and attempted to steer towards it; in this situation the swing was much greater. Going back to the film, it seemed to me that the mechanism being used by the 15-year-old boy was qualitatively different from that being used by the youngest child; and, to take Bruner's point, that this is a mechanism perfected not in the context of learning how to catch balls but in the general business of living and moving about where we learn to use our peripheral vision to orient in space.

CONNOLLY: I am sure this must be what happens in the case of the slip fielder. He just does not have time in catching a cricket ball to focus on it. Similarly if you look at animals which are very skilled like the swallow which can fly through thin railings, it cannot be done by a succession of fixations.

KAY: I should like to come in on that, I really think this is a question where one can show that probability comes in. I agree with Hinde, peripheral vision is probably very relevant. In the case of the little 2-year-old girl I want to argue that this is of little use to her. The ball may be coming towards her but as far as she is concerned it may be going up or it may be going down. She hasn't yet got this degree of predictability and she cannot get the necessary information. If I take a piece of chalk in my hand and make to throw it towards one of you, you all know that it is going to leave my hand at a certain speed but it is quite different for a young child. I might in fact do a sudden flick and the chalk may leave my hand at a relatively high speed. All these effects are much less certain for young children and to this extent it is much more difficult for them.

HOWARD: As Kay was talking it struck me that there were certain problems with the concepts which he was using; in particular, channel capacity, the implication being that an increasing channel capacity develops. In addition we have taken Connolly's notion of sub-routines and assume that these develop, we have also assumed that there must be a relationship between these two concepts. Channel capacity can only be defined in terms of a population or repertoire of information. From the things we are discussing I think it must be in terms of an internal repertoire only. In other words if it is defined in terms of the internal repertoire, channel capacity is a distinct thing from a number of sub-routines. However, externally they are not quite so distinct. Now, does the channel capacity actually develop or does the child acquire an increasing repertoire of sub-routines? How can we test for this difference? In talking of adults we make certain assumptions and then we look at children fumbling with their slow responses and the poor co-ordination which they show, and we tend to say, well, that is because they are children. I cannot ski and if you tried to put me on skis I am sure I would not look any better than the young child playing with the ball. Is there a difference? Are we talking about the development of children into adults or are we talking about the development of skills? It seems to me that these are two quite different things. In what sense is the child fumbling because he is a child, as distinct from the fact that he has not yet learnt this particular skill? In what sense does he fumble in a way that I would not fumble if I were presented with something quite new? I think there are three possibilities that we might explore as a means of explaining this. One of them is that the child has less channel capacity, not merely sub-routines. How do we demonstrate this? Another explanation might be in terms of the fact that he has fewer sub-routines, and this is quite distinct. An explanation in these terms clearly appeals to many of us. Now, perhaps I can bring out a third possibility which I should like to call a super-routine. It is not merely a collection of sub-routines and their juxtaposition into different patterns that marks real development—rather the development of something qualitatively different at this particular stage, what I would call a super-routine.

CONNOLLY: I am not clear how you would differentiate a sub-routine from a super-routine in any way other than in terms of size. I can see that one might prefer to use the term super-routine for a fairly extensive piece of behaviour, but how is one going to be able to distinguish between them objectively and empirically?

HOWARD: I take your point but I cannot provide an answer at the moment. Let us consider the other two alternatives for a moment. I think what one should do is to set up experimentally an artificial population of bits of information and then one might really be able to test whether there is a limitation on channel capacity. It is essential to define the information populations with which we are concerned, and it is only against this that we can talk about channel capacity. We need to know what the child's alternatives are, from his point of view not from the experimenter's. I wonder how much we do develop our channel capacity, the channel capacity of an adult is pretty meagre when he is given a novel situation. I wonder if we do reach the magic number seven? And I wonder how far below this the child is?

CONNOLLY: I suspect the child is not very much below it. Some of what you said surprised me greatly because it seemed to smack of the distinction between performance and ability. When you begin to talk about the difference between the acquisition of skill and the development of the child this seems to me to raise all kinds of issues over again.

HOWARD: Well certainly, unless you want to operationalize these distinctions.

BRUNER: But development is such an averaging concept across the manifestations of skill in different situations. I think we could get into a rather odd situation if we begin to talk about the relationship between skill and development. We are talking about a curious kind of thing, the relationship between the specific measure and a generalized measure which includes the specific. I think it might make things terribly confusing.

LEFFORD: Coming back to the notion of mechanism, I wonder if there are not two problems here. I think the distinction which Connolly drew between hardware changes and software changes could be a very valuable guide to us. We want to know something about both the basic mechanisms involved and the functional capacity or the functional nature of these mechanisms at different stages or levels of development. Perhaps the first job is to define these mechanisms at a particular level, and then to find the factors involved in the modification of these mechanisms during the course of development. This approach might well be applied to sub-routines.

INGRAM: I do not think it is possible to discuss the development of the motor skills that we have been describing without invoking the concept of learning readiness. Whether we are talking about small children carrying trays of coffee cups or trying to catch balls, we don't expect newborn babies to catch balls if they are thrown to them. You can say that they have not got the sub-routines that are needed for this process but there is more to motor activity than this. Perhaps there is an analogy with the situation of learning to speak or learning to read or learning to write; the child has to be at a certain stage of development before he is able to achieve these functions.

BRUNER: It is interesting how closely this relates to Lefford's earlier point. If you take the analogy of language learning, it has turned out to be the case that this is discontinuous in the sense that each time you sample the child's language you have to write a grammar appropriate to that stage. Then comes the question, can you write something about the nature of the transformation rules whereby the child went from the grammar, let us say, of pivot/open class to the grammar which then decomposes the open class into the modifier and stem?

INGRAM: It is stepwise, and this is why we are in difficulties. I think it is because we are regarding the child's motor development as a sort of continuum.

BRUNER: This is one of the issues which has already been joined, as to whether we should regard it as a continuous process. We all know from a close examination of skill that what the classical textbook say, that motor skills are continually perfected, is misleading. Now comes the question whether we can write something about the meaningful steps, the "ratchets" in this particular system. When children move up one notch on such a ratchet they do not usually slip back except under conditions, as Kay was suggesting, of time pressure.

KAY: I have a great deal of sympathy with the point which Howard was making. To me you can only measure channel capacity in a particular set of circumstances. If you select those circumstances such that you know from experience that a lot of prior knowledge of sub-routines is necessary, you get a measure of very poor performance and therefore a measure of limited channel capacity in the child. Obviously one could select other tasks, take a game such as "Snap" for example. Most children seem to enjoy this game immensely, perhaps because of its motor expressiveness. If you watch children doing this, one might well be tempted to say, "Here is an example of an extremely brilliant sub-routine". They can do it much faster than adults can, if I am the adult in question at least. Now this is a picture recognition situation, you put down a card and if you see that your card is identical to the one which has immediately preceded it then you shout "Snap" as quickly as you can. I would expect that in a situation such as this the channel capacity of a 6- or 7-year-old child will be every bit as good as an adult's. Here is a situation which has been very well practised, the recognition of two cards. Quite a lot of information is being transmitted in this situation, there are between 20 and 30 cards from which to select. If on the other hand one takes a more representative sample of children's motor performance, you will probably find that the channel capacity is considerably less than that of the adult. Now all I am saying here is that the channel capacity is variable. You would expect it to vary, it varies in the case of the adult. You can do such things as writing with a pencil much better than other people of your age can do, they in turn, however, may be much better at certain other skills. In most cases I suspect we would find that the channel capacity of the child is rather less than that of the adult. But one can get well practised skills of a limited kind and in such a situation I think we might find the channel capacity was very high.

HOWARD: I can imagine a number of situations where children would probably be much better than adults at learning a skill. I don't know that they are quicker at learning to ski but I would not be surprised if they were.

CONNOLLY: Learning to ski I think is probably a very good example. A 7-year-old would probably learn to ski much more quickly and more easily than a 30-year-old.

HOWARD: That is what I suspected, because the adult has got too many sub-routines already.

BRUNER: He also has a certain amount of interference.

HOWARD: Interference, exactly. He has learned too much already. His problem is unlearning, or not using things which he may think appropriate to skiing. In many ways a child is unfettered and we should count this an advantage to the child, the fact that he has learned less and that he is better off for having learned less. Here then is an example where the repertoire of skills that an adult may acquire could well be to his disadvantage in certain situations.

BRUNER: I am rather worried by one overtone which has crept in here, for example, when we talk about learning how to ski as compared with learning something else. Learning something like parallel skiing is learning a convention. Everyone who skis knows how to ski in some way. The interesting thing is to describe their particular pattern of skiing. A good skiing instructor can give one a hilarious imitation of the various kinds of skiing styles exhibited by beginners. They are all skiing, all exhibiting skill. It is not a question of learning the skill as opposed to not learning the skill, it is rather a question of to what extent one acquires a particularly stylish technique.

HOWARD: I cannot agree there. I think the point which you are making applies to all skills. There are certain conventions defining the outcomes. In any skill you define the outcome, there is always a goal to it and this is where we find our measure of success. I think, too, there is always an element of convention, I do not think skiing is any worse in this respect than any other skill.

Response Speed, Temporal Sequencing and Information Processing in Children[1]

KEVIN CONNOLLY

University of Sheffield

I. INTRODUCTION

THE MOTOR BEHAVIOUR of young children is relatively poor when compared with that of the adult, often not because they are unable to perform the necessary movements but rather because they are too slow. When we observe children engaged in tasks such as writing, catching a ball or eating with cutlery, it appears that they are unable adequately or rapidly to integrate the necessary sequence of sub-skills which go to make up such activities. Watching children of different ages perform simple laboratory tasks, for example, fitting pegs into holes, has led me to the view that one of the principal changes in skill development is concerned with the temporal sequencing of these sub-units. The transition between components is altogether smoother and more rapid in older children, there is less redundancy (in information-theory terms more redundancy) in their performance, every movement counts towards the achievement of the whole task. By analogy with the aims of a mathematician they appear to have achieved a more elegant and parsimonious solution to the problem than previously.

Research on human performance traditionally fragmented the problem into studies of sensory efficiency on the one hand and motor performance on the other. An appreciation of the importance of what takes place between the reception of signals by the sense organs and the initiation of responses by the muscle groups has emerged since the work of Craik (1947, 1948). Craik considered the human operator as a link in a communication channel; receiving, processing and transmitting information from a display (input) to controls (output). In this way

---

[1] The author is grateful to Miss Susan Stuart-Harris for valuable assistance, the Spastics Society for a generous research grant and to the many teachers and children for their co-operation in these studies.

an individual is regarded essentially as a self-regulating servo-mechanism. The efficiency with which this information transfer is accomplished is one of the important limiting features of skilled behaviour.

The speed and fluency with which children come to combine the various sub-units which go to make up common, yet complex, everyday behaviours may well reflect the rate at which they are able to transmit information. In addition, changes in their properties as information-handling systems are likely to affect their motor performance. Since Hick (1952) first applied Shannon and Weaver's (1949) mathematical theory of communication to the study of human performance a great deal has been achieved. Reviews by Welford (1960) and Smith (1968) serve to illustrate this. The experiments reported below are, I think, among the first to apply to developing organisms some of these notions which have proved valuable in studying adult motor performance.

II. EXPERIMENT 1

INFORMATION PROCESSING BY CHILDREN OF DIFFERENT AGES

Several methods have been used to investigate the relationship between the information load of a task and the time required for its execution. In choosing an experimental method to study information processing in children it was necessary to find a task which children of various ages could do and which would not be unduly boring for them. Crossman (1953) used, with considerable success, a card-sorting technique and the method employed in this experiment was a modification of that.

1. Subjects

Six groups of ten subjects, five males and five females in each, took part in the experiment. The ages of the various groups are given below:

Age group	Mean age		Age range			
	Years	Months	Years	Months	Years	Months
6	6	3	5	10	6	9
8	8	3	7	10	8	8
10	9	11	9	5	10	7
12	12	3	11	10	12	9
14	14	6	14	0	14	9
Adult	23	7	20	8	30	11

The children were drawn from two schools, one primary and one secondary. Both schools drew children from the same catchment area in Sheffield. Children with physical handicaps were excluded from the sample which was otherwise selected at random.

2. *Materials*

Stimulus cards were made up by sticking squares of coloured paper (1·5 × 1·5 inches) on to blank playing cards. Four experimental conditions (A, B, C and D) were used, and these are detailed below.

Condition A

Four packs of cards, two colours, 12 cards of each colour in a pack.

1. Red : Dark Blue
2. Yellow : Pale Blue
3. Black : Pink
4. Green : Brown

Condition B

Four packs of cards, four colours, six cards of each colour in a pack.

1. Red : Green : Black : Brown
2. Yellow : Pink : Dark Blue : Pale Blue
3. Yellow : Pale Blue : Green : Brown
4. Black : Red : Pink : Dark Blue

Condition C

Four packs of cards, six colours, four cards of each colour in a pack.

1. Red : Dark Blue : Yellow : Pale Blue : Green : Brown
2. Pink : Brown : Dark Blue : Green : Black : Yellow
3. Brown : Pink : Pale Blue : Black : Red : Dark Blue
4. Yellow : Pink : Black : Pale Blue : Red : Green

Condition D

Four packs of all eight colours, three cards of each colour in a pack.

The conditions therefore gave 2, 4, 6 and 8 choices corresponding to 1, 2, 2·585 and 3 bits of information respectively. A pack of 24 blank cards was used to obtain movement times in each of the four conditions, that is with two, four, six and eight locations.

Cardboard trays, 10 × 8 × 1 inches, were arranged in a semicircle around the subject. Fixed to the back of each tray and slotted in at right angles to the tray were white cards, 8 × 8 inches, on to which were stuck coloured squares, 3 × 3 inches, corresponding to the colours used in the various packs. These cards served to signal the appropriate trays to the subject.

3. *Procedure*

The 24 cards in each pack were arranged in predetermined random orders which were constructed from random number tables. The 16 packs were presented to each subject in a latin square order, thus:

A	B	C	D
D	A	B	C
C	D	A	B
B	C	D	A

The subjects were required to sort a pack of cards into the appropriate trays as quickly as possible. Only the appropriate trays (dependent upon the conditions) were ranged on the table in front of the subject, who stood throughout the experiment. Each pack of cards was given to the subject face downwards and he held the pack in this manner turning over one card at a time until the sort was completed. Before beginning the experiment each subject was asked to name the various colours, this obviated any artefacts which might have arisen from undetected colour blindness or ignornace of the colour names. The instructions given to the subjects were as follows:

> "What I want you to do is very easy. I just want you to play a game with me. First can you tell me the names of all these colours? (pointing to the colour cues fixed to the trays). I'm going to give you a pack of cards like this. Now, you see each card has a coloured square on it which matches one of these (indicating cue cards on the trays). I want you to turn over each card one at a time and put it into the right tray as quickly as you can. Look, I'll show you (demonstration). Can you do that? Good! Now sort this pack for practice. Start as soon as I say 'Go'."

The precise phrasing of the instructions was modified slightly for the older children and the adults such that they did not appear absurd. The 16 packs were then sorted. The time taken to sort each pack was recorded on a stop watch and the number of errors noted. When the packs had been sorted the children were given a few minutes rest. They were then asked to sort packs of 24 blank cards into two, four, six and eight trays going systematically round in each case. The cue cards were removed whilst the blank packs were being distributed. Four blank packs were sorted under each of the four conditions. Again the time to sort each pack was recorded on a stop watch.

4. Results

The data obtained consisted in response times and error rates in sorting packs of 24 cards when the amount of information per card was varied. In addition, movement times were obtained for each condition by having the subject sort packs of cards under zero information load.

TABLE I. DECISION TIME PER CARD
UNDER VARYING INFORMATION LOAD

Age	Information load in bits			
	1	2	2·58	3
6	1·000	1·180	1·570	1·719
8	0·808	0·988	1·230	1·320
10	0·609	0·743	0·934	1·130
12	0·520	0·672	0·860	1·090
14	0·522	0·706	0·850	1·100
Adult	0·338	0·475	0·660	0·730

The mean decision times per card for the various age groups under different information loads are given in Table I. These times were obtained for each subject by subtracting the movement time from the total response time and dividing by 24. Table II shows the mean movement time per card for each age group under the four experimental conditions. From these two tables it is possible to reconstitute mean response times per pack for the various groups. The younger children show a significantly higher within-group variance than the older subjects, a log transform was therefore performed on the raw scores.

TABLE II. MOVEMENT TIME (SECONDS) PER
CARD IN THE DIFFERENT EXPERIMENTAL
CONDITIONS

Age	Choice condition			
	2	4	6	8
6	0·806	0·855	0·873	0·881
8	0·637	0·678	0·659	0·683
10	0·511	0·578	0·590	0·582
12	0·493	0·522	0·527	0·511
14	0·441	0·459	0·457	0·453
Adult	0·393	0·412	0·402	0·390

A two-factor analysis of variance was then carried out on the transformed scores. The results of this analysis are summarized in Table III. The main effects of age, experimental conditions and the interaction between these two, all show significance at less than the 1 per cent level.

TABLE III. ANALYSIS OF VARIANCE ON LOG OF DECISION TIMES FOR THE SIX GROUPS OF SUBJECTS

Source	SS	DF	MS	F	p
Between subjects	4·838	59	—	—	—
A Age	3·936	55	0·787	47·15	<0·01
Subjects within groups	0·902	54	0·017	—	—
Within subjects	2·837	180	—	—	—
B conditions	2·537	3	0·846	564·63	<0·01
A × B	0·057	15	0·004	2·55	<0·01
B subjects within groups	0·243	162	0·001	—	—

These effects can be seen clearly in Fig. 1, where decision times are plotted against entropy per card expressed as $\log_2$ number of choices (binary digits). The curves order quite neatly with age, only the 12- and 14-year groups showing overlap. Figure 2 shows linear regression lines of the form $Y = A + b \log_2 X$ fitted to this data. There is a suggestion of a gradual steepening of these lines as we go down through the age groups. Certainly the slope of the line fitting the data from the 6-year-olds is greater than that fitting the adults' data. The intercepts and slope coefficients of these lines are given in Table IV. From the coefficients giving the slopes of the lines it appears that the significant interaction effect found in the analysis of variance is contributed largely

TABLE IV. CONSTANTS FROM LINEAR REGRESSION OF THE FORM $Y = A + b \log_2 X$ FITTED OVER DATA FROM TWO, FOUR, SIX AND EIGHT CHOICES FOR THE VARIOUS AGE GROUPS

Age	Intercept A	Coefficient b
6	0·5706	0·3712
8	0·5197	0·2641
10	0·3104	0·2516
12	0·2019	0·2719
14	0·2139	0·2705
Adult	0·1171	0·2020

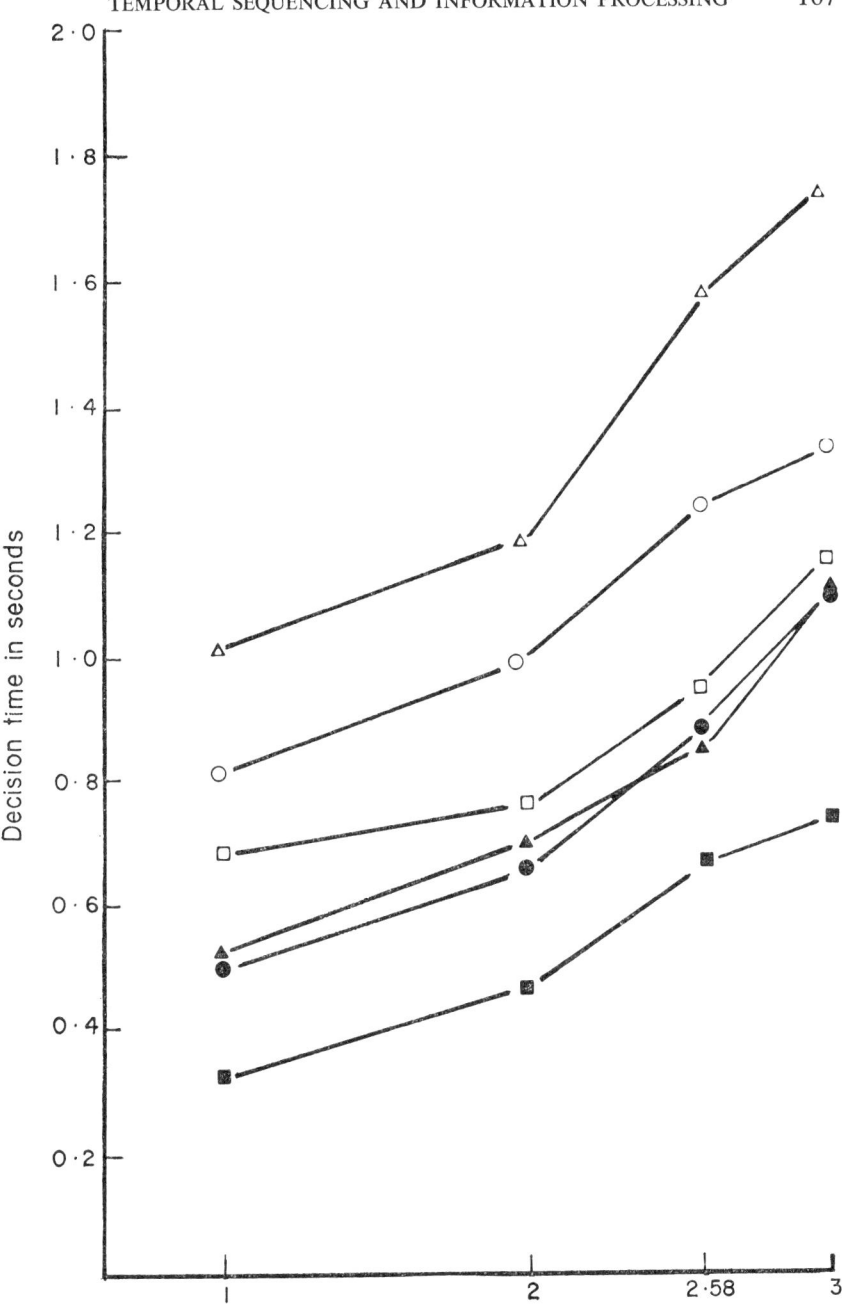

FIG. 1. Decision times plotted against entropy per card (binary digits) for the various age groups. (△, 6 years; ○, 8 years; □, 10 years; ▲, 12 years; ●, 14 years; ■, adult.)

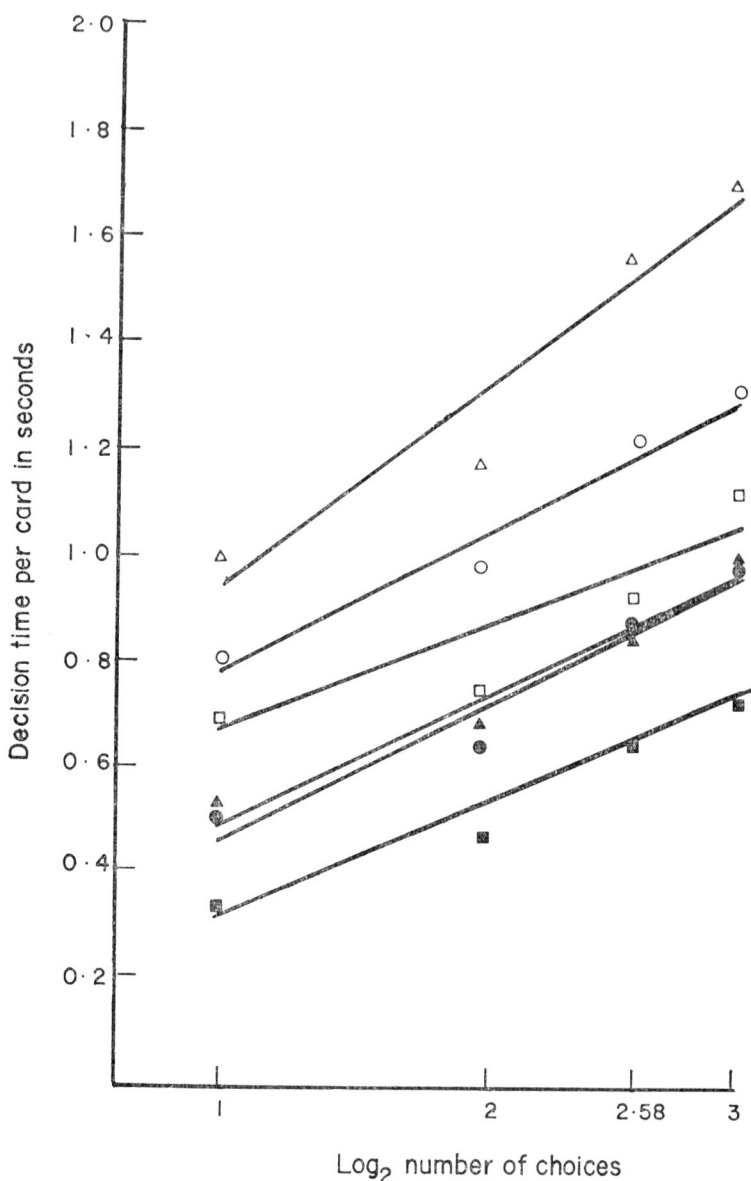

FIG. 2. Linear regression lines of the form $Y = A + b \log_2 X$ fitted to choice time data from Fig. 1. (△, 6 years; ○, 8 years; □, 10 years; ▲, 12 years; ●, 14 years; ■, adult.)

by the youngest children. A further examination of Fig. 1 shows that the decision times rise steeply for the younger children above an information load of two bits. Between one and two bits of information per card the lines showing the performance of the various groups of children are remarkably parallel. A further analysis was therefore carried out. Regression lines of the same form were fitted to the data for four, six and eight choices only. The values of the two constants from the second regression analysis are given in Table V. In this case the intercept

TABLE V. CONSTANTS FROM LINEAR REGRESSION OF THE FORM $Y = A + b \log_2 X$ FITTED OVER DATA FROM FOUR, SIX AND EIGHT CHOICES FOR THE VARIOUS AGE GROUPS

Age	Intercept A	Coefficient b
6	0·1071	0·5472
8	0·3570	0·3268
10	−0·0332	0·3835
12	−0·1676	0·4122
14	−0·0876	0·3851
Adult	−0·0350	0·2589

values are clearly meaningless but the b coefficients giving the slope of the lines are perhaps more informative. This analysis suggests that there are two principal transition stages; the first between the 6- and 8-year groups and the second between the 14-year and adult groups. The high variances within the groups preclude any statistical analysis of the b coefficients and the data must therefore be treated with caution.

Figure 3 shows the movement times for each of the age groups in the various experimental conditions. There is quite clearly a close relationship between chronological age and movement time, the younger the child the greater the movement time. What is particularly striking about these data is that the movement times for two, four, six and eight categories are remarkably flat. In this case, with zero information load on the children and where movement sequences are entirely pre-programmed, there is no increase in the time required to distribute cards between eight as compared with two spatial locations.

The error rates of the various groups of subjects under the different experimental conditions are low, as shown in Table VI. This low error rate may suggest that none of the groups were functioning at near

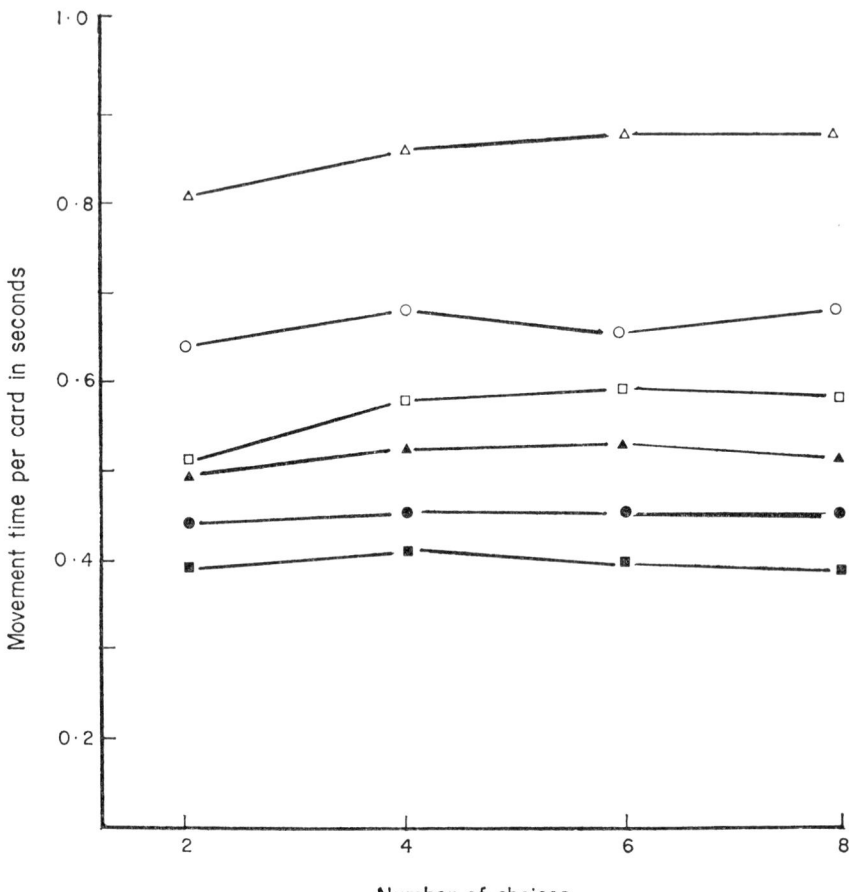

FIG. 3. Movement time as function of number of response locations for the various age groups. (△, years; ○, 8 years; □, 10 years; ▲, 12 years; ●, 14 years; ■, adult.)

capacity level. Bearing in mind that the subjects were essentially unpractised and that for the younger children to obey two instructions, viz. speed and accuracy, is difficult, this observation is not surprising. What is interesting about the error scores is the finding that the highest error rate was, for all groups, the two-choice condition. This comes out clearly in Table VII where the errors in the various conditions are expressed as a percentage of the total error.

A further way to express the information-processing abilities of the various age-groups of subjects is given by the rate of gain of information

TABLE VI. MEAN NUMBER OF ERRORS PER PACK MADE BY THE DIFFERENT GROUPS OF SUBJECTS IN THE VARIOUS EXPERIMENTAL CONDITIONS

Age group	Number of choices				Total
	2	4	6	8	
6	3·2	0·7	0·5	1·2	5·6
8	2·0	0·9	1·0	0·5	4·4
10	1·7	0·8	1·0	1·0	4·5
12	3·8	0·6	1·7	1·1	7·4
14	2·9	0·6	0·9	1·1	5·5
Adult	2·4	0·9	1·6	1·8	6·7

TABLE VII. PERCENTAGE OF TOTAL ERRORS IN EACH OF THE EXPERIMENTAL CONDITIONS FOR THE VARIOUS AGE GROUPS

Age	Number of choices			
	2	4	6	8
6	58	12	9	21
8	46	20	22	12
10	37	17	23	23
12	52	8	24	16
14	53	10	17	20
Adult	35	14	23	28

TABLE VIII. RATE OF GAIN OF INFORMATION (BITS PER SECOND) AS A FUNCTION OF AGE

Age	Number of choices			
	2	4	6	8
6	0·991	1·694	1·643	1·745
8	1·238	2·024	2·097	2·272
10	1·642	2·691	1·762	2·655
12	1·923	2·976	3·000	2·752
14	1·915	2·832	3·035	2·727
Adult	2·958	4·210	3·909	4·109

which they each achieve. The rate of gain of information was computed by dividing the amount of information per card by the decision time per card (Kay and Szafran, 1963). The results of this for the various groups are shown in Table VIII. Except for the two-choice condition there is close agreement between the rates within each age group. The low rates obtained in the two-choice conditions are probably an artefact and relate to the maximum speed of movement which a subject can accomplish in this task. In the two-choice condition the movement times account for a much greater proportion of the total response time than in the other conditions. The best estimate of rate of gain of information as a function of age is therefore given by the average of the information transmitted by each group when sorting into four, six and eight categories. This gives transmission rates as follows. Adults, 4·07 bits/second; 14-year group, 2·86 bits/second; 12-year group 2·90 bits/second; 10-year group, 2·70 bits/second; 8-year group, 2·13 bits/second and the 6-year group, 1·69 bits/second. Information transmission, measured as a rate of gain of information, increases with increasing age, the only exception being between the 12- and 14-year old group. The 12-year old group have a slightly higher rate of gain than the 14-year old group. This apparent disparity can probably be accounted for by reference to the error rates for the two groups. The total mean error rate for the 12-year-old group is higher than that for the 14-year-olds, which suggests that the 12-year-olds were giving more emphasis to speed, as against accuracy, than the 14-year-olds.

5. *Discussion*

Bearing in mind that the subjects in the different age groups had relatively little practice at the task, 384 responses in all, the results are remarkably clear. The time taken to sort a pack of cards decreased significantly with increasing age and increased significantly as entropy increased. The significant interaction between age and information load indicates that the slope of the line relating decision time to information differs between the various groups. From the linear regression lines fitted to the data this appeared to be due largely to the substantial increase in decision time as information load was increased in the youngest group of children.

The low error rates do suggest that the subjects may not have been performing at their maximum capacity. Had this been the case rather sharper differences between the age groups would probably have emerged. What is clear from the data is that information-transmission rates, measured as the rate of gain of information, increase steadily with age and continue beyond the 14-year level. This increase in information-transmission rate is all the more striking when one appreciates that age is a continuous and not a discrete variable. The approximate 2-year difference between successive groups was chosen arbitrarily. Had 3-year intervals been taken and the age range extended down to 4 and up to 19 the trend would almost certainly have been even more clearly marked.

The movement times obtained for each of the age groups across the four experimental conditions are extremely interesting. Under a zero information load, when in fact the response is entirely pre-programmed, the children are able to distribute cards between eight locations as quickly as between two. This observation reinforces the view that the information-processing abilities of children are an important limiting factor on the sequencing of the sub-units which go to make up basic motor skills. A further interesting feature about the movement time data is the relationship between speed of movement and age, the younger the child the slower the movement even when it is pre-programmed. We are now back to the observation that the speed of motor performance increases with age, though in addition we now know that this is true of movement speed itself irrespective of perceptual constraints. This is consistent with a considerable body of evidence showing that even simple reaction time decreases with increasing age (Goodenough, 1935; Jones, 1937). I think this finding points to the need for physiological and biomechanical studies of motor performance in children.

A study by Morin and Forrin (1965) explored the effects of the amount of prior experience on the slope of the function relating choice reaction time to stimulus uncertainty. Their subjects were asked to name stimuli as they were flashed on a screen and the results indicated that prior familiarity with material, such as numbers, leads to no increase in response time when the degree of uncertainty is increased. The results for symbol-naming are, however, similar to the data reported above for a motor task, both age and entropy have a significant effect.

This experiment investigated information-processing in its simplest form. By varying certain of the experimental conditions, differences between children at various ages may emerge and throw light on the mechanisms which lead to the more efficient processing of the information encoded by the sense organs. For example, continuous as distinct from discrete, information handling tasks may show greater differences between children at different stages of development. Stimulus-response compatibility effects may also be greater in children than they are in adults.

III. EXPERIMENT 2

THE EFFECTS OF IRRELEVANT STIMULI ON INFORMATION-PROCESSING BY CHILDREN

Young children often appear to be less task-oriented than the adolescent and the adult. The young child is also generally considered to be poor at selectively focusing his attention; he appears to take information from his environment in a rather indiscriminate fashion. This undifferentiated nature of perceptual and cognitive functioning in young children has been discussed by several authors (Witkin *et al.*, 1962).

If we think of the child's central nervous system as a single communication channel of limited capacity, then where the information in the display exceeds that which the organism can process there will be a state of information overload. (Channel capacity refers to the amount of information which can be transmitted per unit time, usually bits per second; Crossman, 1964). Broadbent (1958) has suggested that adults deal with this problem by filtering out the irrelevant information in the display and processing only that which is necessary to perform the task. Many empirical studies have offered support for this concept of selective filters. Experiment 1 has shown that more efficient information-processing develops with age and it is possible that one important feature contributing to this is the establishment of filtering mechanisms.

Several investigations have been conducted into the effects of irrelevant stimuli on the information-processing abilities of adults. Archer (1954) postulated that the effects of irrelevant stimuli would manifest themselves not only in longer reaction times but also that such effects would increase as the amount of relevant information increased. He found that response times increased linearly as a function of relevant information load but also that they were independent of irrelevant information. In a subsequent study designed to investigate various stimulus-response mappings, Morin, Forrin and Archer (1961) confirmed this and showed that reaction time was related to response information. Stimulus information did not appear to be a crucial determinant of reaction time since irrelevant information had no significant effect on performance. This finding, that reaction time was determined by the amount of information transmitted by a subject, was further explored by Fitts and Biederman (1965). Using Posner's (1964) system of classification they compared information conservation tasks (stimulus information = response information) with information reduction tasks (stimulus information > response information). Their results showed that an important factor in determining the efficiency of performance was stimulus-response compatibility. There was some suggestion that perceptual demands do play a part, but nevertheless response time was largely determined by the amount of information transmitted.

Experiment 2 was designed to examine the efficiency of the selective filtering mechanisms in younger children by investigating the effects of irrelevant stimuli on a card-sorting task.

1. *Subjects*

The results of the previous experiment suggest that substantial changes in information handling take place between the 6- and 10-year groups. This age range was therefore chosen for further study. Three groups of ten subjects, five boys and five girls in each, took part in the experiment. The mean ages and age ranges of the groups are shown below.

Age group	Mean age		Age range			
	Years	Months	Years	Months	Years	Months
6	6	3	5	10	6	7
8	8	1	7	9	8	2
10	10	4	9	11	10	8

2. *Materials*

Stimulus cards were made by sticking spots of coloured paper (5 mm diameter) on to one half of packs of blank playing cards. Each card had six spots of colour and two arrangements of these spots were used. In the first condition the stimuli were ordered in a straight line about one quarter of the way down the card. In the other the spots were stuck randomly over one half of the card face. The following colours were used: yellow, pink, pale blue, green, red, dark blue and black. Of these yellow, black, red and green were used as cue colours being chosen on the grounds that they were, subjectively to adults, the most discriminable. As before, the cards were made up into packs of 24. Twelve cards in each pack contained a signal and 12 did not. The probability of a card carrying a signal was therefore 0·5, so that the average information to be transmitted in each case was one bit.

3. *Procedure*

The procedure was essentially similar to that employed in experiment 1. The children held a pack of cards face downwards in their non-preferred hand and turned them over one at a time. The cards were sorted into two trays, one of which carried a cue card matching the relevant stimulus colour the other merely carried a blank card. Each child sorted four packs of 24 cards for each of the ordered and random arrays of stimulus material. An A B B A design was used to determine the presentation order of the two conditions. The instructions given to the subjects were:

> "What I want you to do is very easy. I just want you to play a game with me. First, can you tell me the names of all these colours (pointing to a card containing a sample of the colours). Now I'm going to give you a pack of cards with a lot of coloured spots on each card. If a card has a spot which matches this (indicating cue card on tray) I want you to put it in there. If it doesn't then put it in the other tray (indication). Turn each card over one at a time and put it into the right tray as quickly as you can. Can you do that? Good! Just practise on this set. Now remember to be as quick as you can. Start as soon as I say 'Go'."

The time to sort each pack was measured with a stop watch. In addition the time to distribute a blank pack of cards was measured. The number of errors made by the children (incorrect sorts) was also recorded.

4. Results

The mean times for the three age groups to sort a pack of 24 cards under the two experimental conditions of an ordered or random stimulus array are shown in Table IX. There is no indication of a difference between the two, either in terms of response time or error rates.

TABLE IX. RESPONSE TIMES IN SECONDS FOR THE THREE AGE GROUPS OF CHILDREN TO SORT PACKS OF CARDS WITH ORDERED AND RANDOM STIMULUS ARRAYS. MEAN ERROR RATES PER PACK FOR EACH AGE GROUP ARE ALSO SHOWN

Age group	Ordered			Random		
	Mean time	S.D.	Mean errors/pack	Mean time	S.D.	Mean errors/pack
6	57·38	11·40	1·5	57·99	11·37	1·5
8	44·77	9·88	1·4	46·07	11·05	1·6
10	34·14	4·17	1·3	34·43	4·68	1·7

To examine the effects of irrelevant stimuli on information-processing, it was necessary to compare the results from this experiment with those obtained in experiment 1 for the relevant age groups in the two-choice condition. These groups from the two experiments are comparable with respect to information transmitted. The mean choice times per pack are shown in Table X. The presence of irrelevant information in the stimulus array increases the choice time at all three age-levels though the increase is much less in the case of the 10-year olds.

TABLE X. MEAN CHOICE TIMES TO SORT PACKS OF 24 CARDS UNDER CONDITIONS OF NO NOISE AND NOISE. PRESENCE OF NOISE (IRRELEVANT STIMULI) INCREASES THE CHOICE TIME PER PACK BY THE AMOUNT SHOWN IN THE DIFFERENCE COLUMN. ALL TIMES ARE IN SECONDS

Age group	No irrelevant stimuli	Irrelevant stimuli	Difference between conditions
6	23·822	29·375	5·55
8	19·355	25·586	6·23
10	14·868	18·124	3·26

These data were subjected to an analysis of variance, the results of which are shown in Table XI. The main effects of age and conditions are both highly significant, $p < 0.001$. The presence of irrelevant stimuli

TABLE XI. RESULTS OF ANALYSIS OF VARIANCE ON SCORES FOR THE THREE AGE GROUPS UNDER CONDITIONS OF NOISE AND NO NOISE

Source	SS	DF	MS	F	p
A age	1031·970	2	515·9852	23·761	<0·001
B conditions	377·0092	1	377·0092	17·361	<0·001
$A \times B$	24·31078	2	12·15539	0·5597	N.S.
Within cell	1172·632	54	21·71541	—	—
Total	2605·916	59	—	—	—
A at B_1	400·8711	2	200·4355	9·230	—
A at B_2	655·4098	2	327·7049	15·090	—
Subjects within cells	1172·632	54	21·7154	—	—
B at A_1	53·0073	1	53·0073	2·441	N.S.
B at A_2	194·1268	1	194·1268	8·939	<0·01
B at A_3	154·1791	1	154·1791	7·099	<0·01
Subjects within cells	1172·632	54	21·7154	—	—

clearly increases the difficulty level of the task inasmuch as information transmission rate is significantly reduced. The interaction between age and conditions is non-significant. However, in examining the simple main effects which are shown in the lower part of the summary table it appears that at the 10-year level, the difference between the two conditions is not significant. This is factor B at A_1; at first sight this is somewhat puzzling, but it probably reflects the high within-cell variance. In order to check this, t-tests were carried out between the two conditions for each of the three age groups. The result of these t-tests indicate that the presence of irrelevant stimuli significantly increased choice time for the 6- and 8-year old groups ($p<0.05$) but the value of t fails to reach the 5 per cent level for the 10-year old children.

5. *Discussion*

The finding that an ordered, as distinct from random, array of the stimuli does not affect choice time is interesting but not central to my principal concern. It is of course possible that, for adults, reducing the area which must be scanned would make the task easier. The single most striking finding of this experiment is that the presence of irrelevant stimuli increases, very significantly, the time taken to transmit one bit of information by young children. This is not the case for the adult subjects as shown by the several investigations cited above, which indicate that decision times are a function of the amount of information transmitted and not the information content of the stimulus array.

The results from the analysis of variance regarding the interaction of age and conditions are equivocal, due probably to violating the assumptions regarding the homogeneity of variance. This might not have been the case had the same subjects been used in the two experiments. There are, however, practical difficulties to contend with regarding the length of time that young children will willingly spend in performing tasks such as these. It is also important to bear in mind that the age groups were selected almost arbitrarily. Had 12- or 14-year-olds been used rather than the 10-year group the interaction effect might well have emerged unambiguously. The findings of other investigators working with adult subjects certainly point in this direction.

The results of this experiment do indicate an important qualitative difference between the properties of young children and adults as information-handling systems. Within the framework of Broadbent's (1958) theory, the data suggest that the selective filtering mechanisms have not yet come into effective operation in the younger children.

IV. EXPERIMENT 3

THE EFFECTS OF PROGRESSIVELY INCREASING THE NUMBER OF IRRELEVANT STIMULI

The results of experiment 2 show that the presence of irrelevant stimuli in the display significantly increases the decision time for 6- and 8-year-old children whereas the increase for the 10-year group is not significant. If these results are interpreted as providing evidence for the establishment of selective filtering mechanisms, it becomes important to explore the properties of such mechanisms as development proceeds.

The total amount of information in the stimulus array, as distinct from the amount of information to be transmitted, may affect performance only when it exceeds a threshold. The increase in decision time may in fact only appear when the total ensemble reaches a given size. Should this be the case then we might expect that the critical ensemble size will be related to the efficiency of the selective filters and so to age. Experiment 3 was undertaken to investigate this possibility by progressively and systematically varying the number of irrelevant stimuli.

1. Subjects

Three further groups of ten subjects, five boys and five girls in each, took part in the experiment. Their mean ages and age ranges are given below. They were drawn from a third school in the same area of Sheffield as those children taking part in experiments 1 and 2.

Age group	Mean age		Age range			
	Years	Months	Years	Months	Years	Months
6	6	0	5	8	6	4
8	7	11	7	10	8	1
10	10	1	9	10	10	3

2. Materials

Packs of stimulus cards were again made up by attaching spots (5 mm diameter) of coloured paper to blank playing cards. Five experimental conditions were used, these related to the presence of one, two, three, four or five irrelevant stimuli on 50 per cent of the cards in each pack. The other 12 cards in each pack carried two, three, four, five or six irrelevant stimuli dependent on the experimental condition. The colours used in the experiment were: red, yellow, blue, green, black, pink and purple. Of these red, yellow, green and purple were used as relevant cue colours.

In each pack of 24 cards 12 carried a signal and 12 did not, the probability of a card carrying a signal was therefore 0·5. In every case the response was a binary sort, signal/no signal, one bit of information was therefore transmitted per card. Four packs of cards were sorted under each of the five experimental conditions. In addition each subject distributed between the two boxes four packs of 24 blank cards in order that movement times could be ascertained.

3. *Procedure*

The procedure was the same as that in experiment 2. A subject held a pack of 24 cards face downwards in his non-dominant hand and turned cards up one at a time. A check was carried out prior to the child commencing the task to ensure that he could recognize, discriminate and identify all the colours used. The instructions given to subects were essentially the same as in experiment 2, modifications being made only where necessary to explain the slightly different nature of the proceedings. Emphasis was, of course, placed on speed.

4. *Results*

Decision times per card were obtained in the manner described previously for each of the age groups under each of the five experimental conditions. The results are shown in Fig. 4. The difference between the age groups is considerable, particularly between the 6- and 8-year-old groups. The systematic addition of irrelevant information is reflected in a progressive increase in the mean decision time per card. This increase is a monotonic function for all three groups except for one point in the 6-year-old's data.

Because of inhomogeneity of variance between the three groups the raw data were transformed into logs before carrying out an analysis. The results from the analysis of variance are summarized in Table XII. The main effects of age and experimental conditions are significant at less than the 1 per cent level but the interaction component fails to reach significance. The absence of any interaction between age and conditions can be seen in Fig. 4. However, there is a suggestion from the F ratios of the simple main effects that irrelevant stimuli have far greater effect on the younger children. The F ratios are as follows: for the 10-year group 5·3, for the 8-year group 12·4, and for the 6-year group 11·1.

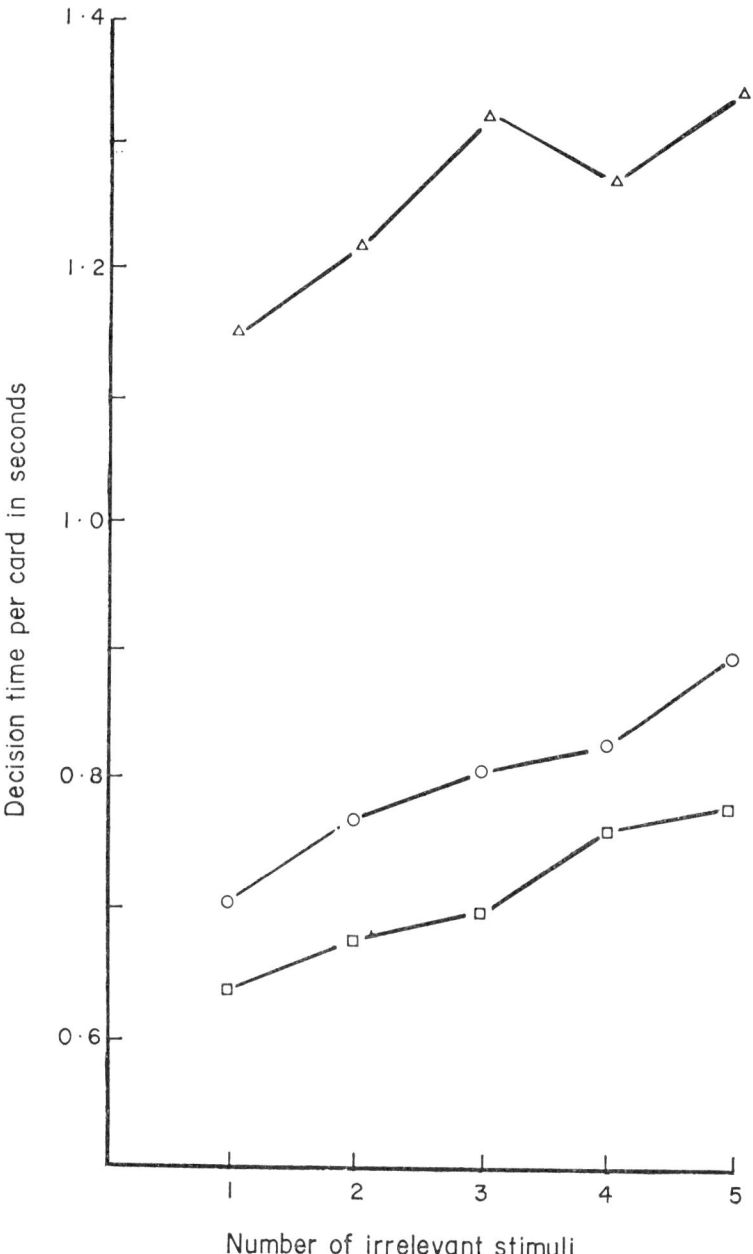

FIG. 4. Decision time as function of number of irrelevant stimuli. (△, 6 years; ○, 8 years; □, 10 years.)

TABLE XII. SUMMARY OF ANALYSIS OF VARIANCE ON TRANSFORMED DATA FROM EXPERIMENT 3. $A_1=6$, $A_2=8$, $A_3=10$

Source	SS	DF	MS	F	p
Between subjects	2·194	29	—	—	—
A age	1·827	2	0·913	67·27	<0·01
Subjects within groups	0·366	27	0·013	—	—
Within subjects	0·074	120	—	—	—
B conditions	0·0347	4	0·008	25·90	<0·01
$A \times B$	0·003	8	0·0004	1·44	N.S.
Between subjects within groups	0·036	108	0·0003	—	—
A at B_1	0·385	2	0·192	64·49	—
A at B_2	0·379	2	0·189	63·49	—
A at B_3	0·403	2	0·201	67·65	—
A at B_4	0·326	2	0·163	54·63	—
A at B_5	0·337	2	0·168	56·52	—
Subjects within cells	0·403	135	0·0029	—	—
B at A_1	0·014	4	0·003	11·07	—
B at A_2	0·016	4	0·004	12·40	—
B at A_3	0·007	4	0·001	5·32	—
Between subjects within groups	0·036	108	0·0003	—	—

5. Discussion

The results indicate that irrelevant stimuli, even when they are few in number, increase decision times for children over the age range studied. There is no suggestion of a threshold related to ensemble size; on the contrary the effects of noise appear to be additive over the whole range. The suggestion from the F ratios of the simple main effects that irrelevant stimuli have a rather smaller effect on older children is consistent with the findings from experiment 2.

Greater differences between children over the age range 6 to 10 in their ability to handle information and select appropriately from a given display might emerge when the amount of information to be transmitted is increased. In this investigation all the experimental conditions imposed a load of one bit on the response mechanism. Were the amount of response information to be increased such that the task demanded of a subject that he perform nearer to his channel capacity, then a significant interaction between age and conditions might well appear with children over this age range. The function relating decision time to the number of irrelevant stimuli would probably be much steeper for a 6-year-old, were he required to transmit three bits of information.

V. EXPERIMENT 4

THE EFFECT OF STIMULUS VARIATION IN TWO DIMENSIONS

Another way in which the information-processing abilities of young children might be affected by the perceptual load imposed is where more than one stimulus dimension is made to vary. In experiments 2 and 3, stimuli varied only in colour. Variation in other stimulus parameters, such as shape or size, although irrelevant may have, along with colour, a multiplicative effect on decision times. Experiment 4 was undertaken therefore to explore further the properties of selective filtering mechanisms in children. Shape was chosen as the other stimulus dimension to be varied. A preliminary experiment was carried out to determine the decision times to sort packs of cards with various stimulus shapes fixed to them. This was followed by an experiment where both colour and shape varied on a single card but only one cue was involved, as before, viz. red independent of shape, or triangle independent of colour.

1. *Subjects*

A further group of subjects in the 6-, 8- and 10-year levels took part in the experiments. Each group was made up of five boys and five girls as before. The children were of comparable socio-economic background to those participating in the previous experiments. Their mean ages and age ranges are given below:

Age group	Mean age		Age range			
	Years	Months	Years	Months	Years	Months
6	6	2	5	9	6	9
8	7	11	7	10	8	2
10	9	10	9	11	10	1

2. *Materials*

Packs of cards were made up by sticking coloured paper cut-outs on to blank playing cards. The area of the various shapes was approximately equal. The shapes used were: circles, triangles, squares, ovals, hearts, bars and ellipses. Of these, circles, triangles, squares and hearts were used as cue shapes because they were the most similar in terms of area and because a pilot experiment showed them to be roughly equivalent with respect to their difficulty of discrimination. A further set of cards was prepared with both shape and colour varying. As in the previous experiments each subject sorted four packs of cards for shape, for colour with shape varying in addition, and for shape with colour also varying.

3. Procedure

The procedure and instructions to subjects were essentially as before, the instructions being modified only to explain that shape, or shape irrespective of colour, or colour irrespective of shape had to be sorted. The cue cards attached to the trays into which the cards were sorted were adjusted according to the task. Before beginning the experiment the children performed a "matching to sample" task to ensure that they could distinguish the various shapes. Each child also distributed four packs of blank cards between the two trays in order to provide data on movement times.

4. Results

A comparison between the response times to sort a pack of 24 cards for colour and for shape is provided in Fig. 6. For all three age groups the total response time to sort for shape is significantly greater than that for colour (Mann-Whitney U-test $p<0.05$). The response times for colour are those obtained in experiment 2. A more detailed breakdown of the data and a comparison between the choice times for colour and shape independently as against the choice times when both are varying is given in Table XIII. The results indicate that when a child is required to sort for colour irrespective of shape the choice time is similar to that

TABLE XIII. MEAN CHOICE TIMES (IN SECONDS) FOR PACKS OF 24 CARDS UNDER CONDITIONS WHERE THE STIMULUS ARRAY VARIES IN ONE OR TWO PARAMETERS

Age group	Sorting for colour		Sorting for shape	
	Only colour varying	Colour and shape varying	Only shape varying	Shape and colour varying
6	24·66	29·37	36·92	42·38
8	25·58	24·10	30·80	38·22
10	18·12	19·29	30·34	29·93

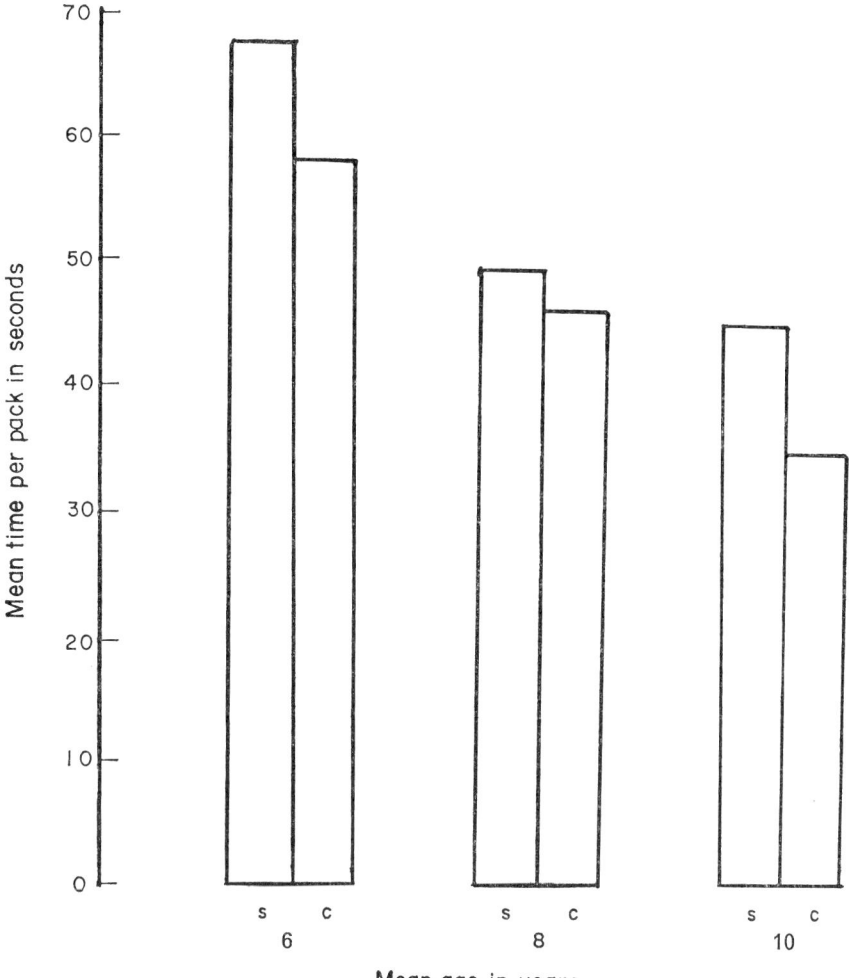

FIG. 5. Comparison of response times in sorting for colour (C) or for shape (S).

when colour alone is varying. This is also the case with shape, the addition of colour as a further variable does not affect the choice time.

5. *Discussion*

This experiment provides a further exploration of the properties of the hypothesized selective filtering mechanisms, and the results indicate clearly that the filters are functioning efficiently in certain ways. When a subject is sorting for colour the presence of information about the shape of the stimuli does not affect performance. In one sense it has been filtered out, the child does not have to process it. This observation could of course be described in other ways: as related to concept formation, discrimination learning perhaps, or the resolving power of the child's conceptual apparatus. By six, shape and colour are easily discriminated stimulus parameters, bolstered probably by the development of linguistic skills. The results from this experiment suggest that an exploration of stimulus-response compatibility effects in children, in various tasks, could well throw more light on the development of efficient information-processing.

VI. SUMMARY AND CONCLUSIONS

Young children are less efficient information-handling systems than are adults or even older children. The results of experiment 1 suggest a close correlation between age and information transmission measured as rate of gain of information. It is also apparent from the data obtained on movement times that developmental changes in the speed of motor behaviour cannot be explained solely on the basis of improved information-handling abilities. Obviously there is more than one kind of mechanism involved and many developmental processes are going on simultaneously.

The curvilinear relationship between the speed of behaviour and age through an individual's life history is interesting. However, it seems intrinsically improbable that the same mechanisms are involved at each end of the life span. In old age various kinds of degenerative physiological and morphological changes are taking place. Crossman and Szafran (1956) have suggested that these changes will lead to an increase in noise in the nervous system and so to a decrease in the signal : noise ratio. In children the very reverse of degeneration is occurring. The growth and integration of the child's central nervous system, which is manifest in his behavioural development, leads to increasing powers of discrimination and therefore a shorter integration-time is required to make fine discriminations. This can be seen by comparing and contrasting the results from experiments 2, 3 and 4.

The investigations reported in this paper have been successful in that they have raised more questions than they have answered. There are several obvious lines of enquiry which could be followed in exploring the development of the hypothesized selective filtering mechanisms. Experimental work on the skilled behaviour of adults also provides a lead, and challenging questions which might be answered by developmental studies (Bilodeau, 1966). It is important to remember that the simple, and in some ways artificial, situations which are devised in the laboratory are far from the real world. Choice reaction times, as measured in experimental situations such as I have described, represent a limiting level of performance rarely, if ever, encountered in everyday life. Most of our common responses are not to coloured spots on cards but to any one of a large number of constantly changing complex stimulus constellations. The child's ability to take in information, make decisions and operate on his environment are affected by many factors. I am reminded in this context of children painting, the grip which is employed may well limit an individual's motor repertoire. Changing the grip, or perhaps the posture, could have enormous effects on the range of motor responses which he can generate.

REFERENCES

ARCHER, E. J. 1954. Identification of visual patterns as a function of information load. *J. exp. Psychol.* **48**, 313–317.

BILODEAU, E. A. 1966. (Ed.) *Acquisition of skill*. Academic Press, London.

BROADBENT, D. E. 1958. *Perception and communication*. Pergamon Press, Oxford.

CRAIK, K. J. W. 1947. Theory of the human operator in control systems. I. The operator as an engineering system. *Brit. J. Psychol.* **38**, 56–61.

CRAIK, K. J. W. 1948. Theory of the human operator in control systems. II. Man as an element in a control system. *Brit. J. Psychol.* **38**, 142–148.

CROSSMAN, E. R. F. W. 1953. Entropy and choice time: the effort of frequency and unbalance on choice-responses. *Quart. J. exp. Psychol.* **5**, 41–51.

CROSSMAN, E. R. F. W. 1964. Information processes in human skill. *Brit. Med. Bull.* **20**, 32–37.

CROSSMAN, E. R. F. W. and SZAFRAN, J. 1956. Changes with age in the speed of information intake and discrimination. *Experientia, Supp.* **4**, 128–135.

FITTS, P. M. and BIEDERMAN, I. 1965. S–R compatibility and information reduction. *J. exp. Psychol.* **69**, 408–412.

GOODENOUGH, F. L. 1935. The development of reactive processes from early childhood to maturity. *J. exp. Psychol.* **18**, 431–450.

HICK, W. E. 1952. On the rate of gain of information. *Quart. J. exp. Psychol.* **4**, 11–26.

JONES, H. E. 1937. Reaction time and motor development. *Am. J. Psychol.* **50**, 181–194.

KAY, H. and SZAFRAN, J. 1963. Motor performance. In G. Humphrey (Ed.), *Psychology through experiment*. Methuen, London.

MORIN, R. E. and FORRIN, B. 1965. Information-processing: choice reaction times of first- and third-grade students for two types of associations. *Child Develop.* **36**, 713–720.

MORIN, R. E., FORRIN, B. and ARCHER, W. 1961. Information processing: the role of irrelevant stimulus information. *J. exp. Psychol.* **61**, 89–96.

POSNER, M. I. 1964. Information reduction in the analysis of sequential tasks. *Psychol. Rev.* **71,** 491–504.
SHANNON, C. E. and WEAVER, W. 1949. *The mathematical theory of communication.* University of Illinois Press, Urbana.
SMITH, E. E. 1968. Choice reaction time: an analysis of the major theoretical positions. *Psychol. Bull.* **69,** 77–110.
WELFORD, A. T. 1960. The measurement of sensory-motor performance: a survey and re-appraisal of twelve years' progress. *Ergonomics*, **3,** 189–230.
WITKIN, H. A., DYK, R., FATERSON, H. F., GOODENOUGH, D. and KARP, S. 1962. *Psychological differentiation.* Wiley, New York.

Discussion

BRUNER: Your hypothesis regarding changes in speed of performance in children is very interesting. You suggest that the speed of overall performance is largely determined by the speed with which the child can integrate the necessary sequence of sub-skills. It would be extremely interesting to do further experiments of the kind you have described and then to go on and require the children to put together different components into a sequence. I think this may well show multiple differences between children of different age groups. I should like to see these experiments done where there is a high degree of contingent constraints based on the outcome of previous moves. Would you agree with this?

CONNOLLY: I entirely agree with what you say. The experiments I have reported are a necessary first stage to what you are suggesting. I think too it would be very interesting to examine the effects of irrelevant stimuli in situations where there is a much higher information load. We have done one experiment of the kind you suggest, where the child has to perform a series of operations. This was a serial assembly task where the child was required to pick a pin out of a hole, transfer it to a target hole, place it in this target hole, come back, pick up another pin and so forth (Connolly, 1968, *Aspects of education*, **7,** 82). The apparatus was designed so that we could measure the four primary components of the task (grasp time, movement loaded time, release time, and return movement time). The results which we obtained did show differences between children and adults. The children, interestingly enough, showed most improvement with practice on the two movement components whereas adults on such tasks, according to Smader and Smith (1953, *J. app. Psychol.* **37,** 308), improve most on the grasp and release components. There are other more subtle differences also.

HINDE: May I ask you about another variable? The probability of getting a signal in your experiment was, I think, 0·5, now if you varied this would you get differences which were age related?

CONNOLLY: This raises a very interesting point. Crossman (1953, *Quart. J. exp. Psychol.* **5,** 41) working with adults has shown that the reaction time is a function of the probability of getting a signal. I think experiments of this kind would give us some information about a child's ability to learn something of the statistical structure of a series. This is particularly important because it may provide us with a way of uncovering to what extent children of different ages can, as it were, "create information". Such experiments could not be done very readily by using the card-sorting technique I have described, but I can think of ways in which they could be done.

BRUNER: I think Neisser's (1966, *Cognitive psychology*, Appleton-Century-Crofts, New York) approach is interesting in this context. He takes what could perhaps best be called a constructionist view. Fundamentally what he suggests is that the individual, in sampling from an array, is constructing a model for holding the information as he goes. As each element comes up he is performing a sort of "goodness of fit" on it with respect to the overall constructive whole. I would like to take this a stage further. In sampling the world, when it is to some extent restricted by what is in the periphery, a person will pick the information up and perhaps say "Oh yes, that's a landscape by Constable" or some such thing. Now this is on the basis of a few features which he detected. It turns out that along the way, as the programme goes into operation, the more he moves towards the confirmation of a general hypothesis the more likely he is to become increasingly selective. That is to say, his filter tightens itself up so that he says, "Ah yes, a gold stubbled haystack in the foreground, that's certainly Constable". It is as if one's pass band filter has become so narrow by this time that one is looking for a specific thing. Neisser, in fact, argues that for the analysis of information processing one must look at what is going on sequentially in this constructive process and not just in terms of what can be called equally probable, equally distributed linear scannings. I think this is Connolly's point too, and I do want to stress the importance of the base line data that we have been provided with. From this we can go on and look at sequential effects.

LEFFORD: I should like to come in here and make an observation. I liked the experiments because they raise certain problems that I have had in understanding my own data. We have been talking so far about understanding the data in terms of the stimulus array and of the response alternatives. In introducing the data Connolly spoke about selective filtering very much in the same way as I spoke about a schema. In order to understand the material he introduced an intra-organismic variable. It seems to me that we have been trying to move away from this and describe the data without introducing such a construct, I wonder why? Why are we so reluctant to postulate some form of intra-organismic variable? The construct of selective filters is an intra-organismic variable which your data show is built up through time. It serves to organize the information which the child has, makes the array less confusing and gradually leads to the development of the adult response. The structure becomes very much a part of the organism and, because of it, it responds more efficiently.

CONNOLLY: I accept your point about the organization of a structure into which a child can fit subsequent experiences, but I am not so sure that selective filter and schema are quite the same thing.

HINDE: It seems to me that the selective filtering is not doing anything more, and not pretending to do anything more, than describe selective responses. I am not so sure about a schema.

PRECHTL: The selective response notion appeals to me very much but might there not be another factor involved? From observations on the growing brain one gets the impression that the younger the child or the infant the more noisy are the channels in the nervous system. If, during the course of the maturation of the nervous system, there is an increase in stability and therefore an increase in the signal to noise ratio then we would expect an increase in the efficiency of performance without necessarily having built in a filter.

CONNOLLY: I thought about this and comparing our data with those obtained from old people there is at first sight a striking resemblance between the performance of the very young and the very old. To account for their findings of a decrement in skilled performance in old people. Crossman and Szafran (1956, *Experientia*, Suppl. **4,** 128) postulate increasing noise in the nervous system, which has the effect, as you suggest, of altering the signal : noise ratio and therefore making the communication system less efficient. I am not very happy about applying this notion of noise in the nervous system at both ends of the age scale for a variety of reasons. First it seems to me intrinsically unlikely that the similarity of results obtained from information processing tasks are due to changes in the same variable in children and in old people. Secondly, is it likely that the signal to noise ratio will still show substantial changes between the ages of 6 and 8? Finally, I am not quite sure how one translates the concept of noise here from the way in which you are using it, which is, I think at the neurological level to the behavioural level. It is a nice word and I use it a good deal but just where does it get us in this context?

LEFFORD: Can I just ask you Prechtl, do you see the noise as being in the nervous system or as being part of the input through the nervous system?

PRECHTL: I think it is in the nervous system. Neurones are very uncertain things, indeed there is a splendid book on the subject (Burns, D. B. 1968. *The uncertain nervous system.* Arnold, London).

BRUNER: I have played with these notions for many years but I am rather worried about concepts such as noise in the nervous system for the following reasons. All too often I think people use a term like this as if it were the only factor involved, and I am quite certain it would be a mistake for us to assume this. Vurpillot's (1968, *J. exp. Child Psychol.* **6,** 632) experiments being a case in point. She worked with children aged from 4 through 9 setting them the task of looking at four houses and saying which one was different. The younger children, as you would expect, were much poorer than the older ones, and it transpired that these children were not in fact encoding sufficient of the information in the display. They would look to see in what way the houses differed; they would compare them, and if at last they found a single feature on which two houses differed then they would respond. In fact they made their judgement without obtaining sufficient data from the array. They had not, if you like, sampled enough to come out with the right answer. This is a qualitative difference in the way in which the children process the information. You see I think simple organisms are not just simple quantitatively; I think they have different modes of coping with things. This is brought out by Connolly's experiments. I do not think any of us doubt that there is noise on both the motor and sensory sides, though the operation of selective filters may be a little too passive. As to Lefford's point, I do not mind internal constructs if they lead us to some external behaviour which I can also observe.

CONNOLLY: I mentioned our observational studies on painting because this is exactly the type of situation where one can see considerable qualitative differences. You see, the way in which a child holds his paint brush may well affect and indeed does affect the movements which he can make. The palmar grasp on the brush makes lateral and vertical arm sweeps much more difficult, whilst the adult grip greatly increases flexibility in the range and ease with which movements may be made.

HINDE: I am bothered by this blanket variable, noise, in this context. There are many things happening as the child gets older. The danger is that in describing them all in terms of a common variable such as noise, we may succeed only in blinding ourselves to other important changes which are taking place.

PRECHTL: I accept your point, using these terms really only makes sense if you know exactly what the signal is in relation to the context.

BRUNER: If this approach makes accessible, a formal, mathematical apparatus for analysis then it would be very valuable.

PRECHTL: I think this construct of noise is very important and this kind of approach is quite the best we have at the moment.

HINDE: But you have gone much farther on this. You said in your initial statement, which you later qualified I think, that the nervous system "Is more noisy".

PRECHTL: Of course, in general, I think this is the case. There appears to be much more disjointed activity in the developing nervous system. Think, for example, of the firing rhythms in hypothalamic units of newborn rabbits, they are much more random, whilst unit activity in the older rabbit in the same area, the hypothalamus, shows quite a different distribution (Hyvärinen, 1966, *Acta physiologica Scand.* **68,** supp. **278,** 67).

The Analysis of Performance

GENERAL DISCUSSION

KAY: When the Roman soldiers invaded Britain they carried on their backs a pack weighing 31 lb. The modern soldier's pack is much the same weight. Apparently it is about the right weight for a soldier to carry around if he is to do the other tasks for which he has been trained. But our example is not typical of what is happening in the world of skills where every day we have instances of old records being broken. The reasons why we are able to establish so many new records in, say, athletics are complicated and do not lie in the initially greater abilities of today's athletes. We have to look to their training and the goals which are set.

My main work has been in the field of adult skills and industry where we have to think continually about the improvement of performance. Today this technological field is presenting us with new challenges, and, in particular, we shall have to train people for skills which they have not hitherto been expected to acquire and to re-train them again in middle life for yet different skills.

This kind of challenge presents psychology with urgent problems but we have already been able to demonstrate that by using specific training techniques we can improve an individual's performance. I have been impressed by the effectiveness of computer-aided instruction when used for training manual skills in our own laboratory. With this technique, we have fed back to the individual operator those signals which were particularly difficult for him to master and have shown marked improvement over normal training performance. It is clear that we can do much in this area but it will depend upon how far we progress in understanding the fundamentals of motor skills. The more I consider the problem the more I return to the old issue of serialization which seems to be the basis of so many high level skills. Miller was so right to talk about "chunks" (Miller, 1956, *Psychol. Rev.* **63,** 81) though that does not tell us how the "bits" are compounded into larger units.

Traditionally skills have been conceptualized along the lines of the three functions shown in the block diagram of Fig. 1. The first stage has to do with the reception of information. Signals are received both from the external environment and from an individual's own actions in the form of feedback. Enough information must be passed from the first stage to the central controlling mechanisms for effective action to be planned. The central mechanisms are responsible for co-ordinating the input with the output if correct timing of response is to be achieved.

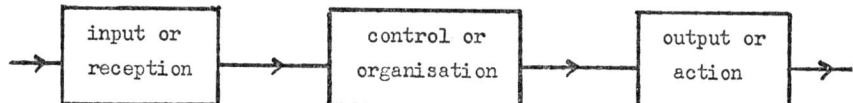

FIG. 1. Basic paradigm for analysis of skill.

The organism is carrying out an elaborate matching exercise between input and output and in order to achieve this co-ordination the central mechanisms must be able to process and to control large units of information. The correct timing of a skill is achieved, in part, by the rapid translation of one particular series of signals before switching to its corresponding effector commands. To some extent this timing involves a continuous switching between the two stages but the secret lies in the size of the unit which the central mechanism can handle. This can be expressed another way by saying the more practised the skill the more direct the coding operation and the larger the unit which the central mechanism can process. The task may, for example, begin with an extremely complex visual display containing thousands of bits of information. But this is quickly compressed at the input stage to those relatively few bits of information which practice has taught the operator are relevant. The input is monitored centrally for sufficient time to extract, say, its rate of change and then a response command is passed from the central mechanisms to the effector system. Here it is elaborated and again, if well practised, predictable feedback signals can be anticipated and quickly processed.

We psychologists tend to speak of a "response" because we are unclear about our units of action but it is a misleading term. In our discussions we have talked much of the tonic-neck-reflex and studied illustrations of it. But these responses are firing an incredible number of motor neurons, illustrating that even relatively simple reflexes are physiologically complex. It is not surprising that we find the problem of serialization so difficult since we are not sure of the units we are trying to put together to form the series but it would seem that one of the most promising ways of exploring the serialization of action is from a developmental standpoint. If we take the newborn and consider which systems are most developed at this early stage of life then it is probable that the early development of skills may well take place by linking new units to already established functions. For example, if we think of a foetus *in utero* then of all its sensory systems the one which is probably the most highly developed is the labyrinth. A baby quickly shows awareness of changes in its position and orientation. We might therefore try to examine how this mechanism is implicated in the various complex behavioural patterns during early infancy. My suggestion is that we look for those "units" in the nervous system which are most developed at that particular stage and which are likely to play a part in the further development of a new skill. In this way, I think, we might get some insight into how units are put together. Now I have not said what a unit is, and I cannot. In the film which I showed you of children catching a ball, even at the youngest level, we were not looking at one skill but at a whole hierarchy. For the 2-year-old child the most difficult element was not so much the catching but the fact that she had to stand and this imposed so many constraints upon her that it gave a whole static rigidity to her performance. The 15-year-old, in marked contrast, could move fluently whilst performing the task, and indeed the flexibility and additional movement which he brought to the skill added greatly to his performance. In many respects it was a more complex skill but it is here, I think, where information theory can be of help to us because it allows for signals becoming redundant as they become predictable or pre-programmed. As long as performance is being continually monitored in such a way that the actions are predictable then I think to this extent it makes sense to talk of hierarchies of skills. The channel capacity is limited but individual signals are put together in a predictable sequence, thereby reducing their total uncertainty or information. Reflecting again on the performance of the 2-year-old, there are a whole lot of signals to be monitored just in order to keep the child standing upright, and similarly with the arm movements. None of these for a young child is predictable, and yet we are asking it to learn another complex skill at the same time. It is not surprising that it fails or makes slow progress.

CONNOLLY: I think the notion of channel capacity is a very difficult one to deal with when considering children. The child is acquiring new modes of behaviour as he develops, in fact he changes his methods of processing information and adopts new ones. Channel capacity is not so much built into the apparatus as it is built into the strategy which the child is using. Might I add, that I think in addition to studying changes in perceptual strategies we should also consider cognitive skills and the manner whereby movements are brought about. I think we must look too, at the way in which internal signals are handled and how such handling changes as the child grows.

WHITE: May I just say that I think the development of visually directed reaching and its emergence from the reflex substrata provides, potentially at least, a very good preparation in which to study a linking of sub-routines. The results which we obtained from experiments designed to enhance the environment in various ways showed clearly, I think, that the development of visually directed reaching could be greatly speeded up. These results suggest that this is a suitable context in which to examine the serialization of skilled responses.

PRECHTL: An essential aspect of the development of skilled motor activity is the programming of anticipatory postural changes, which are carried out prior to the performance of a motor act. Voluntary movements are always superimposed on particular body postures. In reaching and grasping an object lying in front of a subject, shoulder and arm muscles are involved. However, before they become activated, the long spinal muscles contract and a shift in the pelvic position is made in order to shift the centre of gravity in advance of the arm movement. This type of anticipatory motor behaviour has obviously a developmental course. An infant sitting on his knees and reaching out for an object may very well drop on his nose, until he acquires the mechanisms of anticipatory postural adjustment. It seems very likely that the γ-system and probably also the reticular formation play a crucial role in these processes.

There is still another problem which seems to be relevant here. Several years ago Kupfmüller and Poklekowski (1956, *Ztschr. f. Naturforsch.* **11,** 1) and Vossius and Choudhry (1958, *Pflüger's Arch.* **268,** 75) carried out experiments on the control system of goal-directed voluntary movements. They found, when a subject rapidly points with a pen starting from a basepoint to a target area, 10–20 centimetres away from the basepoint but in the same plane, the course of the movement does not follow an ideal, linear control process. While in the first half of the movement, the speed is too high, and it is actually a ballistic movement, the approach to the target area is discontinuous. There are several pauses of 90–120 millisecond duration, during which the visual measurements of the hand position are taken, while the correction of deviations is carried out during each following movement. It can be described in terms of a sampled data control system, because it operates on data obtained at discrete intervals of time.

TWITCHELL: Those little jerks you spoke about when the subject is approaching the target; can they be eliminated by practice or by specific training?

PRECHTL: I do not think that was tried.

CONNOLLY: You would expect this to have the characteristics of a skilled response would you not? That in time practice will improve the performance so that the discontinuous nature of the movement as it approaches the target is reduced to some degree.

KAY: This experiment by Vossius and Choudhry is a curious one. Similar experiments have been done many times, although this particular narrative sounds more detailed than the kind of thing that Fitts was able to do with reciprocal dotting tasks. In one of my experiments (Kay 1961. In F. Geldard, *Defense Psychology*. Pergamon, London) we did investigate the effects of practice on a task very like this. Our principle interest was to investigate changes in information transmission and we found that with practice it was possible to double the transmission rate. Perhaps I should just say that we used serial-assembly tasks in which the subject was required to transfer, one at a time, a set of metal pins which were held in a row of holes. He had to transfer them to another row of target holes at varying distances from the start position. The size of the target hole, relative to the size of the pin, varied from one where the pin had a very snug fit to one having a very considerable tolerance.

HOWARD: I am interested in the effects of various perturbations on skilled performance. We train our subject to move to a target, which is a light, within a particular preset time. If the subject misses the target or does not manage to complete the response within the set time then a signal (buzzer) indicates this. The same applies, of course, if they respond too quickly. When the subjects are responding at the prescribed speed we examine the effects of perturbations on this type of response. In addition to accuracy, velocity and acceleration, we have looked at the effects of adding a weight, and in some cases of requiring that a particular pressure be made during the course of the response. The subject is inclined to throw his arms out at a certain speed, he programmes himself or at least he programmes the response, before he starts; to that extent it is a ballistic response. Perhaps I should add that I do not think there is a really sharp distinction between a ballistic response and a graded one. The usual description of a ballistic response is one which is programmed before it begins and one where there is no possibility of guidance during its execution, rather like a bullet out of a gun. The kind of response which I am concerned with here is one which is programmed before it is begun and also during the movement itself. I do not mean one which is changed as a function of stimulation from without but rather that the programming is still going on during its execution. One might call it a continuously programmed response rather than an initially programmed response.

PRECHTL: How do you know this?

HOWARD: Well, for the moment it is a theoretical distinction. What I am saying is that the response is guided as it is executed but not guided on the basis of changes in the external stimulation. Perhaps I should call it continuous programming and distinguish this from initial programming and also from error guidance. If one experimentally increases the amount of friction involved in movements such as those which I have described, then the subject moves his hand for a given duration of time, exactly as he would have done before the friction was introduced. The subject is doing what he has been trained to do but of course this does not get to the target, not with the increased friction. What I am planning to do is to study the ways in which subjects adapt to these perturbations which are imposed on a skilled movement which the individual has been trained to make. It is a little like the prismatic technique which Held and his collaborators have used. What I am aiming to do is distort the ordering of the limb control system by these various perturbations and then examine the adaption to them.

CONNOLLY: Considerations of this kind might help us to explain the continuous programming and increases in speed of response which are apparent in school-age children, children, that is, of 5 and upwards. Very simple target experiments which we have done with children of different ages (Connolly, Brown and Bassett, 1968, *Brit. J. Psychol.* **59,** 305) show that the characteristic change with age is one of speed with very little apparent increase in accuracy. Do you expect older children to be able to produce a more accurate initial programme or do you think they are able more quickly to correct their programme as they pick out the correct signals?

HOWARD: You might argue that children do not know the physical characteristics of their own limbs, and they first have to learn them. In addition to this they grow and they therefore change all the time; a man's limb is not like that of a child which is changing continuously for many years. It seems to me that the faster the movement and the more ballistic the limb movement the greater the need for accurate pre-programming, if the organism is going to be capable of any accurate intentional behaviour. This pre-programming must be a kind of cognitive map which a subject can use in order to tell the muscles just how they have to contract. I did an experiment which might help to answer the point here. I hung a weight on my arm and used as a skilled task a game of darts. I pre-spotted the target visually, closed my eyes and then threw the dart. In my own situation my aim fell just around the target. I had compensated for the weight. However, this is perhaps not a fair comparison because I was aware of the weight before I started to throw my dart and this may affect the programming. I could feel the weight and therefore had some strong resistance to this kind of perturbation before I began the response. An interesting question is, has a child? I do not know because I have not done the experiment with a child. How old are the children you used in your experiment, Connolly, because I would like to try with children of the same age?

CONNOLLY: I agree entirely, it would be most interesting. In our experiment we had three age groups, 6-, 8- and 10-year-olds.

BRUNER: I feel that these experiments are enormously exciting, in a sense you are introducing a motoric prism and asking questions about adaptation on the motor side. An approach of this kind has many possibilities because fundamentally you have introduced transformations into the motor system and then asked to what extent the subject can make compensatory adjustments. In my observations on young children I have been struck by how the head–eye system ties together. It is interesting how the child learns to handle his head, which is really quite a massive thing. Not only does he have to move it precisely but he has to gear into this system his eye movements so that they too are precise. Perhaps I can describe what typically happens if you hold a baby in a vertical position and watch the way in which he tracks an object moving across his visual field. The first thing that happens when the object moves (the critical distance is about 20° of visual arc and the speed approximately 35° per second) is that he starts off by a flinging response. Whenever the object passes a particular point, there is a lag and then the head is flung to where the object is. I do not think this is a ballistic response, in fact I am sure there is some programming along the way. Typically what happens is that the head moves then the eyes catch up as it were.

Later what happens is that instead of the head taking one big fling in the direction of the object it now moves in essentially a two-stage way. The head moves most of the way towards the object and then the eyes do the rest. It is quite obvious that the error is reduced by this technique, I am thinking here of a child aged about 2 months. What intrigues me about this is that every one of the systems of the body has to learn some way of dealing with transformations in terms of the motoric capacity which it has at that particular time. Consider the hand and arms, how does the child know the length of his arm when it is continually changing as he grows? Obviously there must be something built in, some extraordinary capacity for learning these transformations very quickly. I think the technique which Howard has been talking about may well provide a powerful approach to investigating how a child learns the rules of transformation in space.

KAY: I certainly agree with Bruner that this is an important approach. I think too that there is an everyday corollary of this sort of situation. I am thinking of the way in which we use tools. I can write my name with a very slim pencil; I can write it also, probably just as well, with a fat crayon. Changing the properties of a tool in a skilled situation may be analogous to loading the system in the way in which Howard talked about. The idea of studying manipulations with tools is something which we might follow much more closely in developmental studies. Also if we consider animals, where we have got too little developmental information, it does seem to me this approach could again be used to advantage.

HINDE: Perhaps I could offer an anecdote at this point. Last summer Dr. van Lawick-Goodall showed me a young chimpanzee learning how to fish termites out of a hole. They do it, as you probably know, by breaking off a grass stalk and putting the grass stalk into the hole. The termites then hang on to this and the chimpanzee pulls the grass out. The situation which I observed was of a baby sitting with its mother. The mother was very sophisticated in using this technique and got lots of termites out of the hole. If she failed to get the termites out she would either go and get a longer bit of grass, or just occasionally she would scratch away at the hole with her fingers to make the hole bigger so that she could get her grass stalk further in. The baby could see his mother scratching away at the hole and he could see that the mother was using a blade of grass which was about 6 inches long; the baby was using a bit of grass which was about 1 inch long and utterly ineffective. The baby worked away for about an hour without getting any termites at all and the only thing which he could do to try and improve his performance was to scratch away at the hole: it never seemed to "occur" to him to get a longer piece of grass. This was one thing he apparently could not cope with.

CONNOLLY: May I just say that I do not think the effects of perturbations in the system would be detectable only in very young children. I am sure that we have all worked with school-age children who have been making the graded responses which we have been talking about; any variation in the damping of the system from time to time which the experimenter introduced would, I am quite sure, affect the child's accuracy of response. Also, I suspect, it would take rather longer for younger children to appreciate this and make the appropriate corrections than it would for older children. Comparing, say, 5-year-old children with 10-year-old children, I am sure there would be a difference. This is not, of course, to deny that there are not certain basic parameters built in.

BRUNER: One experiment I should like to do very much is to look at the effects of adding a wrist weight to a child aged about 4 months. It would be possible to vary the weight of the loading as some ratio of the weight of the limb. What I would like to know is what happens to the initial reaching responses which the child shows. If they are correct from the beginning then a terrific capacity to compensate for the loading or the perturbations put on to the system must be available.

ABERCROMBIE: When Kay began this discussion he mentioned two things, helping people to learn skills new to them and preparing people for an unknown future, to learn skills we cannot predict. When he said this I pricked up my ears because this refers to the motto of our research unit, "educating for change". One of the problems which has emerged, and of course others have talked of it before, is this question of integration. We do not really know what is meant by this, but is it not just another way of saying that the skill emerges within a context—the context of the individual? Bernstein (1967, *The co-ordination and regulation of movement*. Pergamon, London) has pointed out that a person's handwriting, for instance, is characteristic, irrespective of the muscles involved. Kay said that he can write with a slim pencil or a fat crayon—his signature will be recognizable though he is deploying different muscles. Presumably the difficulty in training for skills reflects the difficulties of understanding these different associations. Now, as I found to my cost, it is impossible to relax the muscles of my neck unless I relax other muscles in my shoulders and back. Other individuals may have to pay attention to some other part of their body in order to relax their neck muscles. What I am driving at is that the linking of components which we have been talking about is something which is done in a very individualistic way. A person may make many idiosyncratic and variable adjustments which the experimenter or teacher did not know about.

KAY: I think that is a very fair point. I wonder if I can stimulate some discussion on this by taking dart throwing as an example. The problem which intrigues me is, why shouldn't I be able to repeat exactly an action which I have just performed. I grasp a dart, I throw it at the board and all I want to do is exactly the same thing next time, with the same dart if necessary. Funnily enough, this is one of the things which is most difficult to do and yet at the same time it will have about it the particular features of that individual which make it easily recognizable. At this level the business of linking seems to me to be one of identifying the input, certainly identifying the precise transformation and programming the same muscle movement. I would guess that the difficulties of repeating that movement are on the output side of the block diagram I drew. It may relate also to certain neurophysiological properties inherent in the system.

PRECHTL: If you said "Ah" five times and I pick it up on a sound spectrograph, each of the five utterances would appear to be different.

HEFFERLINE: In repeating over and over again what may be a very fine movement, one does not necessarily use the same motor units in the successive instances. In my laboratory when, by means of visual or auditory feedback, we train a person to control the firing of a single motor unit, this is, from the neurophysiological point of view, not an ultimate simplification of motor activity, but a most complex performance, requiring not only facilitation of the required motor unit but also suppression of unwanted ones. Because so subtly balanced, it is of course, unstable. I may have a subject who reliably and repeatedly fires a particular motor unit, starting and stopping it upon command, and who then suddenly loses it. How can he find it again? Well, one thing that seems pretty effective is to tell him to try to remember just how its waveform looked when he saw it on the oscilloscope or perhaps heard it over a speaker. This may bring it back and put him in direct control of it again. If a practiced subject momentarily loses his motor unit, he recovers it very quickly. In one way or another he seems somehow to know where to go and hunt for it.

In skilled movements there is a certain substitutability of effectors, all the way from motor units to whole muscles. If we revert to Kay's example of dart-throwing and analyse the sub-skills involved in it, we see it as an immensely complicated set of more or less equivalent motor patterns, with overlap but not complete identity of components. Perhaps it is not so much surprising that a movement may be performed in many different ways, as it is that we come to do something which is so similar to what we did last time.

TWITCHELL: How similar do you want these movements to be, do you want them to be identical?

KAY: We often say that certain behaviours are identical, but of course this is not true. We know this in the case of something like singing where we can analyse the note (as in Prechtl's sound spectrograph). The notes sound the same but we can demonstrate differences. I was interested in those cases where the individual fails to repeat a response within the defined error of the task. Throwing a dart into the same number would be an example.

HINDE: May I go back to the simple block diagram which was drawn on the board at the beginning of the discussion and ask where the feedback control loops come in.

KAY: Let me first say that my simple diagram was just the bare bones of a model. One could lay out a multiplicity of models to fit particular cases and they would differ from one another in certain respects. In the tracking task there would be external discrepancies between the target itself and the signal which the subject was producing. What I mean by internal signals, speaking now as a psychologist, are the unidentified proprioceptive, kinaesthetic, and tactile stimuli.

In one of his experiments Connolly required a child to pick up an object, a small pin in fact, and place it in a hole. There are a number of interesting things about this experiment. It transpired that it was really rather difficult for the child to release the pin once he had put it in the hole, difficult that is as compared with an adult's performance. Performing a task such as this a child has feedback from his own movements, these are the internal signals which I spoke of, and he will also be able to compare his limb position to the target hole, so he also gets visual feedback. As is the case with so many of these experiments, the aim is to simplify the situation to one which can be adequately handled with the concepts and the equipment available to us. Partly for this reason and partly because I think the development of skill may be particularly rewarding I should like to look more carefully at phenomena such as this in children of different ages. If there are changes in the nature of the internal signals and the ease with which they can be identified it seems to me quite possible that the cognitive strategies which the child brings to bear in carrying out a simple task such as this may very well change substantially and so effect his performance considerably. Fundamentally what I am saying is that we should carry out a detailed and precise analysis of the components of the task. We should if you like look in great detail at the sub-skills which go to make up a whole response.

BRUNER: I agree entirely with this, I do not think that the right hypotheses are just going to jump into our heads, but I do think they may suggest themselves from a much closer look at what the child is actually doing. In fact, the capacity to pause at the right time may be just the thing which will swing a child from one stage to the next. Another example is the relationship between the power grip and the precision grip during development. I think the child must be able to pause as it were between the two in order to grasp something firmly and yet still make fine manipulations. The best example which comes to mind is Connolly's story about his daughter who said, I'll talk to you later as soon as I have put down this tray of glasses. I immediately thought of a situation where I might respond in just the same way as that little girl; when I am in a workshop and I have got the solder on the heated iron and I am just about to begin when someone comes into the shop and wants to talk to me. I do not think this is any different at all. What it is, is that there is a great big assembly going on, an assembly of parts before the execution of a task, and one simply cannot tie this up whilst there are lots of loose ends trailing.

Cognitive Factors in Skill Development

Sensory, Perceptual and Cognitive Factors in the Development of Voluntary Actions

ARTHUR LEFFORD

Yeshiva University, New York

THIS PAPER PRESENTS some findings on the psychological development of the child as reflected in the development of his ability to make differentiated voluntary movements. Evidence will be advanced for the thesis that motor development, at least in some of its skilled aspects, is dependent on prior sensory, perceptual and cognitive developments.

In this study two types of voluntary action, involving the identification of the fingers of the hand as the goal of the action, were observed. The first was a finger–thumb opposition movement: a movement of the thumb and a designated finger of the hand towards each other until they were opposed. The second action studied was a pointing movement indicating fingers designated to the subject by the experimenter.

I. METHODS

The responses of the children were observed as they were demanded under the varying experimental conditions. Firstly, the subjects were required to imitate a finger–thumb opposition movement demonstrated by the examiner's hand. The children could visually regard their own hand under one condition but not under another while attempting to imitate the movement. Secondly, the terminal loci of the movements, the fingers of the hand, were indicated to the subject visually by the examiner pointing to the fingers of the subject's hand. Thirdly, the fingers of the hand were designated to the subject tactually and kinaesthetically by heavily touching the subject's fingers outside his field of vision. While performing the finger–thumb opposition movement the subject was permitted under one condition to see his hand but not under another. Fourthly, the fingers of the hand to be identified were indicated to the subject by the examiner simultaneously heavily touching and pointing to the fingers. Both visual and tactual-kinaesthetic modalities were thus utilized in indicating the terminal loci of the localizing movements. Finally, there were two kinds of pointing responses made by the subjects: pointing to the fingers on their own hand, and pointing to the fingers on a schematic drawing of the hand. In the former response the subject pointed directly to the fingers designated by the examiner. In the latter response the fingers to be identified are designated on the subject's hand, but the subject points to the corresponding fingers on the drawing of the hand.

These variations made up a battery of 12 tests which were administered to each child twice. To compensate for practice effects, the second examination was administered in reverse order. The subjects were nursery and kindergarten children ranging in age from 3 to 6 years. There was a total of 167 subjects, approximately 30 in each half-year interval except in the earliest age group in which there were 15.

The various tasks are indicated in the text by a combination of symbols indicating the sense modalities through which the fingers to be identified were designated to the subjects, and the movements made by the subjects in identifying the fingers. Visual designation of the fingers, tactual and kinaesthetic designation, and simultaneous visual and tactual-kinaesthetic designation are denoted by the letters V, TK, and VT respectively. The finger–thumb opposition movement is represented by the letters FTO; the subject pointing to his own hand is denoted by SELF; and the subject pointing to the drawing of the hand is denoted by MODEL. Responses made outside the subject's field of sight are noted by the sign (nv). The sign "Imit" stands for the imitative FTO responses. A tabulated description of the tasks is given in Table I.

II. FINDINGS

Perhaps the simplest way to present the data is to compare the order of difficulty of the various tasks with age-specific order of development. This can be done by comparing the percentage of subjects who succeeded at making the movement at each age interval. The results presented in Table II show the percentage of subjects who succeeded at the various tasks. A child was considered to have passed on a task when he succeeded in identifying all the fingers of the hand correctly by making the required movement at least once in the two trials given to him.

TABLE I. DESCRIPTION OF EXAMINATION TASKS PRESENTED TO THE SUBJECTS (FTO, FINGER–THUMB OPPOSITION)

Examination task (nomenclature)	Modality in which fingers were indicated to subject	Response required of the subject	Modalities available to guide response
Visual imitation	Visual	Finger–thumb opposition	Visual, proprioceptive
Non-visual	Visual	,,	Proprioceptive
Visual tactual FTO	Visual, tactual-kinaesthetic	,,	Visual, proprioceptive
Visual FTO	Visual	,,	Visual, proprioceptive
Tactual-kinaesthetic FTO	Tactual-kinaesthetic	,,	Visual, proprioceptive
Tactual-kinaesthetic non-visual FTO	Tactual-kinaesthetic	,,	Proprioceptive
Visual tactual on self	Visual, tactual-kinaesthetic	Pointing to self	Visual, proprioceptive
Visual on self	Visual	,,	Visual, proprioceptive
Tactual-kinaesthetic on self	Tactual-kinaesthetic	,,	Visual, proprioceptive
Visual tactual on model	Visual, tactual-kinaesthetic	Pointing to model	Vision
Visual on model	Visual	,,	Vision
Tactual-kinaesthetic on model	Tactual-kinaesthetic	,,	Vision

TABLE II. PERCENTAGE OF SUBJECTS MAKING THE CORRECT MOVEMENTS IDENTIFYING THE FINGERS OF THE HAND

Task		Age interval (years)					
	All	3	$3\frac{1}{2}$	4	$4\frac{1}{2}$	5	$5\frac{1}{2}$
(1) VT FTO	95	73	90	93	97	100	100
(2) VT SELF	90	60	81	97	94	100	100
(3) V SELF	88	40	74	97	100	100	100
(4) V FTO	87	60	74	97	83	97	100
(5) TK(nv)FTO	83	40	65	90	94	94	96
(6) TK FTO	81	53	52	90	89	90	96
(7) TK SELF	57	13	36	57	69	60	92
(8) V Imit	57	40	36	50	57	74	84
(9) V Model	56	0	29	57	57	74	96
(10) VT Model	50	0	23	40	49	71	100
(11) V(nv)Imit	45	13	32	33	43	45	80
(12) TK Model	32	0	16	33	23	52	56
N	167	15	31	35	30	31	25

The tasks in Table II are arranged in increasing order of difficulty and indicate the percentage of all subjects succeeding at the task.

The tasks presenting the least difficulty to the children were those involving finger–thumb opposition movements and pointing to the self where the terminal loci of the actions, i.e., the fingers to be identified, were indicated visually and visual-tactually. No statistically significant differences were found in the distribution of subjects succeeding at the finger–thumb opposition and "pointing to the self" movements when the visual modality and conjoint visual-tactual modalites were used to designate the fingers to the subject. Over 95 per cent of the subjects succeeded at these tasks by the age of 4 years. Even by $3\frac{1}{2}$ years over three-quarters of the subjects succeeded at the tasks.

All of these tasks were found to be significantly less difficult than pointing to the fingers on the model. Why this should be the case is not immediately apparent since the movements themselves are not very different. Actually, it feels more awkward to point with the non-preferred hand than with the preferred hand. This problem will be considered again.

Next in order of difficulty are the finger–thumb opposition tasks in which the terminal loci of the actions have been indicated by tactual-kinaesthetic stimulation. The TK FTO and TK (nv) FTO tasks are not significantly different from the V FTO and V Self tasks. They are, however, significantly different from the VT FTO and VT Self tasks at the third year level. Until the fourth year, the removal of visual cues makes these tasks significantly more difficult, that is, few subjects succeed in making the correct response. By the fourth year there are no significant differences among these tasks; over 90 per cent of the children succeed at them.

The TK Self task is considerably and significantly more difficult than the TK FTO tasks. This is interesting in view of the finding that the V Self and V FTO, and the VT Self and VT FTO tasks are not significantly different. The TK Self task does not appear to follow a similar trend. Considerably fewer subjects succeeded on this task: whereas over 80 per cent of all subjects succeeded at the former tasks, only 57 per cent succeeded on the TK Self task. It is not until the subjects are older than $5\frac{1}{2}$ years that 90 per cent succeed on the TK Self task. This considerable difference in difficulty between the visual and the tactual-kinaesthetic pointing to Self tasks also requires consideration. Such a difference was not found in the FTO movement.

Finally, the most difficult tasks in the battery were those which involved imitating the FTO movements and pointing to the schematic drawing (the model of the hand). There was no significant difference in the number of subjects passing the Visual Model task. The Visual Imitation task was also found not to be significantly different from the Visual (nv) Imitation task. However, at the third- and fourth-year intervals the Chi Square values approached very close to the 5 per cent level of significance. The Non-Visual Imitation task, in which the subject could not see his hand while making the finger–thumb opposition movement and the Tactual on Model tasks were the two most difficult tasks in the battery. While these tasks were significantly different at the third-year level, they were not found to be significantly different beyond the fourth year. The Imitation and pointing to the Model tasks proved to be difficult for the children, and it is not until they are older than $5\frac{1}{2}$ years that more than 80 per cent of them succeed on tasks where the visual modality is used to indicate the fingers. Where heavy touch was used to indicate the fingers, only about half of the oldest children were able to succeed at the task requiring them to identify the fingers on the model by a pointing movement.

Data are available on the course of development for each finger, the detailed treatment of which is voluminous, but not necessary for a discussion of some of the major points.

III. DISCUSSION OF RESULTS

I should like to consider the effect of utilizing different sensory modalities on the effectiveness of the response. For reasons that will become apparent later, the most appropriate comparisons to make in considering the effects of vision and heavy touch are among the finger–thumb opposition tests. The relevant data are found on lines (1), (4), and (6) of Table II. Since the number of subjects within the 6-month age interval at the youngest age level was small, it was necessary for us to study statistically the year intervals. This did some injustice to the developmental characteristics of the data. Using a Chi-Square for correlated proportions test, we found no statistically significant difference between the number of subjects who could correctly oppose each of the fingers indicated to them visually or tactual-kinaesthetically; although only 53 per cent and 52 per cent succeeded at the TK FTO task, and 60 per cent and 70 per cent succeeded at the V FTO task at the 3 and $3\frac{1}{2}$ year age intervals respectively. Both of these tasks were statistically different from the VT FTO task at which 73 per cent and 90 per cent of the subjects at the respective age intervals succeeded. Of the 46 subjects between the ages of 3 and 4 years, only 25 succeeded on the TK FTO task, 32 succeeded on the V FTO task, and 40 succeeded on the VT FTO task. These findings suggest that visual indication tends to be better than heavy touch, and indicates that the addition of vision to heavy touch markedly increases the number of subjects who succeed at the FTO task. It increases the number who succeed beyond what would be expected from the use of vision alone. A possible explanation for this reaction is that the tactual-kinaesthetic stimulation acts so as to mobilize a general orienting response which enhances the effectiveness of the visual stimulation.

These data also have a bearing on the development of the body schema, as first formulated by Henry Head (1920). The FTO response may be considered as an indicator of the child's ability to discriminate among the fingers. The development of this ability is a sign of the development of a body schema. From this point of view the findings reflect the development of visual and tactual-kinaesthetic discrimination of the topography of the hand, reflecting the development of hand and finger body schemata. The data indicate that the topography of the hand and fingers appears to be equally differentiated when visually perceived and when tactual-kinaesthetically perceived. By 4 years of age over 90 per cent of the subjects have fully differentiated hand–finger schemata when perceived in both the visual and tactual-kinaesthetic sensory modes. There is some suggestion from the data that for the younger 3-year-olds visual schemata may be more advanced in development than proprioceptive schemata. I do not know of any other study on children as young as 3 years that concerns itself with the age at which visual and tactual-kinaesthetic schemata of hand and finger topography are established that would affirm or contradict these findings.

I should like next to direct attention to the integration of these sensory schemata of the body topography. Although the data presented offer some evidence for the independent development of visual and tactual-kinaesthetic schemata of the hand and fingers, it is not definitive. Further examination of another aspect of the data suggests more strongly that these schemata are not initially integrated or co-ordinated but only become so in the course of development.

Consider the processes that may be involved in the successful execution of the TK Self task. In this task, the subject localizes his fingers by pointing to the fingers indicated to him by a heavy touch outside his field of vision. The subject responds by pointing to the touched fingers with his contralateral hand. This response movement is guided by his vision. The subject sees the fingers indicated to him by touch and guides his own pointing finger to them visually. This task, therefore, demands that the information conveyed to the subject tactual-kinaesthetically be translated to the visual modality which guides the localizing movement. For this task to be performed correctly it is necessary for the subject to have established some kind of equivalence between the visual and tactual-kinaesthetic body schemata. We believe that the establishment of intersensory integration of the visual and tactual hand schemata may be inferred from success on the TK on Self task. If this is so, then the findings, presented on line (7) in Table II, indicate that it is not until subjects are older than $5\frac{1}{2}$ years that more than 90 per cent of them have developed an integration between the visual and the tactual topography of the hands and fingers. At all age intervals, significantly fewer subjects succeeded at the TK on Self task than at the V FTO, VT FTO, and V on Self tasks. By the first half of the fourth year over 90 per cent of the subjects showed evidence of an intrasensory differentiation of the body topography, but intersensory integration in 90 per cent of the subjects is not evident until they are older than $6\frac{1}{2}$ years. These findings extend an earlier study of intersensory integration into the preschool years (Birch and Lefford, 1967).

There is little in the data to support an hypothesis of an initial synaesthesia from which the individual senses develop. On the contrary the data would seem to support the obverse: that the senses are initially unrelated and that integration is a developmental task. In terms of relevance to the development of motor responses, it must be evident that when the execution of a movement or an action depends on the translation of information from one sensory modality to another, the action cannot be effected until an equivalence between the schemata in the different sensory domains is established. This integration appears to be dependent upon a prior intrasensory differentiation and subsequent integration. When a movement requires precision or skill, the success of that movement depends upon the prior differentiation of the space in which and to which that movement is directed. Earlier we saw that a successful movement on to a specific body part requires a differentiation of the topography of that body part in the sense modality which establishes the goal of the action. This suggests that a skilled or precise action could be defined by the intrasensory differentiations and intersensory integrations upon which it is dependent.

IV. SYMBOLIC REPRESENTATION IN SKILLED MOVEMENT

To recapitulate, so far we have demonstrated with our findings the dependence of skilled movements on intrasensory differentiations and intersensory integration. I would like now to discuss the implications of these findings for the importance of symbolic representations in the ability to make a skilled movement. On the Visual Imitation task the subject had to imitate a FTO movement demonstrated on the examiner's hand. On the Visual on Model and VT on Model tasks the subject was required to point to a schematic drawing of the fingers corresponding to those fingers indicated on his hands. Although the movements involved in these two tasks differ, one involves a pointing movement and the other a finger-thumb opposition movement, the factor they have in common is that the terminal loci of the movements are indicated *indirectly*, and not directly as in previous tasks. That is, the fingers to be opposed, or to which the subject must point, are indicated in a manner requiring the subject to transpose, translate, or displace the information from one object or place to another. In effect, he points to or moves an equivalent or corresponding member, not that which was directly indicated. To succeed at these tasks the subject must not only differentiate that part of his body, but he must understand that the part indicated to him only *represents* the part he must move or indicate. Success at these tasks indicates his capacity to understand such correspondences, representations, or equivalences. This, in effect, demonstrates whether the child can function symbolically with the hand and fingers.

If we compare two FTO tasks involving only the visual modality, the Visual FTO task (line 4, Table II) and the Visual Imitation task (line 8, Table II) we find that the Visual Imitation task is considerably more difficult at every age level. This difference may be attributed to the lack of symbolic or representative comprehension by the subjects who did not succeed at the task. For example, by the 4-year age level 97 per cent of the subjects can visually differentiate their fingers and make the finger-thumb opposition movement; however, only 50 per cent can imitate the demonstrated FTO movement. They fail, I believe, because they lack the ability to establish a correspondence between the fingers on the examiner's hand and their own hand. They lack comprehension of the symbolic equivalence in this respect.

Once the child has grasped the representation or equivalence involved in the imitation task, he can also point to the fingers on the drawings of the hand. When we compared the results of the Visual Imitation task (line 8, Table II) with the results of the Visual on Model task (line 9, Table II) we see a close parallel after the $3\frac{1}{2}$-year age level in the percentage of subjects passing on both tasks. No significant differences were found at any age level. At the third and fourth years, 65 per cent of the subjects succeeded or failed jointly on both tasks, and by the fifth year, 80 per cent responded the same way on either task. This strongly suggests that when the ability for representation operates on one task it also operates on the other task.

To recapitulate, three factors appear to determine the capacity to make successfully the movements studied. They are: the differentiation of the sensory space involved; the co-ordination of the sensory schemata of the different modalities involved in the task; and the capacity to comprehend symbolic representation when it is involved in the task.

The final group of tasks involved the successful integration of these three mechanisms. The Non-Visual Imitation task not only demands that the subject comprehend the correspondence between the examiner's fingers and his own, but that this visually obtained information be translated into proprioceptive schemata which guide the movement of the fingers when they are not seen. This is a difficult task and, until the subjects are older than $5\frac{1}{2}$ years, less than half can perform the task (line 11, Table II). The TK on Model is the most difficult task in the battery. Only 56 per cent of the oldest subjects, $5\frac{1}{2}$ to 6 years of age, succeed at this task, which involves the intersensory translation of information from a tactual-kinaesthetic schema to a visual schema, and the transposition of this information to the corresponding or equivalent representative fingers on the drawing of the hand. Apparently this is not a simple task for a 5-year-old.

Success in making the differential movements required by our tasks appears to depend upon four factors:

(i) The development and differentiation of sensory body schemata relevant to the movement.
(ii) The integration of the separate sensory schemata into a schema of the body part which co-ordinates the separate sensory schemata, thus establishing equivalences among the sensory modalities.
(iii) The development of the symbolic mode when the movement involves indirect representation of the action as in imitation, or indirect representation of the goal of the action.
(iv) The integration and synthesis of all of these processes when required for successful execution of the movement or action.

V. CONCLUSIONS

Finally I should like briefly to relate aspects of these findings to some of Piaget's observations on the development of ordination; to Gerstmann's observations on the neuropathology of the hand; to

Hughling Jackson's theories about the nervous system, and Henry Head's notion of the body schema.

In his studies on the genesis of the concept of number, Piaget (1953) demonstrated that the child must first learn to establish a correspondence between sets of discontinuous items. The ability to establish such a correspondence, independent of the arrangement of the items in visual space, represents an important advance in the child's mental development called conservation of number.

What has this to do with the findings reported? Let us again consider the operations which are involved in making a correct response to the Imitation and Pointing to the Model tasks. As has been shown, the successful completion of the action necessitates the establishment of a correct correspondence of the items in two series; between the fingers on the subject and those on the examiner or on the model. This correspondence can take place only on the basis of some aspect of order or seriation. The fingers could be identified on the basis of middleness, leftness, rightness, third from the thumb, or second from the little finger. If the fingers are identified on the basis of length or size, longer, thicker, bigger, etc., then the child must have the capacity to judge proportions and relationships among proportions, since his fingers and those on the examiner and the model are not the same. It appears that success at the Imitation and Pointing to the Model tasks involves an operation of seriation, the development of a notion of positional ordination among the fingers. Between 75 and 96 per cent of the children ranging in age from 5 years to 6 years were successful at these tasks. This seems to indicate seriation between objects, the fingers, and the beginning of the notion of order. It also appears to take us close to the idea of number since number involves collection of equal elements, which are at the same time an ordered series. Success on the tasks involves at least the beginning of an ordered series in space.

Gerstmann (1957, 1958) reported on a number of observations on finger agnosia, and on the basis of these argued that concomitant with finger agnosia were disorders of finger movement, agraphia, and the cognitive disorders of acalculia and right–left disorientation. The pathology of spatial orientation along with difficulties with numbers and finger movements appeared to him to be clinically related. Gerstmann regarded these symptoms as a reflection of the dissolution of body schemata. However, Stengel (1944) explained the phenomena in terms of a loss of the organization of spatial directionality and spatial relationship. Studies by Benton and Seymour (1951), Benton (1955) and Kingsbourne and Warrington (1963) on the development of finger localization further suggest some relationship between this and certain pathological conditions.

The results reported above demonstrate some connection between the imitation of differential finger movements and the ordering of space. The ordering of space underlies left–right orientation, finger location movements, the notion of number and the naming of the fingers. When the schemata of finger-ordering are impaired or destroyed by insult to the central nervous system it seems reasonable to expect pathology of experience and behaviour which is grounded in such ordering schemata generally. It may be that this is flying too far from the concrete findings; it may be too speculative. Yet it would appear that the loss of ordering schemata, by an insult to the nervous system, results in a loss of those functions which are dependent on such schemata. If this is so, then one might expect that with the loss of the ordering schemata related to the fingers there would be right–left disorientation, acalculia (since numbers are based on ordering) and agraphia (since writing is ordered movement in space). With ordering gone those functions which depend on ordering are also lost.

If this analysis is correct, the study has established a connection between developmental psychology, and neuropathology. The findings reported above reflect the development of a body schema of the fingers and a schema of spatial ordering whilst Gerstmann's observations reflect the dissolution of such schemata. The results also provide evidence for Hughling Jackson's (1887) hypotheses on the relationship between the evolution of the functions of the nervous system and the dissolution of these functions in certain neuropathological states.

I have chosen to interpret the data on finger–thumb opposition as reflecting the development of visual and tactual-kinaesthetic schemata of the topography of the hand. For this notion I am of course indebted to Henry Head (1920) who first postulated the concept of body schemata in explaining the ability of persons to localize their body parts. Although it is assumed that body schemata are the result of a maturational process, the results explicate the concept from a developmental point of view.

REFERENCES

BENTON, A. L. 1955. Development of finger localization capacity in school children. *Child Developm.* **26,** 225–230.

BENTON, A. L. and SEYMOUR, E. 1951. Arithmetic ability, finger-localization capacity and right–left discrimination in normal and defective children. *Amer. J. Orthopsychiat.* **21,** 756–766.

BIRCH, H. G. and LEFFORD, A. 1967. Visual integration, intersensory integration and voluntary motor control. *Monog. Soc. Res. Child Develop.* **32,** 110.
GERSTMANN, J. 1957. Some notes on Gerstmann's syndrome. *Neurology* **7,** 866–869.
GERSTMANN, J. 1958. Psychological and phenomenological aspects of disorders of the body image. *J. nerv. ment. Dis.* **126,** 499–512.
HEAD, H. 1920. *Studies in neurology.* Vol. 2. Hodder and Stoughton, London.
JACKSON, H. 1887. Remarks on evolution and dissolution of the nervous system. *J. ment. Sci.* **33,** 25–48.
KINSBOURNE, M. and WARRINGTON, E. K. 1963. The development of finger differentiation. *Quart. J. exp. Psychol.* **15,** 132–137.
PIAGET, J. 1953. How children form mathematical concepts. *Sci. Amer.* **189,** 74–79.
STENGEL, E. 1944. Loss of spatial orientation, constructional apraxia, and Gerstmann's syndrome. *J. ment. Sci.* **90,** 753–760.

Discussion

PRECHTL: May I ask a rather technical question? What was the hand position of the child in the test? Have you standardized the background muscle contraction? The reason I ask is this; pointing to your thumb is very difficult if your hand is relaxed and your eyes closed. As soon as you contract your hand and move it even a little bit you come near to pointing to your thumb.

LEFFORD: Ours was essentially a clinical procedure and we really didn't develop great precision. The hand was either on the desk where the child was sitting, or the child's hand was supported by the examiner's hand. I can report of the children I examined, that when we touched the child rather heavily we immediately felt the resistance coming back. This may partly answer your question; there was a great deal of resistance; the hand wasn't flaccid.

TWITCHELL: In the case of the 3-year-old children who do the serial oppositions, are they required to do them in order?

LEFFORD: One of the experiments on the Kuhlman–Anderson test requires the child simply to be able to oppose the fingers in order from left to right or right to left. We did not observe whether the child followed the order demonstrated by the examiner. On the basis of previous tests which we have done I think they could do it in either order. A small number of some of the youngest children we examined, two or three out of a hundred, seemed to know what was required of them—they knew that they had to oppose their fingers but they were unable to do it. What they did, inventively, was to grab that finger with their other hand and bring it up to the thumb; it would seem as if they were suffering from some sort of motor disability, which they weren't; these were normal children.

INGRAM: Kinsbourne and Warrington (1963, *Quart. J. exp. Psychol.*, **15,** 132) report this in their dyslexic group, don't they?

LEFFORD: In the terms of the work which they report, we have reduced the age limit well below their age limit.

INGRAM: This introduces another question. These are presumably chronological ages and I would like to know more about your sample therefore; I should also be interested if you would do this on a large group of mentally retarded children.

LEFFORD: Well, I think you would find differences. We used day nursery children, who usually came from upper middle class backgrounds. We had one day nursery in the north-east Bronx which was a day nursery for working mothers, this presumably put them in the lower middle or lower class sociological grouping. We did not separate out those data, but it was my impression that there seemed to be some slowness in development in this group. We are currently repeating a number of these examinations with children who are known to be neurologically impaired. From the preliminary data, which we have obtained to date, it seems to be quite a sensitive test.

TWITCHELL: Have you tried providing tactile/kinaesthetic cues on a graded scale? For example, by giving more pressure, or in moving the stimulus on the finger, or wrapping up the whole finger?

LEFFORD: No. We used heavy touch—to eliminate any differences which may come from differences in pressure sensitivity. I cannot say that it was just tactile stimulation; it was both kinaesthetic and tactile stimulation.

INGRAM: You may even be using muscle stretch in fact.

LEFFORD: Yes, I am aware of that.

CONNOLLY: I wonder if you could pull out these differences, which look as if they are probably there, by imposing some memory constraint on the situation. Let us suppose that instead of immediately requiring the child to point to the finger which you have touched you impose a delay between the stimulus and his response. I am not sure what order of delay you would impose (perhaps 30 seconds), however, this is an empirical question. I wonder whether this may pull the differences out more clearly?

LEFFORD: I hadn't thought of that, you may be right. But I wonder if it would not in a sense complicate the interpretation of the findings in terms of getting into memory trace and decay and such like things.

WHITE: You are already in trouble by the use of verbal instructions with 3-year-olds. I think when you start complicating the situation in terms of response requirements it means you are jeopardizing the validity of the findings.

CONNOLLY: The memory span of very young children may be rather less than ours but young children do remember. You could perhaps make it into a game. I am impressed by how much you can do with very young children if you ask them the right questions. It would be interesting to try and stretch these things a bit further. Just how far can you push it?

LEFFORD: In considering this I was also thinking of your work, because I do not think that the finger–thumb opposition movements demanded simply start *de novo*. There is really a background of the child's total experience with grasping and picking up objects, in which the movement is embedded in other activities.

BRUNER: That is what I was musing about, because I suppose you could make a perfectly good argument that there is a quite well worked out schema present in action. I have in mind an example in terms of the schema, the principle of substitutability in that procedure that we used in studying the development of the precision grip. We had a bead on the top of a little plastic refrigerator box; in some versions of the test we have the bead closer to the edge because we are interested to find out the way in which the child, when holding on with two hands, will detach a finger to reach for this object. What we have discovered is that the child will detach any finger, that is, any one that is close to the object.

LEFFORD: We find the same thing when the child has a "Band-Aid" on his finger, he will sometimes use the other finger for a fine movement, to pick something up.

BRUNER: In so far as there is substitutability in some sense, there is a pretty good schema for action. Here what the child has to do is to turn around on that schema and index it by pointing or by arbitrarily moving his thumb. It seems to me that you are working here on the problem, among other things, of abstraction of the schema for the guidance of an arbitrary indexing operation.

LEFFORD: Well, to get back to the original movement, where the child can oppose, the movement is there. He can oppose successively and serially, it is done to all the fingers, but he cannot do it differentially. What I have described here is really in a sense normative. I would like to know what happens in between the point of this pattern of sequential reaction and the point where the child can go directly to the finger indicated. What happens between these stages?

INGRAM: Luria (1966, *Human brain and psychological processes.*

Harper and Row, London) of course reports this in his book on the brain-damaged adult.

LEFFORD: That they can make the pattern?

INGRAM: That they can do it and that they cannot do it; they cannot do it to instruction, but they are physically able to do it.

TWITCHELL: That is apraxia.

INGRAM: It is a type of apraxia.

LEFFORD: You have many other analogues in a brain-damaged patient, like reciting a list of the days of the week or the month. They can recite the list, but cannot say what comes after Wednesday?

HINDE: My question may be naïve because it comes from an outsider, but I understand that it is an aid to communication between us to talk about a Head type schema. When you talk about 50 per cent or 90 per cent of children having this schema it seems to me that you are reifying it in a way which goes perhaps a bit beyond the needs of communication. What I want to ask is—what exactly does this concept of schema imply, if anything? What predictions does it lead to? Is this a fair question?

LEFFORD: I suppose what I mean is some organization in the nervous system which organizes incoming stimuli. This is strictly an inference or a hypothetical construct that I am using in a sense to explain the data. I have given you the data, and one way in which one could possibly look at it and perhaps think about it is in terms of the Head type schema. Is this a fair answer?

HINDE: Does it permit you to make a prediction outside the immediate context of these experiments, which is different from saying that the subject can transpose from this modality to that?

LEFFORD: The transposition from one modality to another isn't appropriate to the Head schema.

HINDE: Well no, or any of the other sorts of language which you used to describe your experiments.

INGRAM: I don't think we should worry too much about this; Lefford is testing what he is testing.

BRUNER: That may well be all right from the point of view of doing a diagnosis, but from the point of view of trying to understand motor behaviour with language there is trouble. As I understand it, what Hinde is worried about is that you can introduce the notion of a schema so that a schema hypothesized on a set of data can now guide motor behaviour. Or are you not talking about the very thing which you inferred from the motor behaviour and which you are now having guide itself?

INGRAM: I am implying exactly the same—it may worry him or you but it doesn't worry me. I would use this for a different purpose and what excites me about it is that, in the same way that some of the Ozeretsky tests and some of Fog's tests are very valuable, it may be a useful clinical tool.
BRUNER: Valuable for what?
INGRAM: For diagnosing neurological immaturity in older children.
CONNOLLY: They are notoriously unreliable, because they have no meaning in terms of what reliability or validity you can give to them.
INGRAM: I agree, but they are still useful in clinical terms.
BRUNER: Well, that is because you have a very specific job to do, and everybody respects that job. You really have to make a diagnosis as to whether you have got a sick child. But now comes the question which always emerges in a group of this sort, where you have got mixed purposes. To what extent have you diagnostic requirements and to what extent have you requirements of explanation (or I will even say "explication" to make it not so strong)? Do these serve the same purpose? We will have to face that one.
INGRAM: Well I would very much like to see this test standardized.
BRUNER: Why? This is exactly what I would not like to see.
INGRAM: I would like to see the Ozeretsky test standardized, and I would like to see more work on the standardization of the Fog tests.
BRUNER: But why would you like to see this standardization?
INGRAM: Because I could then use them more in the way that a psychologist uses his tests. For example, the Wechsler–Bellevue test.
BRUNER: One could make a very good claim that the standardization of the Wechsler–Bellevue did more to set back the study of intelligence than any single thing that has ever happened in the history of cognitive processes.
HINDE: I was not attacking the notion of schema but I felt that if it was going to help us to understand what was going on then we ought to be able to take it one stage further and say "What is this concept doing?"
KAY: As I understand it, Hinde is challenging us to answer the question, Is this anything more than a description of the working efficiency of the translation process, to which you were giving certain percentages in the data which you presented? This is a good point. In a sense we might try and make it as extreme as possible by saying, "We are studying here the intellectualization of motor skills, the degree of cognitive function that is required in the different forms of processing." Suppose we begin with the motor skill which the subjects can do, and which you can demonstrate at one level. If now we add a number of translations to it

the question is whether a subject can still manipulate the schema. We have a fair amount of data showing that practice does in fact increase this manipulation. For example, we can manipulate the first few letters of the alphabet, ABC, more easily than we can manipulate some of the later ones, presumably because we practise them more. Our concept of them, our schema of them, allows us to manipulate in this way. Now I suspect in the case of the children who can make the appositions but who cannot make the selections, that it is so unpractised that they cannot distinguish between the different components which make up the schema under novel or adverse conditions.

LEFFORD: I can give you some anecdotal observations in terms of the practice effect. We did have a first and a second trial though this is obscured in our data because the child who failed on the first trial and did it on the second was counted as succeeding. It may therefore be that there was a one-trial learning effect. I myself observed one child who didn't do very well; when I came back to work with the other children a few days later, he was somewhere in the nursery, off in a corner, practising the movements. I don't know how much practice is involved but apparently children seem to respond to this sort of thing as something which could be practised.

KAY: Like Connolly (page 219), I would be fascinated to try and tease out some of these problems. Assuming your particular apposition was fairly complex, suppose we took a very much simpler action such as tactile stimulation of that finger. The finger is tickled, or stimulated in some way, and then we get a subject to try and transpose this on to some point. Here the actual units of behaviour (which he is having to transpose) are simpler. I am trying to see exactly where the difficulty arises. Is it on this transposition stage itself? Or maybe it is not the actual translation which presents the problem.

BRUNER: The fact that you could trace the formation of the schema in terms of the incorporation of a set of higher units I think might answer it, from the point of view of the genetic history of the schema.

WHITE: May I put forward an extension of what you have just suggested? Could one make the situation even simpler by using temperature? One could perhaps apply a good deal of cold to one finger, which the child couldn't see, and then make sure he couldn't see the finger again in the test situation. If one could build up the stimulus to a level so that it would not be painful but would nevertheless linger for a few seconds he would not be relying upon a memory effect. I think our ingenuity is the thing which limits the number of ways in which we can get reactions from children.

LEFFORD: May I mention some other observations. We are also interested in observing what kinds of errors they would make. There appears to be a sort of response gradient, if you can call it that. When the children missed a finger they would tend always to go back to the index finger. I think this is the original form of movement from which this action differentiates.

CONNOLLY: Children do this kind of thing when they are counting. I have noticed it with my own children: they begin to count and go "four, five, seven", realize they have made a mistake but do not go back to six and continue from there—rather they go right back to one and start all over again.

BRUNER: One rather nice technique which could be used here is the confusion matrix, the kind that one uses for input/output analysis. You could include the finger which you have just touched and the one which the child responds with, and find out whether there is any clustering; clustering, that is to say, around the index finger. This might be used as an index of the amount of differentiation, when they begin to get away from clustering around the first and index fingers.

CONNOLLY: Are there any mechanical restraints to do with the tendons or finger differentiations in a situation of this kind? One noticed that in Zazzo's (1960, *Manuel pour l'examination psychologique de l'enfant*. Delachaux and Niestle, Neuchatel) test where a child is asked to raise a single finger when the examiner points to it; this is always more difficult with the third finger on the nondominant hand. This is always the last one to be independently lifted.

LEFFORD: We saw that the two middle fingers were identified last, but I don't know of any mechanical restraints operating here.

Vicarious Perceptual Actions: A Study of The Motor Components of Recognition, Immediate Memory and Thinking

VLADIMIR P. ZINCHENKO

Moscow State University

ALL EXPERIENCED RESEARCH workers who have studied the ontogeny of human behaviour would agree that it is impossible to separate the processes of perception, reasoning and performance during the early stages of a child's development. The connection between perception and action in the first months of an infant's life is easily demonstrated; according to Piaget's data (1954) and later confirmed by Bruner (1968), a 6- or 7-month-old child finds great difficulty in differentiating between an image and a motor action. The child's behaviour confirms this if he is observed while looking for an object that has disappeared from his visual field. Gradually perception acquires an autonomy distinct from action, the situation is analogous when we consider the intellect. The ontogenetic ties between perception, reasoning and performance have often been overlooked; as a result thinking is studied separately from behaviour and behaviour is considered apart from perception; skills are studied separately from perception and perception apart from performance. Despite the specialized methods of investigation which have been developed and the vast amount of data accumulated in certain areas of psychology it is important to inquire to what extent it is still helpful to preserve the traditional sharp distinctions between perception, memory and performance.

Recently a gradual blurring of these distinctions has become discernible. A few illustrations may help to explain how it is possible to investigate cognition and performance with a new technique. It is unnecessary to say that this task is closely connected with the great difficulty experienced in integrating the mass of data from research in perception, thinking and action. For the psychologist, the difficulties of thinking in general terms about sensory and motor processes are greatly magnified when we consider the child who is in the process of establishing sensory-motor co-ordination. Progress towards the solution of a problem such as the development of voluntary actions and skills was achieved only after the gap between the study of the alphabet of images and the motor alphabet was bridged. Investigations by Zaporozhets (1960) indicated that the key to the problem of skill development lies in the study of orientation-search and the study of perceptual activity; the latter leads to the formation of perceptual images which control performance. However, close ties between perceptual activity and skills are best observed when skills are in the formative stage. Once they have been established, perceptual actions do not participate in their realization in any very obvious way, and the specific mode of image regulation of skills becomes less and less evident.

Galperin's (1959) work demonstrated that there are different types of orientation-search and different types of perceptual activity at the basis of mental actions. Moreover, there have been a number of publications dealing with the problem of the mutual relations and connections between the exterior, practical activity, and the inner, mental activity. Leontiev has summarized the main features of the attempts made to solve this problem and emphasized the significance of mutual transformations of the exterior, practical and the inner, mental activity. On the basis of psychological and genetic-epistemological research he presents convincing evidence for the connections between external and internal activity.

The development of a perceptual image, and of the actions to be performed, not only precedes the attainment of motor skills but is itself realized by the participation of the motor processes. Other processes, such as those of so-called simultaneous recognition, cannot be considered as special skills (irrespective of arguments about perceptual learning) until a motor alphabet, on the basis of which the above mentioned processes are realized, is discovered and studied.

The examples given above draw attention to the fact that only at the primary stages of development are the interactions between cognition and performance clearly observed. In adult forms, any interactions taking place would only exist implicitly. As Leontiev (1959) stated, the specific attribute of various complex psychological abilities and functions is the way in which, having once been formed, they function in the course of time as a unity and do not reveal their complex and compound nature. These complex psychological processes are characterized by relatively simple immediate actions. Leontiev suggests that complex psychological abilities and functions should be conceived as the result of special functional organs being formed in the course of our individual development. Here he uses *organ* in the sense in which Uchtomsky (1950, p. 299) used it in expressing his idea of "physiological organs of the nervous system". Dwelling on the development of functional organs, Leontiev says that their effector links would be reduced or impeded, and so they come to serve as central controlling processes. This covert form of action (i.e. of perception participating in thinking and thinking participating in action) makes for great difficulty in studying the psychological mechanisms underlying these processes. The question arises as to whether all these difficulties are substantial and also to what extent they reflect inadequate experimental techniques. An alternative view, which we have accepted and chosen to investigate in connection with the activity of the visual system, is that the difficulties reflect primarily the problems of separating the integral activity into its component parts.

Our hypothesis rests on the fact that in the course of development the functions of the visual system are improved and elaborated; changes occur not only in the image alphabet but also in the motor alphabet. A specific system of actions, with its own physical attributes, is equally necessary for simultaneous recognition, recall, reproduction and problem-solving. This hypothesis is connected with the notion of organs. However, the principal theme of the study does not deal with the development of these organs nor with central brain processes; our particular concern is with the effector links of the motor alphabet and whether these vary in complexity. The succeeding sections deal with the background to the hypothesis and its experimental investigation.

VICARIOUS BEHAVIOUR AND ORIENTATION-SEARCH ACTIVITY

The hypothesis about recurring changes of the motor alphabet in the development of psychological abilities and functions arose from work on the analysis of vicarious trial and error behaviour as well as from data on orientation-search activity. The concept of vicarious trial and error (VTE) was introduced by Muenzinger (1938) and refers essentially to the stage reached in development when true performing reactions are replaced by orienting reactions. The latter anticipate the performance of one form of behaviour or another. Vicarious trials and errors have their own motor alphabet which consists in head movements, limb movements and movements of the sense organs, all of them being directed to examining the object or situation. |When these movements disappear the number of trial and error responses diminishes. Vicarious trial and error was studied by Tolman (1939); on the basis of his investigations Tolman concluded that the VTE process itself represented partial errors. Under certain conditions the density of vicarious trials increases until they become an independent aspect of behaviour, directed at the mastery of the situation: such behaviour, according to Tolman, has a "vector of identification" which comes into conflict with behaviour which is directed by the "pragmatic vector". Thus the concept of vicariousness implies that an orientation-search form of behaviour is being established on the basis of performance, and this slowly replaces the initial responses. Analogous description and research were used by Pavlov's school and in more recent work on the ontogeny of orientation-search activity (Zaporozhets, 1960). Poddyakov (1965) traced the ontogeny of orientation-search activity and Galperin drew attention to the fact saying that, contrary to the behaviourists' point of view, Soviet investigators treated the orientation-search activity as a means of determining object relations between phenomena, and also as a channel reflecting those relationships in the brain processes. It is significant to note that in this paper the system of perceptual actions, the exterior form of which is similar to the perceived object and which is directed to the development of the image, should itself represent a derivative of orientation-search activity.

Thus, the perceptual actions rest upon their own motor alphabet (see Zaporozhets *et al.*, 1967; Zinchenko, 1967) and represent a specific self-regulating process which provides feedback adapted to the peculiarities of the investigated object. The performance of this system of actions results in the development of a perceptual image of the object and this image controls subsequent performance and orientation-search behaviour. During development perceptual actions become differentiated from practical performing (motor) actions (including vicarious ones) and acquire their own specific qualities.

A system of stages may be traced in the development of behaviour; practical actions are replaced by orienting ones and these are in turn replaced by perceptual ones. The emergence of each stage makes behaviour more adaptive and increases the chance of learning and of anticipation. During the development of each stage the motor alphabet of the previous stage is employed initially, this is perfected and acquires new features which give rise to the motor alphabet of the succeeding stage. Each new form of action may be considered as vicarious, it extends the previous stage rather than rejects it. The question arises as to whether the system of perceptive actions is the "last substitute". Study of visual system activity, however, suggests that this is not the case. The perceptual, mnemonic and intellectual activities have a complex structure and certain stages may be followed in their developments.

METHOD OF INVESTIGATION

In order to examine the hypothesis, stabilized retinal images were used along with different methods of measuring eye-movements. The methods suggested by Ditchburn and Fender (1955), Pritchard (1961) and Yarbus (1965) served as prototypes for the stabilization technique and they were modified in accordance with the tasks employed. With the technique of stabilized retinal images it was possible to employ a wide range of tests used in the psychological study of vision, though three-dimensional objects and moving objects led to certain difficulties. The three main techniques discussed below were perfected in our laboratory by Vergiles and Zinchenko (1967a, 1967b).

1. *Image Stimulation with an External Light Source*

One of the principal problems with the existing methods of working with stabilized retinal images relates to the limits imposed on the length of the investigation. There was little advantage therefore in comparison with the tachistoscopic technique which increases the effective time of the experiment. We were thus faced with the task of finding conditions under which the image would be stable and visible for longer periods and under which satisfactory experiments would be possible. By a theoretical analysis and by experimental study we developed certain experimental conditions which permitted lengthy observation of stabilized retinal images. This was achieved by alternately switching to light sources of different colours; under these conditions the observer saw the image continuously and without fragmentation.

The stabilization of the image on the retina was attained by means of a sucker; the axis of the sucker's optical system was displaced at an angle of $45°$ to the axis of the body, and the central position of the sucker coincided with the visual axis of the eye. The focal distance of the lenses used in the sucker were 9 mm and 5·5 mm. In the first case the angle of the visual field was $30° \times 30°$, and in the second $60° \times 60°$. In order to increase the sharpness and depth, diaphragms with apertures ranging from 0·8 to 1·5 mm were used. Black and white or coloured photographic negatives were used to provide stimuli. The device consisted of an outer source of light which, passing through the collecting lens, lit the matt-surface screen on the sucker. An obturator was placed between the lit object glass and the collecting lens to help change the luminosity of the matt screen in the course of the experiment. During the experiments the system was arranged in such a way that the lighted screen in the sucker was closer to the eye than the focal length of the lens, a position which permitted the exclusion of light rays from the screen despite any eye movement or rotation. The number of rotations of the obturator when fitted with light filters could be varied from 0·3 to 1·5 per second. This technique, which increased the time during which the stabilized image could be observed, was used to study various perceptual processes; the construction of an image, the recognition processes and the visual examination of objects.

2. *A Stabilization Technique for Studying Changing Images*

In the investigations of perception with stabilized retinal images we took the opportunity of studying changing images, presented either upon the same part of the retina or on different parts, in addition to the tachistoscopic presentation of images. A special sucker, in the construction of which inertialess electroluminescent radiators were used, met these requirements. Electroluminescent plates were placed on the tube perpendicular to one another and a translucent mirror with a reflection coefficient of approximately 50 per cent was placed at the point where their normals crossed. The plane of the mirror was slanted at an angle of 45° to the optical angle of the sucker. When the central radiator was switched on, part of its light passed through the translucent mirror and reached the object glass, the remainder was reflected at an angle of 90°. This also happened when the side radiator was switched on, although in this case it was the reflected ray which reached the object glass. An external light source could be used instead of one of the radiators. This technique is flexible because it is possible to use combinations of differently coloured electroluminescent radiators and it is possible also to control the brightness of their separate parts.

3. *An Electromagnetic Technique for Recording Eye Movements*

When tests were performed without electroluminescent radiators, an electromagnetic record of eye movements was obtained. The principle of the alternation of a directed electromagnetic field, depending on the distance between the radiator and the receiver, is fundamental to the technique of eye-movement recording by an electromagnetic transducer. The radiator, fixed on the sucker, directs the alternating electromagnetic field in the receiving coils, which are connected to pre-amplifiers. The signal, after passing through a smoothing filter, is amplified by d.c. amplifiers and displayed on a cathode ray oscilloscope. Registration is accomplished by image-photo and image-copying; it is also possible to achieve intermediate recording of this registered image on a tape recorder.

The important advantage of this technique is the rapid conversion which may be achieved from one registration scale to another, and also the simultaneous registration on various scales. This technique permits precise registration equal to 0·5 minutes of arc and so relieves the experimenter of the need to adjust the optics in the course of an experiment. But time saved is important when working with suckers. This technique was used for studying perception under stabilized conditions and also under free conditions.

RESULTS: THE PERCEPTION AND RECOGNITION OF STABILIZED IMAGES AND THE MECHANISM OF THE FUNCTIONAL FOVEA

From the psychological point of view there is no essential difference between perception under the conditions of a stabilized retinal image and under free conditions. Under stabilized conditions the subjects successfully solve many problems; learning Japanese hieroglyphics, geometrical configurations, solving maze problems, finding the break in Landolt rings and so on. The solution of these problems under conditions of image stabilization tends to be poorer in quality and takes two to three times as long. It is interesting to note that whilst solving the problems all the subjects formed a clear impression that they were scanning the object.

The results obtained from experiments with stabilized images suggest that some mechanism, which may be likened to foveal scanning of the perceptual field, is involved in the solution of complex visual problems. This mechanism permits the subject to perceive sequentially information received by different parts of the retina. Thus a phenomenon of *ideal attention*, which is not connected directly with the position of the eye, was obtained in these experiments.

The eye movements, which were recorded under conditions of stabilization, correspond closely with the subject's impressions regarding his shifts of attention. If the subjects were instructed not to move their eyes during the experiment they were unable to solve complex search problems and unable to learn geometrical configurations. Under conditions of stabilization of the image therefore the eye movements are markedly reduced when compared with the angular size of the objects presented. By these criteria the movements which take place under conditions of stabilization are similar to the post-tachistoscopic eye movements. I shall return to this comparison below.

As our observations demonstrate, the direction of eye movements under conditions of stabilization is related to the position of the object in the visual field. This provides evidence for suggesting that with varied positions of the eye, the role of different receptive fields of the retina would be changed, i.e. some of them would be activated while the others would be inhibited. From this approach the function of eye movements under stabilized conditions might be regarded as a mechanism of successive and directed activation of various receptive fields, corresponding to those parts of the image which carry information.

Thus a detailed study of the process of image development, visual search, and recognition under stabilized conditions, has demonstrated that all these processes function on the basis of their proper motor alphabet. This alphabet has been called the alphabet of vicarious perceptual actions; and vicarious perceptual actions themselves represent a selective shift of sensitivity in separate parts of the retina, the change being controlled by small eye movements. These movements are made in the zone of 2–4° and may be either drifting or rapid and saccadic. Psychologically the motor alphabet is expressed as an ability to shift attention over the whole field of the stabilized image. A mechanism compensating for the stabilization of the anatomic fovea was found; this we called the "mechanism of the functional fovea".

In contrast to external perceptual actions the extraction of information with the aid of vicarious actions is made not from the object itself but from an after-image which has accumulated in the visual system. It has been shown, by a special analysis, that the perception of a stabilized image is identical with the perception of an after-image. The stabilized image is projected on one and the same part of the retina and its projection is not changed by eye movements; the after-image, which is also stable as regards the retina, behaves analogously. Should the stabilized image and the after-image move in relation to one another the solution of problems under the stabilized conditions (with the techniques we have used) would be impossible. In our view the perception of a stabilized image and an after-image constitute two stages of a single process, whilst the extraction of information under stabilized conditions and from an after-image are accomplished by one mechanism. This mechanism, known as the mechanism of vicarious perceptual actions, ensures that an image is scanned after a tachistoscopic presentation.

An investigation carried out in our laboratory has demonstrated that the so-called simultaneous recognition is arbitrary (Rumyantsev et al., 1968). When the test image was replaced by a noise field, relevant to the test image, the minimal exposure time sufficient for recognition was of the order of 80–100 milliseconds. Lower exposure times reported by other authors might be explained by the fact that the noise field did not secure the effective obliteration of an image on the retina. This is important in the present context because 100 milliseconds is long enough to make the eye movements necessary for the recognition of familiar stimuli. When the noise field is not used the exposure times required are significantly less. In this case eye movements are also necessary, but with their assistance the information is extracted not from the object itself, but from the after-image on the retina.

Perhaps the most convincing and delicate experiment demonstrating the necessity of vicarious perceptual actions was an experiment aimed at an investigation of immediate memory span. In collaboration with Vergiles (Vergiles and Zinchenko, 1967b), we used the stabilization technique which employed an electroluminescent source of illumination. The subjects were presented with tables containing 36 figures, the size of the table was $15° \times 15°$ and each figure was about $1°$. A sucker was fixed on the subject's eye and the brightness of the test field gradually increased. The adaptation of the visual system, under these conditions of test-field stabilization, proceeded more rapidly than the increase in brightness. Hence, in the preparatory phase of the experiment the subject did not see anything, although the full brightness of the test field reached 570 foot lamberts. (This technique is called the method of sub-threshold accumulation of information.) The voltage on the test field was then sharply reduced, and at the same moment the neutral field was switched on; against its background the subject observed the negative after-image of the test table. On the experimenter's instruction the subjects read out the figures in the table: on average they could read 10–12 figures before the after-image disappeared, which is more than double the immediate memory span obtained in tachistoscopic experiments. Like Sperling (1960) we made use of the partial reporting technique and asked subjects to read out figures from different parts of the table. (The subjects were given instructions before the test field was switched on, i.e. in that phase of the experiment when they had not yet become aware of the available stimuli.) It appeared that the subjects were indifferent to what part of the after image they were asked to read from, the span of material reproduced did not change. In fact the subjects seemed to memorize the whole test field in a short time provided that it was stabilized on the retina.

One cannot obtain such good results with tachistoscopic presentation, the visual system is unable to accumulate sufficient stimulus energy during a brief period of time. Under conditions of free visual perception (when the retinal image is not stabilized) the memory span obtained experimentally is substantially lower; this may be explained by the obliteration of the memory span artificially, the process taking place when the subject changes fixation points.

Vicarious perceptual actions are also required to read out information from the after-image without any conscious perception of the image presented. If the subjects are not allowed to make eye movements the results prove to be much more unsatisfactory.

VICARIOUS PERCEPTUAL ACTIONS AND THE MANIPULATING ABILITY OF THE VISUAL SYSTEM

Numerous facts suggest that the visual system is capable of certain "manipulating actions" in righting the distortion of perceived objects. The term "manipulation" is introduced by analogy with manual actions. The question arises as to whether it is possible to obtain any direct proof of this putative "manipulating" ability of the visual system. To test this we used reversible figures:

(a) Necker's cube, $15° \times 15°$ in size, (i) lit from time to time in different colours, (ii) presented against a background of electroluminescent radiators;

(b) Schreider's stairs; and

(c) concentric circles, with the diameters of the outer and inner circle of $10°$ and $7°$ respectively, the distance between the circles and the contour thickness being equal and measuring $1°$.

All these tests involved the use of photographic negatives with a dark field and a bright figure. The images were presented both under stabilized and free conditions, when the sucker holding the object was placed before the eye but was not fixed on the eye. A three-dimensional model of Necker's cube was also used and under free perceptual conditions it was seen as three-dimensional. The last test in this series was the simultaneous presentation of the flat image of a cube with a three-dimensional spiral laid upon it, the contour thickness of the spiral being about 5°. We also used a number of tests to study apparent movement under stabilized conditions.

This cycle of experiments demonstrated that under stabilized conditions the visual system gave the subject a number of images, the majority of which were imperfect and distorted. The most characteristic distortions reported were: (a) the subjects did not differentiate between flat and three-dimensional objects under stabilized conditions; (b) the three-dimensional truncated pyramid and its image looked alike, both as flat or three-dimensional; (c) in another experiment the subjects reversed the figures, e.g. they saw the smaller square either nearer or farther than the larger one; (d) the three-dimensional spiral, crossing the cube's image, was perceived as drawn on the cube's background and their positions were reversed. There were also moments during this experiment when the image took on an unusual form, for instance, two diagonals connecting the large and small squares seemed to be directed towards the subject, while two others seemed to be directed away from him. Analogous phenomena were observed when the subject was presented with a few concentric circles. The Necker cube test under stabilized conditions in combination with the eye-movement records showed that the reversal of the cube's perspective came only when the eye position was shifted. These data amount to some additional evidence of the fact that eye movements, under stabilized conditions, could lead to the shifting of the "functional fovea", and to the appearance of new points of view for the subject, so as to cause the above transformations of the stimuli which were presented.

Under stabilized conditions, when bright lines were flashing at the frequency of 0·6–0·8 cycles per second, the subject received a clear impression of apparent movement from each bright line. Moreover, a dark after-image of this line appeared to move in the opposite direction: the after-image moving closer to the subject while the bright line on the surface receded from him. Then the apparent movement and the after-image of this movement combined into a whole figure, which seemed to be a rectangle rotating around its own axis. On presenting two pairs of flashing lines placed one under the other, the effect of the rotating rectangle persisted, but in this case the subject observed two rectangles rotating in opposite directions around the same axis.

The phenomena described above indicate that, under stabilized conditions, the phenomenal field has a greater number of degrees of freedom compared with the subjective field of the perceived objects. Under stabilized conditions the subject meets with some difficulty in distinguishing the direct from the after-image, the static from the moving object, the real from the apparent movement, the figure from the background, the flat from the three-dimensional object and so on. These phenomena then may be considered as different phases of object observation in one experiment. In the light of the facts obtained we suggest that the term "alternating image" is more correct for the one seen under stabilized conditions than the term "stabilized (fixed) image".

The technique used by us (involving the exclusion of image movement over the retina), paradoxical as it may seem, allowed us to test the ability of the visual system to achieve the visual manipulations of images. The conclusion to be drawn is that under conditions of free perception the possibility of image movement over the retina might at least impede to a considerable degree the analysis of this ability. Thus, eye movements not only take part in the development of an image, but also limit the number of degrees of freedom of the images presented.

It is quite clear that no orientation in this situation is possible with the aid of images that the subjects receive under stabilized conditions. The subject's task is to find and fix the adequate image among many inadequate ones. It seems that the problem of image organization and the problem of movement organization have something in common. In movement organization, control is exercised over excessive degrees of freedom of the body's kinematic links (Bernstein, 1947); in the process of image development, excessive and inadequate variants of the object's image are eliminated. The same mechanism secures the invariance of the image despite the numerous transformations of the stimulus.

The manipulating ability of the visual system discovered by us is of great significance in understanding the process of skill development. From the biomechanical point of view (Bernstein, 1947), there are a large number of degrees of freedom in the body's kinematic links, i.e. the performing aspect of skilled movement, while the visual system represents by itself an essential part of the skill control mechanism. We argue that the control mechanism, in comparison with the performance mechanism, cannot have fewer degrees of freedom, otherwise some degrees of freedom of the performance mechanism would not be controlled. The manipulating ability of the visual system represents a psychological aspect of this superiority in degrees of freedom attributed to the control mechanism of a skill.

In conclusion we may say that the essential feature of vicarious perceptual actions is that they depend on images as their media instead of real objects. The suggested manipulating ability goes beyond the limits of the traditional conception of perceptual functions, and we are thus led to believe that vicarious perceptual actions take part in performing more complex functions such as recall, visualization and problem-solving.

PERCEPTUAL ACTIONS AND THE SOLUTION OF COMBINATORY PROBLEMS

In psychological investigations the process of problem-solving is usually described in terms of visual metaphors, such as "enlightenment", "discovery" and "insight". The early experimental work emphasized the essential contribution made by the visual system in problem solving activities. The adherents of the Gestalt psychology talked about the significance of reconstructing and recentring the phenomenal field. Along with this, the creative act was, as a rule, contrasted with the active performance. The latter was allotted only some preparatory function; but the enlightenment itself, the discovery, was described in full conformity with the introspective data as a spontaneous and unconscious act. The same contrast between the preparatory and the decisive stage may be found in Kohler's (1956) classic study with apes.

In the light of the investigations into vicarious perceptual actions mentioned above, it seemed quite natural for us to try to check whether they took part in the solution process; and whether the vicarious actions made up a motor alphabet of thinking processes, which could be given a material basis. In other words, the thinking processes ought to have their own motor alphabet—just as any model of a real situation—that would allow both perceptual and thought transformations.

The hypothesis was that a real situation is not suitable for transformation; but its image is acceptable, composed either at the stage of "trial and error", or at the stage of the orientation-search perceptual activity accomplished in a purposive way. The real situation cannot serve as an object for immediate mental transformations: one must be detached from it, i.e. be free for a moment; otherwise it will constitute a hindrance to such transformations.

On the other hand the real situation is necessary to control the expediency and adequacy of these transformations; but the material for transformations of this kind should be the object's image, which can be manipulated into new relations with the aid of vicarious actions. If this suggestion is correct, then the preparatory stage of the solution process, in which the conceptions about the nature of the problem are formed, will necessarily be followed by a period of complete detachment from the situation—the stage of image transformations. This activity of image transformation and its reconstruction should be performed with the assistance of a certain motor alphabet, which would differ from the alphabet of orientation-search perceptual actions, by both its biomechanical and its functional parameters.

The function of such a motor alphabet might be performed by vicarious actions of smaller amplitude, occurring either in the form of a drift or in the form of saccadic movements. Quite independently of the process of problem-solving, drift and saccadic movements of small amplitude have often been noted by investigators. The experimental task which we set ourselves was to check these assumptions. In these experiments we employed the technique of instantaneous registration of macro-eye-movements and of movements performed during fixation. The summary of the eye movement behaviour while scanning the stimulus field was recorded on one cathode-ray tube, and the movements during the fixation period were recorded on another which had a greater gain. The movement trajectory was registered with the cathode-ray tube, and the movement components were registered on a polygraph.

The use of oscilloscopes with a memory function permitted the experimenter to observe directly the eye movements and to compare them with the subject's verbal report. Depending on the task and aim of the experiment it was possible either to choose beforehand a registration field for the eye to move over or, after observing the eye movements, to choose a suitable field during the experiment. The visual field was also artificially limited to between 1 and 5° during the experiment by means of a sucker. Thus our technique made it possible to register and analyse the eye movements both at the scanning stage and during moments of seeming inactivity.

The main tasks given to the subjects in the course of the experiments concerned imaginary and simple manipulatory geometrical figures; for example, "Inscribe a star into a hexagon and count up the angles". The eye movements were studied in detail during the solution of the problem, "playing-5"; the various methods of solution have been studied in detail by Pushkin (1965). The problem is solved by the subjects quite quickly (30–60 seconds). We also studied the eye movements accompanying the solution of chess problems, with adults aged from 20 to 30 as subjects.

The experiments afforded confirmation of the data, obtained by many other workers, that whilst the eye is fixating a point there is some drift around the fixation point, as well as saccadic movements which reverse to the fixation point. The region in which both kinds of movements are made does not exceed 20–30 minutes of arc if the subject observes the point over 10–15 seconds. If there is no fixation point and if there is no other visual task, it is possible to observe drift movements of small amplitude occurring in a larger region (up to 40–50 minutes of arc) during 10–15 seconds of recording; saccadic movements were almost completely absent.

With the problem of the mental representation of simple geometrical figures (the fixation point being absent), the drifts may be observed over a considerably larger region, approximately 2·5–3° or more. These drift movements (made in the region of 2·5–3°) were first observed in problems requiring a mental representation of geometrical figures and their manipulation. On the basis of evidence obtained from the previous experiment, the drift movements are probably connected with the formation of an image (mental representation) of the stimulus. Subsequently small saccadic movements (approximately 1°) could be observed during the performance of the main task: the total extent of those movements was also limited within 2·5–3°. The movement trajectories were essentially similar in character to the trajectories observed during the period of greatest eye movement, when large amplitude movements were used to scan the stimulus field.

We may conclude, therefore, that whilst solving a problem the subjects either focused upon the field in which that problem was displayed or they attempted a solution without the aid of this display. Small saccadic movements may be interpreted as vicarious perceptual actions, which are the means of manipulating an image. With the visual field limited, the subjects found it more difficult to scan the problem, this technique therefore allowed us to distinguish more precisely the scanning movements of large amplitude from the vicarious actions of small amplitude; the latter occur even in the absence of an object in the visual field. Under these conditions the duration of fixation became as long as 50–60 seconds. The character of movements in the fixation region remained the same when the visual field was not limited. But in some cases the subjects were helped towards a solution by a narrow field, and in a few cases rapid jumps during fixation were replaced by small drifts (which may be interpreted as a means to aid the recall of the problem conditions which were presented) followed again by rapid jumps of small amplitude.

Finally, in the last series of experiments, "playing-5" was presented to the subjects orally, a problem which completely excluded large scanning movements of the eyes. In this the subjects had before them a neutral, homogeneously lighted field, and we observed an alternation of drift and small saccadic movements, which continued until the final solution was made, or until the subject gave up attempting to solve the problem altogether. Analogous observations were made during the solution of chess problems, in which case the more complicated the problem for the subject, the greater the role played by vicarious perceptual actions. Moreover the drift was predominant in the case of the vicarious actions, when the problems were very difficult.

When the subjects in control experiments were presented with visual problems requiring them to extract letters or figures from tables, or solve maze problems, large eye movements predominated; there was little drift and small saccadic movements were infrequent.

The results of the investigation make it clear that perceptual activities contribute greatly to the process of problem-solving. A more detailed analysis of eye-movement activity, performed in the course of problem-solving, reveals a sequence of stages. In the first stage perceptual actions of large amplitude are observed. It is by these that the subject acquaints himself with the task and develops an image, his own conceptual model of the situation. In the next stage the subject seems to detach himself from the situation, and we observe drifting which indicates that he is visualizing the elements of the problem; this is the point at which the solution of the problem, "by the internal plan", begins. In the same stage the manipulation of the image or of a model is achieved through vicarious actions, such manipulation being purposive and adequate for the task of transforming and reorganizing the image.

Consequently, the image reorganization made by vicarious perceptual actions plays an essential part in the solution and in the elaboration of a system of actions, needed for obtaining a decision or for its execution. In this sense the solution process will, in fact, present by itself an *internalized activity*: an activity "in the internal plan", or an activity with the image of the situation. Enlightenment, insight and discovery are the results of this activity, which, properly, should have its own motor alphabet to justify its being called an activity. The important parts of the situation-image activity performed in the internal plan will be externalized by the system of vicarious perceptual actions, and so will be accessible to investigation.

On the whole the results obtained convince us that there are good prospects for investigating the various motor alphabets which are involved in simple information processes, as well as those involved in the more complex ones. It is hoped that the technique developed for the investigation of motor alphabets will help place on a firm experimental basis such problems as the "development of functional organs"

(Leontiev, 1959); the development of "physiological organs" of the nervous system (Uchtomsky, 1950); the "theory of schemata" (Oldfield, 1954); and finally, the development of motor skills. They all appear to be different ways of designating the same problem.

REFERENCES

BERNSTEIN, N. A. 1947. *On movement organisation*. Medgiz Publ, Moscow.
BRUNER, J. S. 1968. The growth of representational processes in childhood. *Voprosy Psikhologii*, 135–146.
DITCHBURN, R. and FENDER, D. 1955. The stabilized retinal image. *Optica Acta* **2**, 128–133.
GALPERIN, P. Y. 1959. The development of investigation in mental action formation. *Psychological Science in the U.S.S.R.* Vol. 1. Acad. Pedagogical Sciences, Moscow.
KOHLER, W. 1956. *The mentality of apes*. Humanities Press, New York.
MUENZINGER, K. F. 1938. Vicarious trial and error at a point of choice. A general survey of its relation to learning efficiency. *J. genet. Psychol.* **53**, 75–86.
LEONTIEV, A. N. 1959. *Problems of mental development*. Publ. Acad. Pedagogical Sciences, Moscow.
OLDFIELD, R. C. 1954. Memory mechanisms and the theory of schemata. *Brit. J. Psychol.* **45**, 14–23.
PIAGET, J. 1954. *The construction of reality in the child*. Basic Books, New York.
PODDYAKOV, N. N. 1965. Development of dynamics of visual perceptions in children of pre-school age. *Voprosy Psikhologii*.
PRITCHARD, R. M. 1961. Stabilized image on the retina. *Scient. Amer.* **204**, 72–76.
PUSHKIN, V. N. 1965. *Operative thinking in large systems*. Energiya Publ, Moscow and Leningrad.
RUMYANTSEV, D. A., VERGILES, N. Y. and VUCHETICH, G. G. 1968. On the problem of recognition time in the obliteration of test objects by a noise field. *Proceedings of the 3rd Congress of U.S.S.R. Psychologists' Society*. Vol. 1. Prosvetsheniye Publ, Moscow.
SPERLING, G. 1960. Information available in a brief visual presentation. *Psychol. Monog.* **74**.
TOLMAN, E. C. 1939. Prediction of vicarious trial and error by means of the schematic sowbug. *Psychol. Rev.* **46**, 318–336.
UCHTOMSKY, A. A. 1950. *The dominant as a factor of behaviour*. Collected works, vol. 1, p. 291–309. Leningrad.
VERGILES, N. Y. and ZINCHENKO, V. P. 1967a. The problem of the image adequacy. *Voprosy Filosofii*, **4**, 56–65.
VERGILES, N. Y. and ZINCHENKO, V. P. 1967b. A functional model of the sensory link of the visual system and a possible mechanism of short-term visual memory. *Voprosy Psikhologii*, 144–147.
YARBUS, A. L. 1965. *The role of eye movement in the visual process*. Nauka Publ, Moscow.
ZAPOROZHETS, A. V. 1960. *Development of voluntary actions*. Acad. Pedagogical Sciences Publ, Moscow.

ZAPOROZHETS, A. V., VENGER, L. A., ZINCHENKO, V. P. and RUZSKAYA, A. G. 1967. *Perception and action.* Prosvetsheniye Publ, Moscow.
ZINCHENKO, V. P. 1967. Perception as an action. *Voprosy Psikhologii*, 3–7.

Conditioning and Motor Control

Feedback Control of Covert Behaviour[1]

R. F. HEFFERLINE, L. J. J. BRUNO,
AND J. E. DAVIDOWITZ[2]

Columbia University, New York

BEHAVIOUR IS COVERT when invisible and overt when plain to see. Some behaviour obviously becomes covert simply by reduction from its previously overt magnitude or intensity. When Jacobson's (1932) subjects, wired up for electromyographic recording, were asked to imagine activities, such as cranking an old-fashioned ice cream freezer, the patterns of muscle potentials recorded were essentially miniatures of those obtainable from the overt activity. On the other hand, to locate and examine by means of instrumentation covert behaviour which perhaps has never been identified with an overt counterpart presents a problem of quite a different order of magnitude.

A measure of the problem may be taken from the description of covert activity offered by Davis, Buchwald and Frankmann (1955): "somatic responses abound. One has but to observe them on a set of recording instruments to believe that they are by far the most numerous responses of the organism. It is clear that any overt response, vocal utterance, or bodily movement, is surrounded by a wide penumbra of them, and it may not be too bold a guess to say that, whenever there is any evidence of a stimulus affecting the individual, something in his periphery or viscera is set into motion. Not infrequently these may be seen when there is no other means at hand for detecting that the person has been stimulated" (p. 1).

While the complexity of the covert substrate may give pause to the faint-hearted, this aspect of the problem might be expected to yield to modern instrumentation and a modicum of ingenuity. More problem-

---

[1] The work described here was supported by NIMH grants M–2961 and MH–13890, by Columbia University grants from the Higgins Fund and from the Institutional Scientific Research Pool, and by a Public Health Service post-doctoral fellowship to J. E. Davidowitz.
[2] Now in the Department of Ophthalmology, New York University Medical Center.

atical in fact is the diversity of analytical concepts whose embodiments have been relegated to the covert substrate. Theorist and experimenter alike have looked to behaviour called covert, implicit, or incipient, for the correlates of meaning, perception, thought, consciousness, emotion, and fractional anticipatory goal responses, to mention a few. Although theory and data have occasionally shown a satisfying congruity (cf. Davis, 1940, 1952), more often, as Davis and his co-workers (1955) put it, "disappointments have been severe, and more of them are probably to come" (p. 1). It would seem, then, that to sift the covert substrate in search of somatic correlates is, at best, imprudent: there is no guarantee that a concept derived analytically has a physical manifestation, nor, should one exist, is there necessarily an optimal systemic location.

The uncommitted investigator may well have qualms about plumbing the covert substrate; and reports that autonomic responses tend to be peculiar to the individual (Lacey et al., 1953; Lacey and Lacey, 1958; Malmo et al., 1950) offer no reassurance. Nevertheless, a deliberate, if uncommitted approach can be made to the study of covert behaviour. If nothing else, it is generally conceded that the covert substrate may have particular relevance as a determinant and a support of overt behaviour: "we would say that confronted with problems about the last of a chain of events [an overt response], we propose the study of [covert] events immediately before it, and of similar events which are not followed by the same conclusion" (Davis et al., 1955, p. 2). In short, while the concepts of psychological theory may be inadequate to guide our study of the covert substrate, we can navigate, nevertheless, using the landmarks provided by overt behaviour.

Our approach to the covert substrate has typically employed a two-stage technique. In the first stage, an overt response, such as the key-press in the traditional reaction-time experiment, is selected for study, and electrophysiological methods are used to record its covert precursors. Our purpose at this point is to establish covert-response/overt-response correlations which may then be elaborated in the next stage. In the second stage, a covert response, for example, electromyographically measured tension, is chosen from among those which were correlated with the overt key-press, and the parameters of the covert response are manipulated in order to determine its effect on the reaction-time response. Our two-stage technique forms the basis for a programme of research in which covert behaviour becomes the independent variable.

Of particular importance to such a programme are the methods by which an experimenter can come to control the occurrence of covert responding. In general, these involve the use of exteroceptive feedback, of which two types have been distinguished historically: pay-off or reinforcement, as used in conditioning approaches to behaviour; and augmented sensory feedback, as more commonly applied in human engineering approaches to behaviour modification. The remainder of this paper describes our applications of reinforcement and augmented feedback to the problem of controlling covert responses of the skeletal musculature.

I. CONTROL THROUGH REINFORCEMENT

Although the similarities between classical and instrumental conditioning are many (Kimble, 1961, pp. 78-98), and are probably more compelling than the differences (Miller, 1969; Schoenfeld, 1966), the two varieties of conditioning continue to be distinguished, at least at the procedural level. While classical conditioning makes the reinforcing stimulus (and the response it elicits) consequent upon the prior presentation of a conditional stimulus, instrumental conditioning makes the reinforcing stimulus consequent upon the prior occurrence of a response. Of course, both classical and instrumental procedures have long been used to generate and control overt responding in the skeletal musculature (cf. Bekhterev, 1913; Thorndike, 1911) but rarely have the procedures been applied to behaviour at the covert level. In principle the effects of a reinforcement procedure should be the same regardless of the level of behaviour. The distinction between covert and overt behaviour, is, after all, an arbitrary one which refers to the visibility or magnitude of the behaviour, and not to its functional properties. Since, within limits, the mechanism of muscular contraction is the same no matter what the magnitude of the response (cf. Lippold, 1967), the effects of reinforcement should be the same to the extent to which they depend upon that mechanism. Although, as we shall presently see, this seems to be the state of affairs with regard to the effect of instrumental procedures, an additional factor—that is, the nature of the evoked myogenic response—may be important in relation to the outcome of classical procedures.

When one recalls, with Sperry (1952), that except for neurohumoral and glandular responses "the entire output of our thinking machine consists of nothing but patterns of motor co-ordination" (pp. 297-298), it is not surprising to find that the muscular response evoked by even the simplest of stimuli is in fact rather complex. Although the data are at best incomplete, it seems reasonable to distinguish two components of the evoked myogenic response: an alpha or early component which appears at the forearm within 50 milliseconds of stimulus onset, and a beta or late component whose forearm latency is greater than 50 milliseconds.[3] The alpha response, whose discovery awaited the advent of computer-averaging techniques (Bickford et al., 1963; Bickford et al., 1964; Katzman, 1964; Rapin, 1964), appears relatively difficult to habituate, while the beta response, which has been described most extensively by Davis and his collaborators (Davis, 1948a, 1957; Davis and Buchwald, 1957; Davis et al., 1955; Davis and Van Liere, 1949), seems to habituate quickly, at least over the middle range of stimulus intensities. Both alpha and beta responses are found throughout the skeletal musculature, and occur irrespective of the sensory modality stimulated. For each, the magnitude of the evoked response generally increases with stimulus intensity, and with increases in the pre-stimulus level of muscle tension. While the alpha response may be interpreted alternatively as a stimulus-detection or motor-tuning reaction, the beta response appears to be a component of both the orienting reaction (Lynn, 1966, pp. 1–13; Sokolov, 1963a) and of the defence-startle reaction (cf. Landis and Hunt, 1939; Lyn,, 1966, ibid.; Sokolov, 1963b). Most importantly, it may be presumed that both alpha and beta responses will be evoked by both conditional and unconditional stimuli under a classical conditioning procedure.

1. *Classical Conditioning*

The relevance of evoked myogenic responses becomes apparent as we turn to those studies in which electromyography has been used to assess covert responding under classical procedures. Of particular interest are the data of Van Liere (1953) who measured masseter and forearm tension while presenting paired tones of moderate intensity. Van Liere's conditional stimulus was an 850 Hz tone of 43 db whose offset preceded the unconditional stimulus of 1,000 Hz and 70 db by 40 milliseconds. Each tone lasted about 2 seconds and each initially evoked the beta response (the alpha response was not measured). After 15 training trials intermixed with four extinction trials, the magnitude of the beta response to the conditional stimulus had increased above that initially recorded, and was greater than that measured in subjects who had received 20 presentations of the conditional stimulus

[3] The alpha and beta responses distinguished here are not necessarily the "a" and "b" responses described by R. C. Davis and his co-workers: Davis's "b" and our beta are generally the same, but Davis's "a" sometimes falls into our alpha and sometimes into our beta category. The latency of Davis's "a" is variously given as less than 0·1 second, at least 0·2 second, etc. The problem lies in the fact that our alpha description is based on computer-averaged records, while Davis's "a" comes from measurements made from film or by electronic integrator over 0·1 second periods.

alone. Of themselves, the results are hardly conclusive since the usual sensitization and pseudo-conditioning control groups were not run. Taken together with the earlier work of Hilden (1937) and Hunter (1937), however, an important suggestion begins to emerge: "conditioning may merely be the process of raising certain neuromuscular reactions above a certain threshold so that a previously defined response can be measurably elicited" (Van Liere, 1953; p. 323). The suggestion is corroborated by Hilden's observation that the conditional hand withdrawal to a light paired with shock "was built up as a graded muscular contraction, increasing in degree until the overt response appeared" (p. 193), and by Hunter's conclusion that light-shock pairing administered to rats while recording from the gastrocnemius muscle "may bring into activity individual [motor] units not before excited by the light or it may serve to increase the frequency of spontaneously firing units" (p. 623).

To this point, the electromyographic evidence indicates that the classical procedure rather than generating new responses *per se* operates upon the beta response pattern evoked by the conditional stimulus and escalates its magnitude until an overt conditional response is produced. Additional evidence for this possibility comes from the classical paradigm called "anticipatory instructed conditioning" (Grant, 1964, pp. 3–8). In effect this paradigm represents a reaction-time experiment with a constant foreperiod: the subject is requested to clench his fist or to close a key either to the offset of the conditional stimulus or to a reaction signal which follows it after a fixed delay. That the procedure is capable of producing overt conditional responses is made clear by the elaborate precautions taken in reaction-time experiments to forestall premature or anticipatory responses (cf. Woodworth and Schlosberg, 1954, p. 9). At the covert level "the effect of telling the S to respond . . . [is] to enhance in a particular locality, a response which occurs anyway" (Davis, 1948b; p. 755). For conditional stimuli of threshold (Davis, 1950), of moderate (Davis, 1948b) or of strong intensity (Dawson and Davis, 1957), the effect is the same: beta responses occur whenever a stimulus is presented, but their magnitude is greater when an overt response is required. In the muscles which execute the response, their magnitude tends to increase with the number of repetitions of the conditional stimulus (cf. Davis, 1940). Interestingly enough, covert conditional responses are also observed when the unconditional response is not initiated by the subject but instead is elicited by passive limb movement (Doehring, 1957; Sokolov, 1963b, p. 155).

The importance of the beta response to the classical procedure is emphasized by Sokolov's comparison of anticipatory instructed conditioning with and without prior habituation of the conditional stimulus (1963b, pp. 247–255). Sokolov paired a 1000 Hz, 70 db tone with verbal instructions to "raise your hand", and observed that acquisition proceeds much more slowly with, than without, habituation, and that conditional motor responses develop only after the orientation reaction has re-appeared. (Here, the orientation reaction was represented by the galvanic skin response and not by the beta response. Electromyographic recordings were obtained, however, and they showed, as expected, that covert responses appeared on a number of trials before an overt response emerged.) Sokolov inferred from this experiment and from others like it that the occurrence of an orientation reaction is essential to the development of a conditional motor response.

The trend which characterizes the data taken under classical procedures is that, contrary to the view expressed by Pavlov (1927) and by many psychologists after him, the conditional stimulus does not come to substitute for the unconditional stimulus: the conditional is not a duplicate of the unconditional response (cf. Notterman *et al.*, 1952), but rather appears to be an elaboration of the beta component of the response evoked by the conditional stimulus when it is presented alone.[4] Of course, this trend can only be taken to refer to skeletal responses, and even so, much work remains to be done on evoked myogenic responses and on the classical procedure, before firm conclusions can be drawn.[5] Still, the implication of the trend is intriguing. It would seem that both classical and instrumental procedures make the reinforcing or unconditional stimulus temporally contiguous with the occurrence of a prior response. In the classical case the response in question is evoked by an identifiable (and programmed) stimulus; in the instrumental situation "no correlated stimulus can be detected upon occasions when it [the response] has been observed to occur" (Skinner, 1938, p. 21).

2. *Instrumental Conditioning*

If in fact conditional responses develop from the pattern of behaviour set in motion by imposing a conditional stimulus, we are left to

[4] At this time little is known of the role, if any, which the alpha component plays in conditioning. There is evidence (Luschei *et al.*, 1967) that the alpha component undergoes a transformation when a reaction-time response is called for, but the functional significance of this change is best described as obscure.

[5] Extrapolating from the current analysis, we are led to expect the elaboration of conditional responses whenever the conditional stimulus evokes an orientation reaction. In fact, multi-variable recordings show that conditional responses may develop concurrently in several different systems (cf. Liddell, 1934; Moore and Marcuse, 1945; Zeaman and Smith, 1965).

conjecture on the mechanism by which a covert beta response, whose magnitude is measured in tens of microvolts, is potentiated to an order of magnitude which is sufficient to produce observable movement. To put the problem differently, we can ask whether the effect of reinforcing a covert response is to strengthen responses of that and similar magnitudes, or whether reinforcement operates to call out successively larger versions of the response. To answer this question we turn now to studies of instrumental conditioning carried out in our laboratory using both positive and negative reinforcement (Hefferline and Keenan, 1961, 1963; Hefferline et al., 1959).

The experimental arrangements were similar in each of the studies. The subject sat in a reclining chair within a dimly lit, shielded enclosure. An intercom provided communication with the experimenter, and a one-way mirror permitted observation of the subject. After preparation of the skin, surface electrodes were applied to the thenar eminence formed by the muscles of the thumb, and to the hypothenar eminence formed by the muscles of the little finger (Brash, 1951, pp. 504–507). A ground electrode was attached to the ear lobe, and additional sets of dummy electrodes were applied to confuse the subject about the actual recording site. Action potentials appearing between the thumb and little finger muscles were differentially amplified by a factor of one million, and then rectified and displayed on a vacuum-tube voltmeter. A permanent record of the rectified signals was made using either magnetic tape or a recording light-beam galvanometer. The system, which had a time-constant of 0·1 second, was calibrated at the beginning and end of each session.

The response in each study consisted of a ballistic deflection of the voltmeter needle or photorecorder beam which rose sharply above and then returned quickly to the resting tension level. Response magnitudes were categorized according to peak needle or beam excursions, and frequency distributions for most of our subjects were compiled after their sessions by examining the tape or photorecorder records. At the beginning of each experimental run, a response magnitude which occurred not more than once in 1 or 2 minutes was selected for later reinforcement. This response was always much smaller than that which produced observable movement in our least responsive subject (about 300 microvolts).

When the effect of positive reinforcement was under study the subject was informed that "we are measuring your ability to relax ... After 30 or 40 minutes numbers will begin to appear on the lighted box in front of you. These numbers represent your total score. For each increase in score you will receive a nickel." When negative reinforcement was used, some subjects were told that the study concerned the effects on body tension of noise superimposed on music; others were told that a response, so small as to be invisible, would temporarily turn off the noise, or, when the noise was not present, postpone its onset; and still others were informed that the effective response was a tiny twitch of the left thumb.

Each session began with a 10-minute baseline period during which the spontaneous rate of responding was determined and a criterion response magnitude was selected. In the subsequent conditioning period (60 minutes or more), the experimenter pressed a key which produced the reinforcement whenever a criterion response was observed. For subjects receiving positive reinforcement, the experimenter's key-press advanced the displayed score by one digit, representing another nickel earned. For subjects working under a negative reinforcement contingency, the key-press turned off for 15 seconds the aversively loud 60 Hz hum which, during conditioning, was superimposed on the music presented via earphones throughout the entire session. When the noise was already off, a key-press postponed its resumption for 15 seconds. For all subjects the experimental run terminated with 10 or more minutes of extinction during which criterion responses no longer produced reinforcement.

Similar results were obtained for both positive and negative reinforcement contingencies; typical results for the positive contingency are shown for four subjects in Fig. 1. The frequency histograms display the distributions of response magnitude which were obtained in the last 10 minutes of each experimental phase, with the reinforced value shown in solid black. Prior to conditioning, the frequency distributions are skewed markedly towards the high-amplitude end. Conditioning tends to normalize the distributions: in all cases, the reinforced value becomes the most frequent, and in three of the four cases the non-reinforced amplitudes fall off more or less symmetrically from this peak. Despite this radical shift in the shape of the distribution, a brief period of extinction sufficed in three cases to restore the initial skewing.

Comparable data were taken using the negative contingency except from those subjects—informed of the effective response—who kept so busy producing voluntary thumb-twitches that the small, reinforceable type of response had little opportunity to occur. Although other data showing the effect of instrumental contingencies on covert electromyographic responses are not available for comparison,[6] our data

---

[6] Two other instances of instrumental conditioning of electromyographic responses have

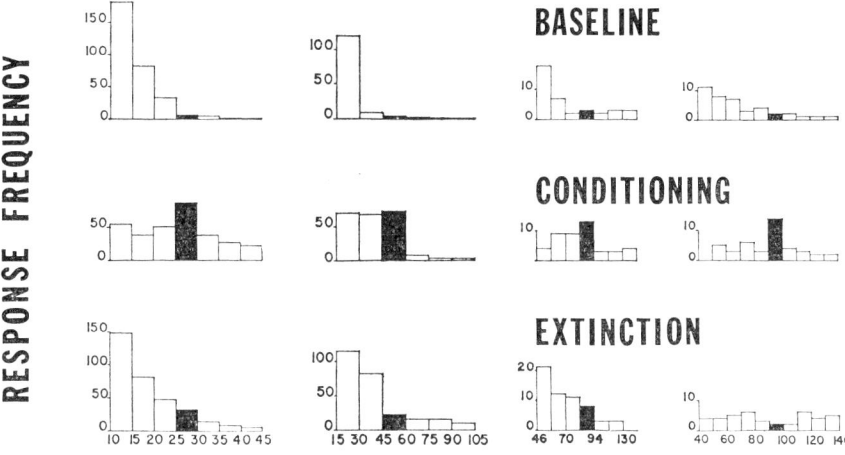

AMPLITUDE CLASSES (microvolts)

FIG. 1. The effect of positive reinforcement on covert response magnitude; reinforced value shown in black (Hefferline and Keenan, 1963. Reprinted with permission of *J. exp. Anal. Behav.* Indiana University).

compare favourably with the results obtained in a variety of species when an intensive response dimension has been studied at the overt level. When upper and lower limits for the criterion response were established, the modal response category approximated the criterion category in studies of force, effort, and duration of response (Birch, 1964; Herrick, 1964a, 1964b; McMillan and Patton, 1965; Notterman and Mintz, 1965, pp. 105–108). When all responses above a criterion value were eligible for reinforcement, the modal response approximated the minimal reinforced value (Goldberg, 1959; Herrick, 1963; Margulies, 1961; Notterman and Mintz, 1965, pp. 20–80). We are led to conclude, then, that at the covert, as at the overt, level the effect of instrumental reinforcement is to produce a response whose magnitude approaches the value specified by the reinforcement criterion.

3. Classical Conditioning Revisited

In contrast to the conclusion just drawn, we put forward a suggestion about the effect of classical reinforcement, viz., that it appears to call

---

come to our attention. Black (1965, 1967) showed that training to respond (and not to respond) given under nearly complete curarization affects the subsequent extinction of a previously acquired overt avoidance response. Fetz (1969) reports: "By integrating and reinforcing rectified electromyograms, we were able to train animals to contract specific muscles" (p. 957).

out successively larger versions of the beta or orienting response evoked by the conditional stimulus. This difference in outcome emphasizes the relevance of distinguishing between classical and instrumental conditioning on a procedural basis. While we have noted that the reinforcing stimulus in each procedure appears to follow contiguously upon a response, it is only in the instrumental case that a response, and thus a criterion response magnitude, is in fact required.

The importance of the requirement may perhaps be made clear by observing the effect of reinforcement when the requirement is removed. The reference experiment is a model of simplicity (Skinner, 1948): a hungry pigeon, previously trained to eat grain from a hopper, was placed in an experimental box and the hopper was operated for 5 seconds at 15-second intervals *"with no reference whatsoever to the bird's behaviour"* (p. 168). The effect of the procedure, which will be recognized as the temporal paradigm of classical conditioning (cf. Kimble, 1961, p. 48), was to generate stereotyped responses which were "so clearly defined that two observers could agree perfectly in counting instances" (Skinner, 1948, ibid.). The responses, however, were topographically different from bird to bird: while one bird turned counter-clockwise about the box, another developed a head-tossing response, still others produced pendulum-like motions of the head and body, etc. The important point here is that the particular form and magnitude of the behaviour generated in the absence of a response requirement is largely a matter of chance: "The bird happens to be executing some response as the hopper appears; as a result it tends to repeat this response" (Skinner, 1948, p. 168).

Our analysis of the classical conditioning procedure suggests that if Skinner had arranged to present a stimulus just before each hopper activation, the response topography strengthened would have been predictable in part from a knowledge of the orienting responses evoked by the stimulus. In fact, this experiment has recently been carried out (Brown and Jenkins, 1968). The authors used a box in which a response key was set into the wall about 5 inches above the grain-bearing hopper. After an inter-trial interval which averaged 60 seconds in length, the response key was lit for 8 seconds, and then, as the light was extinguished, the hopper was operated for 4 seconds (classical delayed conditioning paradigm: Kimble, 1961, ibid.). Under this regimen, ten out of 12 pigeons came to peck steadily at the key when it was lit, and to peck quite infrequently when it was dark. That most of the subjects came to make topographically similar responses—that is, key-pecks—is attributable in large part to the introduction of the light as a conditional stimulus. Brown and Jenkins report that "the bird notices the onset of the light and perhaps makes some minimal motor adjustment to it. The temporal conjunction of reinforcement with noticing leads to orienting and looking toward the key" (p. 7), and it is from "looking toward the key" that pecking eventually emerges (cf. Brown, 1968).

The implication to be drawn from Skinner's experiment and from that of Brown and Jenkins is that the effect of reinforcement in the absence of a response requirement—that is, the effect of non-contingent or classical reinforcement—need not be regarded as fundamentally different from instrumental reinforcement except in the factors which specify which responses will be strengthened. Of course, in an instrumental procedure the response to be strengthened is specified by the reinforcement criteria. In a classical procedure, however, the determining factors may be identified with the available stimuli and with the responses which they occasion. While we noted that the topography of the final performance in Skinner's experiment was "largely a matter of chance" it seems reasonable to infer that the performance developed from the "set of responses which frequently occur 15 seconds after reinforcement" (Skinner, 1948, p. 171). Similarly in Brown and Jenkins' study, it seems safe to assert that pecking was eventually elaborated from the orienting responses initially activated by the onset of the key-light.

Thus, taking together the results of the pigeon experiments and those obtained electromyographically, we can tentatively identify the topographical determinants of a response generated under classical reinforcement with the stimuli antecedent to that response. We are left, however, without a clear notion of the factors which determine response magnitude. With regard to this problem, Brown and Jenkins observed that it was not the initial orienting reaction to the lighted key which was strengthened, but rather a succession of increasingly more "effortful forms" which culminated in the emergence of key-pecking. In explanation, they appealed to "the species-specific tendency of the pigeon to peck at things it looks at" (1968, p. 7). While this may be a fully appropriate explanation for the pigeon, another, still more general, account is needed since the data taken electromyographically also indicated a tendency for the initial orienting or beta response to increase in magnitude under continued reinforcement.[7] Since our inclination is to believe that the strengthening effect of a reinforcing stimulus is specific to the magnitude of the response it follows, the problem becomes one of identifying the

---

[7] It may be of interest to note that the classical procedure which Brown and Jenkins used on the pigeon will also produce key-pressing when applied to monkeys, although this response "would not otherwise have been generated" (Sidman and Fletcher, 1968, p. 308).

variable which, independently of reinforcement, potentiates response magnitude in the classical procedure. Although several candidates for this variable present themselves—viz., extinction, motivation, arousal—we prefer not to choose among them without further directed research on the problem.

II. CONTROL THROUGH AUGMENTED FEEDBACK

Although our review of reinforcement control emphasizes problems and not principles, it seems clear that, where precise behavioural control is sought, there is much to be gained by using an instrumental rather than a classical reinforcement procedure. Analytically, at least, two factors seem to contribute to the efficiency of instrumental procedures, most obvious of which is their application of the reinforcement "where it will do the most good"—to the class of behaviour which we are in fact trying to strengthen. Perhaps a less obvious but still important factor is the sensible provision of more frequent reinforcement for the subject who uses whatever resources are available to him to increase the precision of his performance. By resources we mean the wealth of information usually available to a subject about his own behaviour from afferent channels—visual, auditory, and somaesthetic—as well as from efferent sources. To see how this sensory and motor information might be helpful, we can view the situation under instrumental reinforcement as a sort of psychophysical procedure in which the response attributes which are reinforced establish a kind of "standard" which it is the subject's task to try to "match" by adjusting his behaviour until its attributes coincide with those of the "standard" response. Clearly, the subject who "matches" best will procure the greatest number of reinforcements, and this will surely be the subject whose behaviour is best controlled by the information he has about its attributes.

To take this line of reasoning a step further, it makes sense to assume that a subject provided with an extra measure of information might achieve an even more noteworthy performance, especially if that "extra measure" were a variable stimulus whose values reflected exactly those of the dimension along which the criterion performance is defined. In particular, we would expect a stimulus of this kind (which presumably augments the sensory feedback naturally consequent upon responding—hence the name for the procedure[8]) to be especially effective when applied to the problem of controlling covert muscular responses. In this

---

[8] Our own preference is for a name which underlines the operational aspects of the procedure, e.g., "selective feedback".

case, the responses are typically so slight as to provide the subject with little information via the usual sensory and motor routes, and indeed their minuteness makes it unlikely that the subject has ever learned to attend to them at all.

1. *Meter Feedback*

We looked into the possibility of using augmented feedback to improve a covert instrumental performance while studying the effects of negative reinforcement (Hefferline *et al.*, 1959; cf. *Instrumental Conditioning* above). Subjects in the feedback group were told that a tiny thumb-twitch would temporarily turn off the noise superimposed on the music, or, when the noise was already off, the twitch would postpone its onset. In addition the subjects were provided during the first half-hour of conditioning with a meter which was driven by the activity recorded between the thumb and little-finger muscles. While the meter, whose readings were identical with those used by the experimenter to determine criterion or reinforced responses, did not enable the subjects to achieve direct control of the criterion response, it seems to have provided a basis for rapid responding within a range which included the reinforced size. The feedback group obtained many more reinforcements than other groups without feedback who had been informed to varying degrees of the nature of the task and of the response required. Most interestingly, this effect continued throughout the second half-hour of conditioning, when the meter had been removed. It would seem that by providing feedback we not only provided an "extra measure" of information, but we also made more distinctive the information naturally available to the subject.

That augmented feedback might provide an effective means of teaching a subject to attend to the response information he already has seems to be true not only for "phasic" responses, like those we examined under instrumental reinforcement, but also for "tonic" or steady-state responses of the sort encountered in a pursuit or tracking procedure. Using an experimental arrangement similar to that described above, we monitored the electromyographic activity recorded between an electrode placed on the jaw over the belly of the masseter and another placed over the temporal bone just far enough back to avoid eye-blink (Hefferline, 1958). The subject was seated comfortably in a reclining chair and a feedback meter was positioned in front of him at eye-level. He was told, as he relaxed with jaw sagging, that "what you are to do is to close your mouth by the smallest amount you can. This will make the needle rise on the scale . . . We want you to try to make the needle go to midscale—to the position where it is standing straight up—your meter will go dead ... What we want you to do during this next 10 seconds is to keep *our* meter at midscale ... " After this "you are in a 10-second rest period and can do whatever you want ... " A session consisted of 30 cycles, each containing three 10-second periods, the first with feedback, the second without feedback, and the third a rest period; the transitions between 10-second periods were marked for the subject by lights and by a tone.

The rectified electromyograms taken under this procedure were fed to the subject's meter and to an Esterline–Angus recording milliammeter which had been critically damped to give peak-to-peak readings. A backing current was run through both meters in order to offset the noise of the amplifying system (c. 2 microvolts) as well as the "noise" contributed by the subject himself at his resting level (another 2 or 3 microvolts). The current allowed us to display to the subject and to record permanently the action potentials occurring within a 5-microvolt range above the offset noise level.

The subject's performance appeared on the Esterline-Angus records as a series of excursions or sweeps of the pen, each varying in amplitude and duration. Taking each pen-excursion as a behavioural unit, we constructed a performance measure by subtracting the starting value of each excursion from the maximum value, dividing by 2, and adding this figure to the starting value. We took the constructed measure, which gives the "midpoint" of each pen-excursion, to represent the subject's success in approximating the criterion meter deflection. Mean values of this measure are shown, by session, for one of our subjects in Fig. 2A. The values have been normalized so that 0·0 is the "noise" level for a relaxed subject and 1·0 is an increment of 5 microvolts above "noise" at the electrodes. Deviations on either side of 0·5, or midscale deflection, represent rather consistent over- or undershooting of the criterion value during a particular session.

Performance with feedback shows no improvement. We take this to mean that the requisite skills were already highly developed and were effectively brought into play during the first session. In contrast, performance without feedback began with marked undershooting, which was gradually corrected on succeeding days. By the fourth session, performance is indistinguishable from that with feedback and remains so thereafter. Although for both conditions the average length of the pen-excursions tended to decrease with practice—indicating a developing ability to restrict overshooting and to make more subtle corrections—no consistent change in the variability of pen-excursion midpoints was

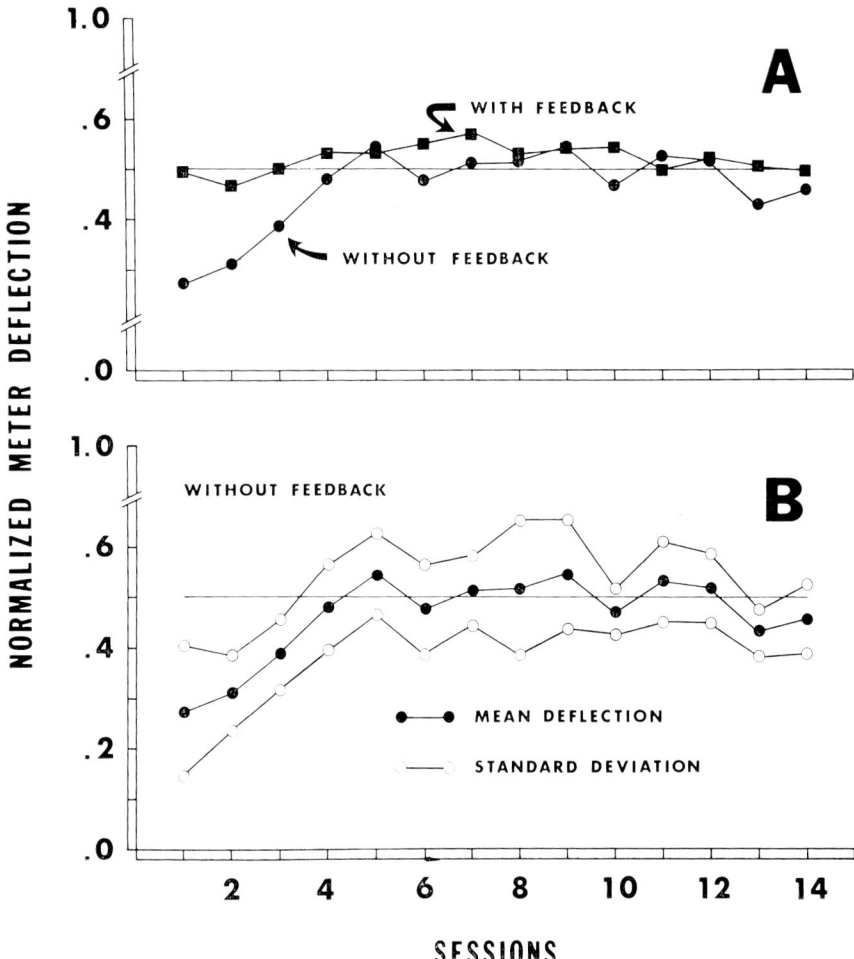

FIG. 2. Performance of a subject trying to maintain a midscale (0·5) meter reading with and without visual feedback. Each point is based on 150–200 pen-excursion midpoints (Hefferline, 1958. Reprinted with permission of The New York Academy of Sciences).

observable. This can be seen in Fig. 2B, where the midpoint means taken without feedback have been replotted with an envelope representing plus and minus one standard deviation. Standard deviations with feedback were of the same order of magnitude and also without systematic trend.

The data do not, of course, suggest that the sight of the meter had become irrelevant; they do, however, indicate a learned ability to sustain without feedback a response magnitude initiated while the meter was available. While the subject may have learned to keep the needle at midscale wihout feedback by learning to discriminate exceedingly small changes in response magnitude—and the data on pen-excursion length indicate he did learn this—he may have acquired a tension scale. In support of this possibility are the data obtained from another group of subjects whose task it was to keep the needle at 0·3, 0·5, or 0·7 during feedback periods, and to approximate scale values not previously practised (0·2, 0·4, 0·6, or 0·8) during periods without feedback.

Under this multiple-value task, performance with feedback was similar to, but less accurate than, that of subjects trained with only a single scale value. Performance without feedback showed a tendency to overshoot low values and to undershoot the high ones. Produced values approached the required values with practice, but never consistently matched them; instead, produced magnitudes appeared to be a power function of required values, with an exponent of about 0·5.

The finding that a power function describes the data taken without feedback may not of itself be surprising (cf. Stevens and Galanter, 1957), but the ability of our subjects to produce and discriminate response magnitudes in the range from 0·0 to 5·0 microvolts is indeed quite remarkable. Recent work from our laboratory (Bruno, 1968) indicates that subjects asked to scale tension magnitudes typically do not discriminate amplitudes smaller than 20 or 30 microvolts, that is, not without explicit training. While it seems fair to say that our subjects learned to attend to or discriminate response magnitudes outside of the usual range of experience, whether they learned the form or exponent of the produced magnitude function (cf. Irwin et al., 1967) or whether these were determined by the response-system under study (cf. Stevens, 1961) remains an interesting question for further study.

2. Feedback and Response Discrimination

An important result of our feedback studies was the finding that a covert performance developed with augmented feedback can, after sufficient exposure, be maintained when the feedback meter is withdrawn.[9] Since we accounted for the outlasting effects of feedback in terms of the development of a response discrimination, it became relevant to establish directly that a covert muscular response can, in fact, acquire discriminative control of behaviour (Hefferline and Perera, 1963).

Our plan was to train the subject, although he might remain otherwise

[9] The informal reports of Hardyck, Petrinovich, and Ellsworth (1966) and of Whatmore (1968) tentatively generalize this result to other muscles and to other forms of visual and auditory feedback.

unresponsive to an occasional twitch in the muscle of his left thumb (abductor pollicis brevis), nevertheless to "report" its occurrence within 2 seconds by pressing a key with his right index finger. In order to circumvent the problems of "self-instruction", we disguised the purpose of the experiment by representing it to the subject as a reaction–time task. After the first session, during which the subject had only to sit back and relax for the duration of the hour, he was informed that his task in each succeeding session was to press the key with his right index finger whenever he heard the moderately loud tone (1000 Hz; 0·5 second) which we would occasionally superimpose on the constant, random masking-noise. He was told that each correct key-press would advance his score, as shown on a digital display, and would be worth two cents at the end of the session. What the subject was not told was that our aim was gradually to transfer discriminative control of the overt key-press from the tone to the covert thumb-twitch.

Throughout the experiment we monitored electromyographically both the thumb-twitch and the covert activity in a muscle associated with key-pressing (extensor carpi radialis brevis). The twitch and the covert key-press, or the "sub-key press" as we termed it, appeared on separate traces of our dual-beam oscilloscope as sinusoidal deflections of less than 75 microvolts amplitude, peak-to-peak. Our purpose in recording the sub-key was two-fold: since it represents a fractional version of the response that we intended to bring under the control of the thumb-twitch, we hoped, (a) by training the sub-key press to occur within 2 seconds after a twitch (see below), to have "partially" trained its overt counterpart, and (b) by measuring the sub-key press, to obtain a "covert" index of the course of the discrimination (cf. Fink and Davis, 1951).

In fact, two discrimination indices were computed: "detected thumb-twitches" (those followed within 2 seconds by sub-key presses) and "correct sub-key presses" (those occurring within 2 seconds after a thumb-twitch). The indices summarize the conditional relations between the thumb-twitch and the sub-key press, each of which occurred about 600 times per hour throughout the experiment. Evidence for the formation of a discrimination required a concurrent increase in both indices—that is, since the absolute rates of the thumb-twitch and the sub-key press remained stable over sessions, we required that most twitches should come to be detected and that most sub-key presses should come to "report" twitches.

As shown by the first point on each curve in Fig. 3, the relative frequency of detected twitches and of correct sub-key presses was approximately 0·15 in the first session, when no contingency was imposed (the curve for detected thumb-twitches has been displaced upward by 0·2). The subsequent break in each curve indicates that relative frequencies could not be gathered in session 2. In this session, as indicated by the schedule of contingencies in Fig. 3, we triggered the tone as quickly after each thumb-twitch as was manually possible. Our aim was to generate incipient or sub-key presses in the interval between the twitch and the tone. We thought of this interval as comprising the fore-period of a reaction-time experiment in which the discriminable or "stimulus" aspects of the twitch played the role of the warning signal,

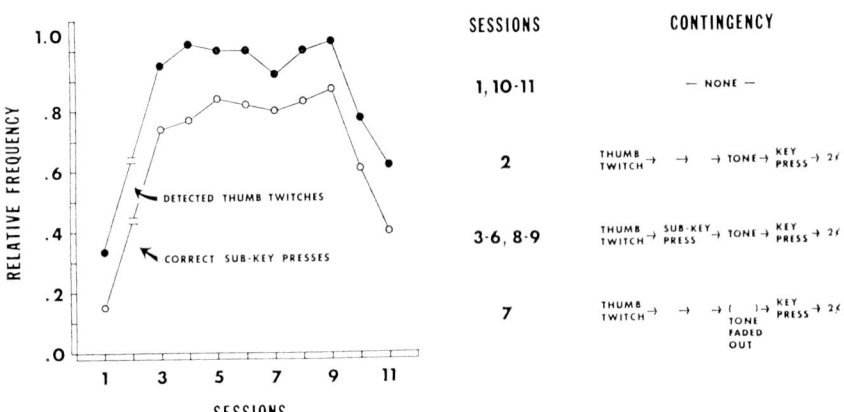

FIG. 3. Procedure and results for a subject trained under augmented feedback to report covert twitches of the left thumb by pressing a key with his right index finger. Results are for covert sub-key presses except in session 7 where they are for overt presses. The curve for detected thumb-twitches has been displaced upward by 0·2. Both curves computed from raw data reported by Hefferline and Perera (1963).

and the tone, of course, functioned as the reaction stimulus.[10] As we mentioned earlier in discussing anticipatory instructed conditioning, Davis in a similar situation found that covert key-presses do, in fact, develop during the fore-period (1940).

In sessions 3–6 we modified our "reaction-time" paradigm to *require* that sub-key presses occurred in the fore-period: the tone was presented only after those thumb-twitches which were followed within 2 seconds by a sub-key press. In other terms, we changed from non-contingent to

[10] If, instead, the response aspects of the twitch are emphasized, then the session 2 contingency appears to be a variety of the observing response experiment described by Wyckoff (1952).

response-contingent presentation of the tone. The effect was an unmistakable increase during session 3 in both detected thumb-twitches and in correct sub-key presses (cf. Fig. 3), and this was maintained with only slight additional increases in sessions 4–6. Presumably, the tone was not only a feedback stimulus for the thumb-twitch, but it exerted as well a reinforcing function for those sub-key presses it followed and a discriminative function for the subsequent overt key-press.[11]

In session 7, each time the twitch and sub-key press occurred together the tone was reduced in intensity, so that after 20 presentations it was completely gone. Of course, as the tone became faint, the subject complained over the intercom that it was "getting hard to hear"; he was told to continue to respond to those tones he did hear. Our hope was that by fading out the exteroceptive stimulus we could transfer discriminative control of the overt key-press from the tone to the twitch (cf. Terrace, 1963). We expected this process to be facilitated by the fact that the twitch had already come to exert discriminative control over a portion of the overt response, viz., the sub-key press. Fading out the tone was marked by small reductions in both indices of the discrimination, although this was not observed in other subjects. What is remarkable, however, is that the curves for session 7 were computed using overt key-presses, and not sub-key presses as in all other sessions: with the tone faded out, 72 per cent of the thumb-twitches were followed within 2 seconds by an overt key-press, and 80 per cent of the key-presses "reported" the occurrence of thumb-twitches. Although we would say that the subject was detecting thumb-twitches and this indeed was what we were paying him to do, when questioned at the end of the experiment the subject said that he still heard the tone.

The apparent discrepancy between our account and the subject's is not, however, difficult to resolve when we recall that our instructions to the subject had explicitly equated, at least within the experimental context, the status of two responses—the overt key-press and the verbal report "I heard it". We had, in effect, told the subject to report with a key-press the same events which ordinarily he would report by saying "I heard the tone". If we assume, with Schoenfeld and Cumming (1963), that what is reported is the occurrence of a mediating event, and not the occurrence of the stimulus *per se*, then it makes sense to presume that the effect of our procedures was to enable the thumb-twitch to enter

---

[11] To generalize this observation, we assume that where the discriminated and the discriminative responses are all sub-classes of the same behaviour, and not isolated as in this experiment, part of the efficacy of augmented feedback lies in its ability to function in both reinforcing and discriminative capacities.

significantly into the control of those events originally evoked primarily by the tone, with the result that the twitch, via the mediating events, acquired discriminative control of *both* the key-press *and* the verbal report. Loosely put, the verbal report was, in fact, no more "hallucinatory" than the key-press.

Our analysis is in keeping with the results of the final sessions of the experiment. In sessions 8 and 9, we reinstated the tone after joint occurrences of the twitch and the sub-key press. Although this had little effect on the discrimination indices, we found that the subject responded to his thumb-twitch with a key-press that came faster than our reaction time in presenting the tone. The subject claimed that he sometimes heard the tone twice in rapid succession. Apparently the events evoked by the twitch and those evoked by the tone were not appreciably different; indeed, they both gave rise to the same verbal report. In the last two sessions, both the tone and the payoff were withheld, and the discrimination indices decreased towards their baseline values. Here again, the key-press and the verbal report showed evidence of being jointly controlled: the subject pressed the key, and later reported that he had heard the tone, not more than four or five times in each of the last sessions.

Our results clearly establish that a covert muscular response can acquire discriminative control of behaviour through an augmented feedback procedure. The combination of these with our earlier results gives, we think, reasonable grounds to assume that augmented feedback facilitates the development of discriminations based on the properties of covert responses, and that it is these response discriminations which ultimately sustain a covert performance when feedback is withdrawn. Assumptions apart, we are nevertheless without clear evidence on a question whose status is belied by the term "augmented sensory feedback"—namely, whether it is afferent information which is augmented, as the term implies, or whether as recent reports suggest (Festinger *et al.*, 1967; Festinger and Kirkpatrick, 1965; Merton, 1964; Taub and Berman, 1968), it is efferent information which is just as likely to be involved. On this point, we can only suggest that a study of the interactions between exteroceptive feedback and behaviour might well provide a convenient model from which to make further assessments of the mechanisms of response discrimination.

3. *Waveform Feedback*

Our work with reinforcing and feedback stimuli has convinced us that covert muscular contractions are indeed amenable to external control; moreover, that the performance obtained may be remarkably precise. For example, in some of the records taken from subjects attempting to approximate a midscale meter deflection "the pen virtually stands still for short intervals and . . . it appears that the subject is discriminating muscle changes that, as reflected at the electrodes, are of the order of one-hundred millionth of a volt" (Hefferline, 1958, p. 757): yet, no matter how exquisite the control displayed, the muscular origin of the performance was always, in part, unknown. To return to our example, the placement used in the meter deflection study was capable of recording not only masseter activity, as intended, but also, in attenuated form, the activity of nearby, and some not so nearby muscles,

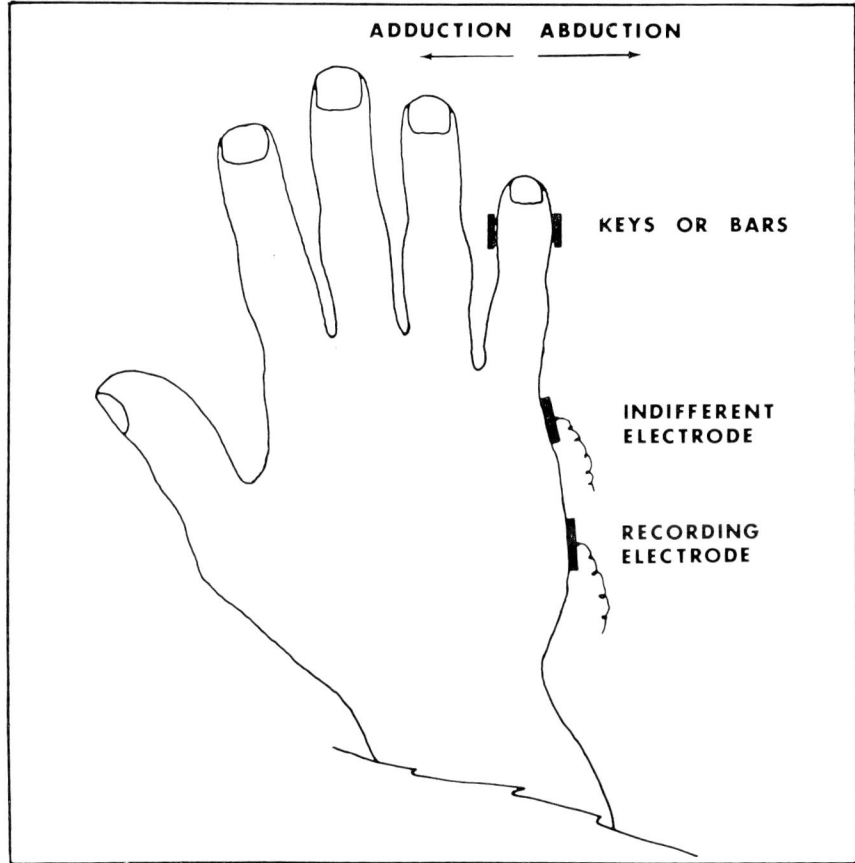

FIG. 4. Electrode placement used to record the EMG associated with inward (adductive) and outward (abductive) movements of the little finger.

among them, those innervating the tongue, lips, scalp and neck. To be sure, the widespread pick-up encountered at the masseter is not peculiar to the placement, but rather is characteristic of the electromyogram (EMG) taken with surface electrodes (cf. Basmajian, 1967, p. 25; Lippold, 1967; Norris, 1963, p. 62). This property clearly poses a problem when the object is to quantify and, through a feedback display, to control the activity of a specific muscle. The remainder of our paper describes a solution to the problem of widespread pick-up based on the finding that the muscle of origin may be identified by the durations of the EMG waveforms recorded at the surface of the skin (Davidowitz, 1963).

Figure 4 illustrates an electrode placement which gives convenient waveform data. The recording electrode is centred on the belly of the hypothenar eminence, a muscle group formed by the three short muscles of the fifth finger: abductor digiti minimi, opponens digiti minimi, and flexor digiti minimi brevis (Brash, 1951, p. 504–507). The indifferent electrode is seated at the base of the fifth finger, and the ground electrode, not shown in Fig. 4, is clipped to the lobe of the ipsilateral ear. The recording and indifferent electrodes were silver/silver-

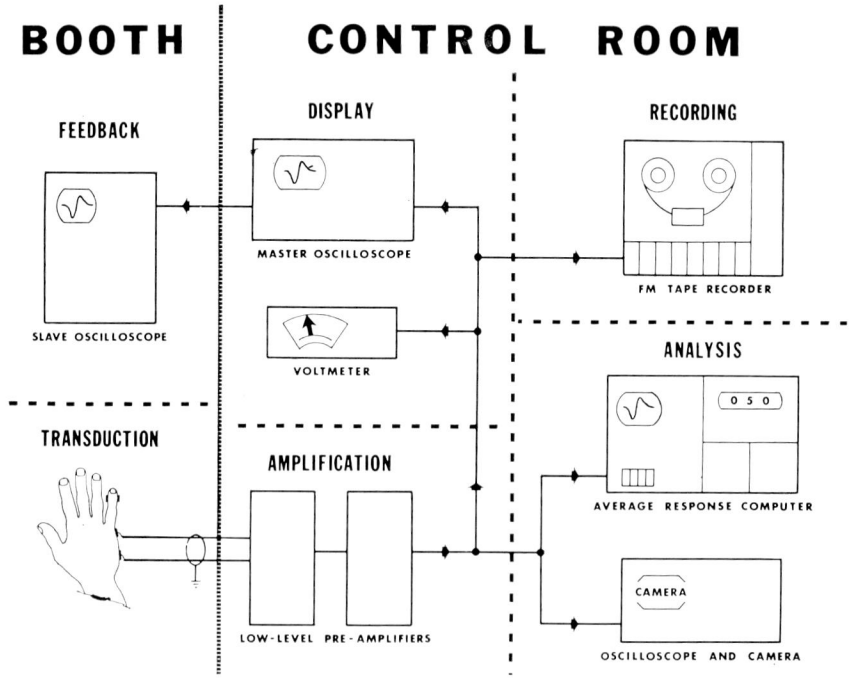

FIG. 5. Equipment configuration used in waveform experiments.

chloride pellets encapsulated in plastic (Beckman), while the ground electrode was formed of two silver discs set into the jaw of a spring-loaded clip assembly. The electrodes were filled with jelly and applied after the skin had been scrubbed with acetone and then abraded with emery cloth. They were re-applied when pair-wise resistances, measured with a battery-operated multimeter, differed by more than 10 per cent, or were greater than 3,000 ohms. In some cases, the skin beneath the electrodes was pricked with a pin to lower contact resistance.

As shown schematically in Fig. 5, a cable running between the subject's booth and the adjoining control room connected the electrodes directly to cascaded low-level pre-amplifiers. Signals appearing between the recording and indifferent electrodes were differentially amplified and then filtered to attenuate frequency components below 8 and above 1,000 Hz. An analogue voltmeter, and a master oscilloscope provided with triggered sweep-circuits, were used to display the amplified signals, while a FM tape system recorded them continuously. Outputs from the master oscilloscope were available to drive a slave oscilloscope providing visual feedback to the subject. On-line or playback analysis was performed using an average response computer (Technical Instruments CAT 1000) or a triggered oscilloscope and camera system.

Our method of waveform analysis is illustrated in Fig. 6. The "raw" data of the method are displayed in the top portion of the figure, where the EMGs taken during weak (C), moderate (B), and strong (A) contraction are depicted as they appear in conventional recordings. The "typical electromyograms" show the activity photographed from the face of an oscilloscope during a single slow sweep of the beam from left to right. With increasing degrees of contraction, the single motor unit pattern shown in (C) gives way first to the mixed pattern (B), in which individual units may still be recognized, and then to the high-voltage interference pattern obtained when many different units have been called into play (A). As regards the single motor unit pattern of (C), the "hypothetical electromyogram" in the middle portion of the figure shows how this pattern would appear if the sweep-speed were increased about ten times. To save space, the records of several single sweeps have been placed side-by-side, with the "quiet" segments deleted. What remains are three biphasic, roughly sinusoidal waveforms of relatively constant duration and amplitude. The waveforms are sufficiently similar to allow the "paste-and-scissors" method of waveform comparison to be replaced by electronic means. The dotted lines illustrate the process. The EMG is fed in parallel to the beam of an oscilloscope and to its joint slope and voltage detector (trigger) circuits. The latter

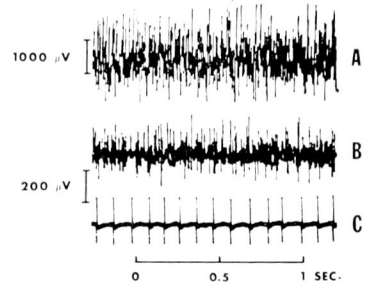

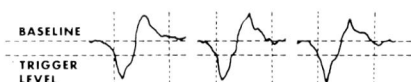

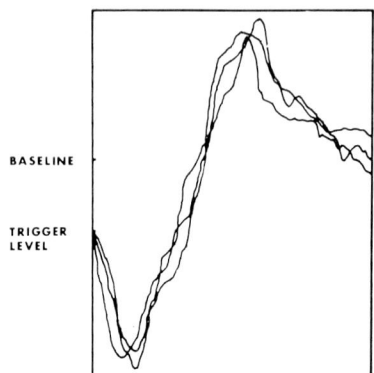

FIG. 6. A comparison of the EMG display obtained when the oscilloscope beam was free-running (top, middle) and when it was triggered (bottom). See text for details.

are adjusted so that the initial component of each waveform crosses the "trigger level" in a negative-going direction at the point indicated by the left hand dotted line in each vertical pair. A trigger pulse derived at this point initiates a single, brief sweep of the beam which is timed to end at the right hand line, at about the point when the second or positive component of the waveform returns to the "baseline" voltage level. Since the sweep circuits are inhibited except after receipt of a trigger pulse, a film exposed to the face of the oscilloscope long enough to record multiple instead of single sweeps will superimpose photographically only the portions of the electromyogram which fall between the dotted vertical lines. The resulting "superimposed oscilloscopic display" is represented in the bottom portion of the figure; a similar display may be observed visually on oscilloscopes equipped with medium- to long-persistence phosphors. In addition, an "average" waveform display may be obtained by using the trigger pulse which initiated the sweep to initiate the storage cycle of a summating computer. In this case, the cycle length, like the sweep duration, is timed to include a single EMG waveform. Although the method of waveform extraction has been described with reference to the single motor unit pattern, it is also applicable to the more complex mixed and interference patterns. For these, the trigger level is set well away from the baseline so that the final display excludes all but the high-amplitude waveforms in a given sample of activity.

A simple demonstration will serve to illustrate our basic waveform findings. The subject was tested in a reclining chair with his right hand resting palm-down on a board which held two microswitches (keys). The tip of his fifth finger was placed between the keys, as shown in Fig. 4, and he was instructed to close one or the other key—each operated at a static pressure of about 25 g—and to hold it closed by pressing against it lightly for about 30 seconds. The EMG taken from the hypothenar eminence under this procedure typically included waveforms of short and long duration. These are characterized in three ways in the panels of Fig. 7. The upper panels, taken by computer summation, indicate the central tendency of the waveforms; the middle panels, taken by multiple-sweep photography, represent, by the dispersion and intensity of the traces, the variability about the mean for the same data. The lower panels in the figure were made with a tape-recorder technique in which the trigger pulse derived from the waveforms, in effect, moved back in time so that the full waveforms were included in the computer average. The left hand panels show the waveforms taken as the subject maintained an inward (adductive) pressure just sufficient to keep the key closed. The peak-to-peak duration of the waveforms is about 2 milliseconds.[12] In comparison, the duration of the waveforms associated with the minimal outward (abductive) pressure necessary for key closure is about 6 milliseconds, as shown in the right hand panels.

The apparent correspondence of short and long waveforms to

---

[12] We have used peak-to-peak rather than total duration because the initial deflection from the baseline is not available when waveform displays like those in panels A–D of Fig. 7 are examined.

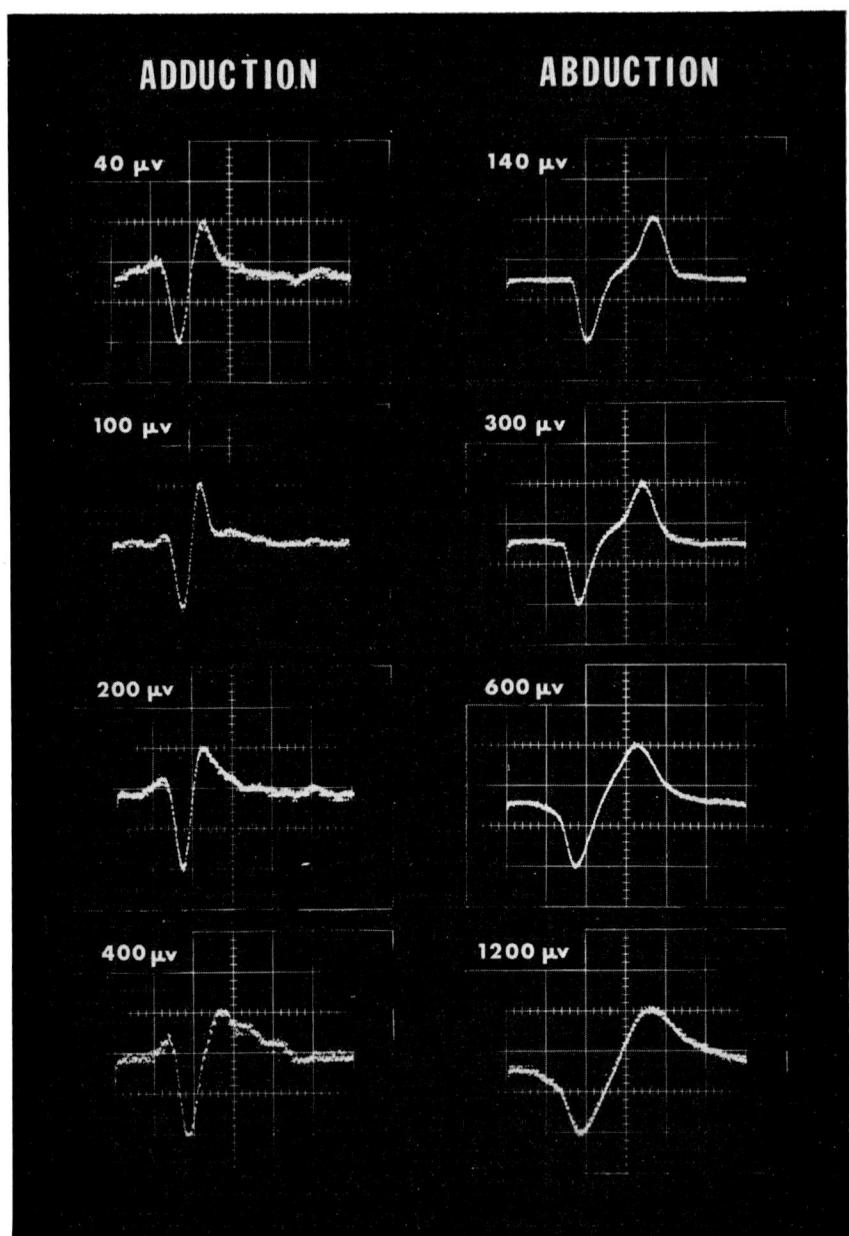

FIG. 7. Waveforms extracted from the EMG taken at the hypothenar eminence during sustained inward (adductive) and outward (abductive) pressures of the fifth finger. Each horizontal division shows 3·1 milliseconds of activity. With negativity downward, the amplitudes are 50 microvolts per division for adduction, 100 microvolts per division for abduction. Fifty waveforms make up each computer-averaged (A, B, E, F) and each photographically superimposed (C, D) display.

adductive and abductive pressures was further examined by requiring the subjects in the key-pressing procedure to work at various levels of effort. An oscilloscope placed in front of the subject displayed a vertical line whose length was controlled by both the amplitude of the EMG waveforms and by the magnification of the amplifier used to display them. The subject was asked to keep the line at the same, pre-determined length throughout each trial. On successive 30-second trials, the magnification of the subject's display was gradually reduced, so that progressively higher amplitude waveforms were needed to produce a line of the required length. When the subject could no longer maintain a criterion display, a maximum amplitude waveform was recorded. The display magnification was then increased, so that progressively lower amplitude waveforms were required. When the subject was no longer closing the key, he was told to "move as if to close the key", and to maintain the criterion display on each trial. After a minimum amplitude waveform had been recorded using one key, a set of trials using the one which operated in the other direction was begun. Both sets rarely required more than two 30-minute sessions.

The waveforms presented in Fig. 8 are characteristic of those obtained from most subjects under the variable pressure procedure. The top and bottom rows, show, respectively, the minimum and maximum amplitude waveforms recorded for an individual subject; representative waveforms taken from the same subject at intermediate pressures are displayed in the two middle rows. The correspondence of short (3 milliseconds) and long (8 milliseconds) waveforms to adductive and abductive pressures is unmistakable: although the shapes of the averaged waveforms change slightly with amplitude—in part, this reflects the increasing variability associated with increasing waveform amplitude—the peak-to-peak duration remains relatively constant. In general, short waveforms (1·5–3 milliseconds) were recorded over the range of amplitudes from 20 to 600 microvolts, and these were associated with adductive pressures of the fifth finger. Long waveforms (5–8 milliseconds) were recorded from 80 to over 2,000 microvolts, and these occurred during sustained abductive pressures. Although the waveforms extracted from the EMG differed in other respects (discharge rate, amplitude, long-term variability), it was the different durations that consistently related the waveforms to the directions of movement of the fifth finger.[13]

---

[13] It should be noted that two additional waveforms appeared—quite infrequently—during abductive pressures. One was about twice the duration and of the same polarity as the common "long" waveform. The other was shorter and smoother in shape, but of opposite polarity.

ADDUCTION   ABDUCTION

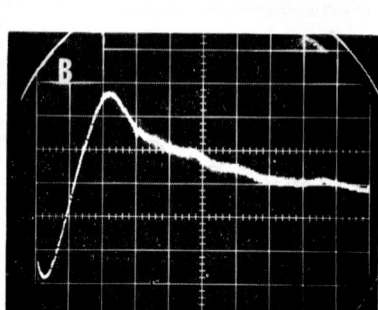
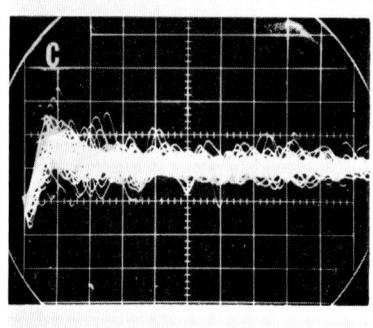
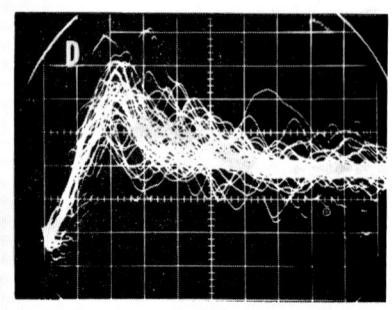
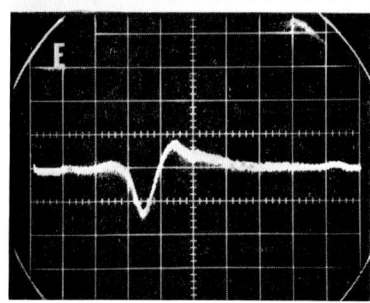
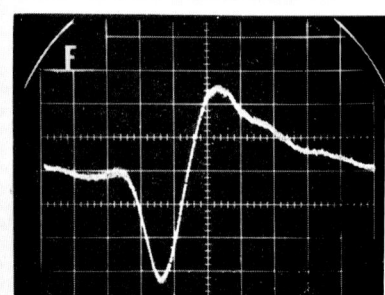

FIG. 8. Computer-averaged waveforms taken at four adductive and four abductive levels of pressure. Amplitudes are peak-to-peak measures based on the average of 50 waveforms. Horizontal calibration is 31·2 milliseconds.

Since anatomical and electromyographic evidence both indicate that different muscles are active during adduction and abduction of the fifth finger (cf. Basmajian, 1967, pp. 187–204; Hollinshead, 1960, pp. 189–196), the obvious implication of our results is that short and long waveforms originate in different muscles. To be sure, it was a relatively simple matter to confirm the implication. Surface electrodes were placed on the hypothenar eminence as shown in Fig. 4; concentric needle electrodes (Adrian and Bronk, 1929) were arranged around the recording electrode in a diamond configuration, each needle penetrating to a depth of 1·2 cm. During abduction, the surface and bipolar needle derivations showed concurrent activity, and at low effort levels, long surface waveforms and motor unit needle potentials occurred synchronously (cf. Harrison and Mortenson, 1962). However, during adduction, only short surface waveforms were obtained, except when volume recordings were made across the tips of two needles. The long waveform, then, appears to originate in the hypothenar muscles, as expected. In contrast, the short waveform seems to be volume-conducted from a more distant muscle—presumably the third palmar interosseous (cf. Basmajian, 1967, *ibid*; Hollinshead, 1960, *ibid*)—although it has not yet been convenient to verify this.

To this point, our results suggest that the duration of the surface waveforms collected at the hypothenar eminence may be used to identify activity in the muscles of the hand which adduct and abduct the little finger, and this seems to hold for all degrees of sustained isometric contraction. We offer the results, however, not as conclusive evidence but rather in illustration of a more general finding, namely, that waveform duration, once it has been correlated with other indices of muscular activity—observable contraction, movement of the appropriate joint, needle activity in the muscle—may be used to identify the activity of a specific muscle at all levels of effort.[14] Our finding is limited by two factors, electrode placement and the posture of nearby joints, both of which appear, in part, to determine waveform duration, but neither of which offers serious problems for a waveform methodology.

In application, the waveform finding makes it possible not only to identify, but also to train the activity of a specific muscle using the surface EMG: the same on-line waveform display which provides the experimenter with a "continuous" validator of the muscle potential

---

[14] Our finding does not apply to most needle recordings. Although the mean duration of needle potentials does differ from muscle to muscle, and is stable for a given muscle at weak and strong effort, it must be determined from at least twenty different locations, since the individual durations from placements within the same muscle may differ by a factor of five or more (Buchtal, 1957).

record can also provide the subject with a unique form of augmented feedback. Unlike most feedback stimuli, the waveform display can tell the subject both about response magnitude (waveform amplitude) and about response topography (waveform duration). Or, when the sensitivity of the vertical amplifier is adjusted to compensate for magnitude changes, the display can convey topographical information alone. Feedback of this sort is useful when the object is to generate a full-scale performance through development of its miniature counterpart. For example, by training subjects to make increasingly higher amplitude versions of the adductive and abductive waveforms taken from the hypothenar eminence, we were able to teach them to make overt movements of the fifth finger, in some cases without their observation of the response.

In this study, the active electrodes were placed as in Fig. 4, but additional dummy electrodes were placed on both hands to confuse the subject about the actual recording site. The EMG was fed back to the subject on a slave oscilloscope triggered in real time by the hypothenar waveforms (cf. Fig. 5). After the shapes and characteristic durations of the short and long waveforms were described to the subject, he was asked to watch for their occurrence on the slave oscilloscope. With the display magnification at nearly 10^6, low-amplitude waveforms, representing single motor unit responses, were quickly obtained. These were pointed out to the subject—"that's it; good"—and he was encouraged to make them, and to learn to produce one duration and then the other on command.[15] With about half an hour of practice, most subjects came to control both types of waveforms. Although able to stop and start waveform production upon command, the subjects could not report how they did this. When asked how they controlled the response, five of the fifteen subjects made no association at all with the fifth finger.

These five subjects were then selected for further study. They were given waveform displays of progressively lower magnification, and were instructed to "do the same thing, only more so" in order to maintain a constant waveform display on the slave oscilloscope. In this way, the subjects were gradually trained to make short and long waveforms of increasingly greater amplitudes. Although they had never been instructed to move the fifth finger, the subjects each came to make visible inward and outward movements of the finger during the production of high amplitude short and long waveforms, respectively, and most

---

[15] The procedure will be recognized as a variant of that used by Harrison and Mortenson (1962) and by Basmajian (1963). For an extensive review of motor unit training, see Basmajian (1967), pp. 103–115.

subjects eventually became aware of the finger movements. However, in a post-session interview, one still had nothing to report about the fifth finger, and another reported only that the finger "felt nervous".

Of course, the inability of some subjects to report verbally on what, in fact, were gross excursions of the finger was an incidental result stemming from our attempt to subvert the subject's tendency to self-instruction. The main result was the development of specific overt responses through feedback training based on the waveform parameters of the surface EMG. The result emphasizes, we think, the potential usefulness of the waveform technique both in therapeutic applications, where the object may be to develop or refine a specific muscular performance, and in psychological applications, where the study of set, of motor theory, and of response bias may call for the ability to control and to identify the covert and overt forms of an isolated response.

REFERENCES

ADRIAN, E. D. and BRONK, D. W. 1929. The discharge of impulses in motor nerve fibres. *J. Physiol* **67,** 119–151.

BASAMAJIAN, J. V. 1963. Control and training of individual motor units. *Science* **141,** 440–441.

BASAMAJIAN, J. V. 1967. *Muscles alive: their functions revealed by electromyography.* Williams & Wilkins, Baltimore.

BEKHTEREV, V. M. 1913. *Objective Psychologie.* Teubner, Leipzig and Berlin.

BICKFORD, R. G., GALBRAITH, R. F., and JACOBSON, J. L. 1963. The nature of the average evoked potentials from the human scalp. *Electroenceph. Clin. Neurophysiol.* **15,** 922.

BICKFORD, R. G., JACOBSON, J. L., and CODY, D. T. R. 1964. Nature of average evoked potentials to sound and other stimuli in man. *Ann. N.Y. Acad. Sci.* **112,** 204–223.

BIRCH, J. D. 1964. Differentiation of response characteristics during multiple fixed ratio extinction. *Psychol. Rep.* **15,** 495–502.

BLACK, A. H. 1965. Cardiac conditioning in curarized dogs: the relationship between heart rate and skeletal behavior. In W. F. Prokasy, (Ed.), *Classical conditioning.* Appleton-Century-Crofts, New York.

BLACK, A. H. 1967. Transfer following operant conditioning in the curarized dog. *Science,* **155,** 201–203.

BRASH, J. C. (Ed.), 1951. *Cunningham's text-book of anatomy.* Oxford Univ. Press, London.

BROWN, P. L. 1968. Auto-shaping and observing responses (R_0) in the pigeon. *Proc. 76 Annu. Conv., APA,* 139–140.

BROWN, P. L. and JENKINS, H. M. 1968. Auto-shaping of the pigeon's key peck. *J. exp. Anal. Behav.* **11,** 1–8.

BRUNO, L. J. J. 1968. Unpublished observations.

BUCHTAL, F. 1957. *An introduction to electromyography.* Scandinavian Univ. Books, Copenhagen.

DAVIDOWITZ, J. 1963. Termainal report. NIMH post-doctoral fellowship MH-17827.
DAVIS, R. C. 1940. Set and muscular tension. *Ind. Univ. Sci. Ser.* No. 10.
DAVIS, R. C. 1948a. Motor effects of strong auditory stimuli. *J. exp. Psychol.* **38** 257–275.
DAVIS, R. C. 1948b. Responses to "meaningful" and "meaningless" sounds. *J. exp. Psychol.* **38**, 744–756.
DAVIS, R. C. 1950. Motor responses to auditory stimuli above and below threshold. *J. exp. Psychol.* **40**, 107–120.
DAVIS, R. C. 1952. The stimulus trace in effectors and its relation to judgement responses. *J. exp. Psychol.* **44**, 377–390.
DAVIS, R. C. 1957. Response patterns. *Trans. N.Y. Acad. Sci.* **19**, 731–739.
DAVIS, R. C. and BUCHWALD, A. M. 1957. An exploration of somatic response patterns: stimulus and sex differences. *J. comp. physiol. Psychol.* **50**, 44–52.
DAVIS, R. C., BUCHWALD, A. M., and FRANKMANN, R. W. 1955. Autonomic and muscular responses and their relation to simple stimuli. *Psychol. Monogr.* **69**, No. 405.
DAVIS, R. C. and VAN LIERE, D. W. 1949. Adaptation of the muscular tension response to gunfire. *J. exp. Psychol.* **39**, 114–117.
DAWSON, H. E. and DAVIS, R. C. 1957. The effects of an instructed motor response upon somatic responses to a brief tone. *J. comp. physiol. Psychol.* **50**, 368–374.
DOEHRING, D. G. 1957. Conditioning of muscle action potentials resulting from passive hand movement. *J. exp. Psychol.* **54**, 292–296.
FESTINGER, L., BURNHAM, C. A., ONO, H., and BAMBER, D. 1967. Efference and the conscious experience of perception. *J. exp. Psychol. Monogr.* **74**, No. 637.
FESTINGER, L. and KIRKPATRICK, C. 1965. Information about spatial location based on knowledge about efference. *Psychol. Rev.* **72**, 373–384.
FETZ, E. E. 1969. Operant conditioning of cortical unit activity. *Science* **163**, 955–958.
FINK, J. B. and DAVIS, R. C. 1951. Generalization of a muscle action potential response to tonal duration. *J. exp. Psychol.* **42**, 403–409.
GOLDBERG, I. A. 1959. Relations of response variability in conditioning and extinction. Unpublished doctoral dissertation, Columbia Univ.
GRANT, D. A. 1964. Classical and instrumental conditioning. In A. W. Melton (Ed.), *Categories of human learning*. Academic Press, New York.
HARDYCK, C. D., PETRINOVICH, L. F., and ELLSWORTH, D. W. 1966. Feedback of speech muscle activity during silent reading: rapid extinction. *Science* **154**, 1467–1468.
HARRISON, V. F. and MORTENSON, O. A. 1962. Identification and voluntary control of single motor unit activity in the tibialis anterior muscle. *Anat. Rec.* **144**, 109–116.
HEFFERLINE, R. F. 1958. The role of proprioception in the control of behavior. *Trans. N.Y. Acad. Sci.* **20**, 739–764.
HEFFERLINE, R. F. and KEENAN, B. 1961. Amplitude-induction gradient of a small human operant in an escape-avoidance situation. *J. exp. Anal. Behav.* **4**, 41–43.
HEFFERLINE, R. F. and KEENAN, B. 1963. Amplitude-induction gradient of a small-scale (covert) operant. *J. exp. Anal. Behav.* **6**, 307–315.
HEFFERLINE, R. F., KEENAN, B., and HARFORD, R. A. 1959. Escape and avoidance conditioning in human subjects without their observation of the response. *Science*, **130**, 1338–1339.

HEFFERLINE, R. F. and PERERA, T. B. 1963. Proprioceptive discrimination of a covert operant without its observation by the subject. *Science* **139**, 834–835.
HERRICK, R. M. 1963. Lever displacement during continuous reinforcement and during a discrimination. *J. comp. physiol. Psychol.* **56**, 700–707.
HERRICK, R. M. 1964a. Lever displacement during a discrimination differentiation. *J. comp. physiol. Psychol.* **57**, 139–146.
HERRICK, R. M. 1964b. The successive differentiation of a lever displacement response. *J. exp. Anal. Behav.* **7**, 211–215.
HILDEN, A. H. 1937. An action current study of the conditioned hand withdrawal. *Psychol. Monogr.* **49**, No. 217.
HOLLINSHEAD, W. H. 1960. *Functional anatomy of the limbs and back*. 2nd ed. Saunders, Philadelphia.
HUNTER, W. S. 1937. Muscle potentials and conditioning in the white rat. *J. exp. Psychol.* **21**, 611–624.
IRWIN, R. J., ELAMPIED, N. M., and DOUGLAS, B. 1967. Estimates of flicker can be taught. *Psychon. Sci.* **9**, 479–480.
JACOBSON, E. 1932. Electrophysiology of mental activities. *Amer. J. Psychol.* **44**, 677–694.
KATZMAN, R. 1964. The validity of the evoked response in man. *Ann. N.Y. Acad. Sci.* **112**, 238–240.
KIMBLE, G. A. 1961. *Hilgard and Marquis' conditioning and learning*. 2nd ed. Appleton-Century-Crofts, New York.
LACEY, J. I., BATEMAN, D. E., and VAN LEHN, R. 1953. Autonomic response specificity: an experimental study. *Psychosom. Med.* **16**, 8–21.
LACEY, J. I. and LACEY, B. C. 1958. Verification and extension of the principle of autonomic response-stereotypy. *Amer. J. Psychol.* **71**, 50–73.
LANDIS, C. and HUNT, W. A. 1939. *The startle pattern*. Farrar & Rinehart, New York.
LIDDELL, H. S. 1934. The conditioned reflex. In F. A. Moss (Ed.), *Comparative psychology*. Prentice Hall, New York.
LIPPOLD, O. C. J. 1967. Electromyography. In P. H. Venables and Irene Martin, (Eds.), *A manual of psychophysiological methods*. Wiley, New York. Pp. 245–297.
LUSCHEI, E., SASLOW, C., and GLICKSTEIN, M. 1967. Muscle potentials in reaction time. *Exp. Neurol.* **18**, 429–442.
LYNN, R. 1966. *Attention, arousal and the orientation reaction*. Pergamon, New York.
McMILLAN, D. E. and PATTON, R. A. 1965. Differentiation of a precise timing response. *J. exp. Anal. Behav.* **8**, 219–226.
MALMO, R. B., SHAGASS, C., and DAVIS, F. H. 1950. Specificity of bodily reactions under stress: a physiological study of somatic symptom mechanisms in psychiatric patients. *Res. Publ. Assoc. nerv. ment. Dis.* **29**, 231–261.
MARGULIES, S. 1961. Response duration in operant level, regular reinforcement, and extinction. *J. exp. Anal. Behav.* **4**, 317–321.
MERTON, P. A. 1964. Human position sense and sense of effort. In *Symposia of the Society for Experimental Biology*. Number XVIII. *Homeostasis and feedback mechanisms*. Cambridge University Press.
MILLER, N. E. 1969. Learning of visceral and glandular responses. *Science* **163**, 434–445.
MOORE, A. U. and MARCUSE, F. L. 1945. Salivary, cardiac, and motor indices of conditioning in two sows. *J. comp. Psychol.* **38**, 1–16.
NORRIS, F. H. 1963. *The EMG*. Grune & Stratton, New York.

NOTTERMAN, J. M. and MINTZ, D. E. 1965. *Dynamics of response*. Wiley, New York.
NOTTERMAN, J. M., SCHOENFELD, W. N., and BERSH, P. J. 1952. Conditioned heart rate responses in human beings during experimental anxiety. *J. comp. physiol. Psychol.* **45**, 1–8.
PAVLOV, I. P. 1927. *Conditioned reflexes*. (Translated by G. V. Anrep.) Oxford University Press, London.
RAPIN, I. 1964. Evoked responses to clicks in a group of children with communication disorders. *Ann. N.Y. Acad. Sci.* **112**, 182–203.
SCHOENFELD, W. N. 1966. Some old work for modern conditioning theory. *Cond. Reflex* **1**, 219–223.
SCHOENFELD, W. N. and CUMMING, W. W. 1963. Behavior and perception. In S. Koch (Ed.), *Psychology: a study of a science*. Vol. 5. McGraw-Hill, New York. Pp. 213–252.
SIDMAN, M. and FLETCHER, F. G. 1968. A demonstration of auto-shaping with monkeys. *J. exp. Anal. Behvav.* **11**, 307–309.
SKINNER, B. F. 1938. *The behavior of organisms*. Appleton-Century, New York.
SKINNER, B. F. 1948. "Superstition" in the pigeon. *J. exp. Psychol.* **38**, 168–172.
SOKOLOV, E. N. 1963a. Higher nervous functions: the orienting reflex. *Ann. Rev. Physiol.* **25**, 545–580.
SOKOLOV, E. N. 1963b. *Perception and the conditioned reflex*. Macmillan, New York.
SPERRY, R. W. 1952. Neurology and the mind-brain problem. *Amer. Scient.* **40**, 291–312.
STEVENS, S. S. 1961. The psychophysics of sensory function. In W. A. Rosenblith (Ed.), *Sensory communication*. M.I.T. Press and Wiley, New York.
STEVENS, S. S. and GALANTER, E. H. 1957. Ratio scales and category scales for a dozen perceptual continua. *J. exp. Psychol.* **54**, 377–411.
TAUB, E. and BERMAN, A. J. 1968. Movement and learning in the absence of sensory feedback. In S. J. Freedman (Ed.), *The neuropsychology of spatially oriented behavior*. Dorsey, Homewood, Illinois.
TERRACE, H. S. 1963. Errorless transfer of a discrimination across two continua. *J. exp. Anal. Behav.* **6**, 223–232.
THORNDIKE, E. L. 1911. *Animal intelligence*. Macmillan, New York.
VAN LIERE, D. W. 1953. Characteristics of the muscle tension response to paired tones. *J. exp. Psychol.* **46**, 319–324.
WHATMORE, G. B. 1968. Dysponesis: a neurophysiologic factor in functional disorders. *Behav. Sci.* **13**, 102–124.
WOODWORTH, R. S. and SCHLOSBERG, H. 1954. *Experimental psychology*. rev. ed. Holt, New York.
WYCKOFF, L. B. 1952. The role of observing responses in discrimination learning. Part I. *Psychol. Rev.* **59**, 431–442.
ZEAMAN, D. and SMITH, R. W. 1965. Review and analysis of some recent findings in human cardiac conditioning. In W. F. Prokasy (Ed.),*Classical conditioning*. Appleton-Century-Crofts, New York. Pp. 378–418.

Discussion

CONNOLLY: In speaking of one of your earlier experiments you mentioned you had used a fading technique, having established control, I think, by using a simple auditory signal. When you fade out the auditory signal do you begin to get errors as well as correct responses?

HEFFERLINE: There were no errors. So far as the subject was concerned it was as if the situation was exactly the same except that he was having to work a little harder to hear the signals.

CONNOLLY: Were the signals presented at regular time intervals?

HEFFERLINE: No, this couldn't be the case since we had to wait for the subject himself to initiate the sequence. It was his thumb-twitch, made without his knowledge at irregular intervals, which gave the experimenter his visual cue on the oscilloscope to present the tone as quickly as he could. He did this for 500 instances before slightly modifying the procedure. Now, for four additional sessions of 500 instances each, he delayed presentation of the tone until he saw on the second trace of the dual-beam oscilloscope activity which indicated the subject's anticipatory readiness to press the key after his thumb had twitched. If he saw such activity, the experimenter immediately presented the tone and recorded a "hit". If, on the other hand, he saw no such activity within two seconds, he recorded a "miss".

INGRAM: Was the 2 seconds period arbitrary?

HEFFERLINE: Yes, in order to test for the development of the discriminatory property of the response in the key-pressing muscle, we had to determine first of all the operant level for both the thumb-twitch and a similarly minute response of the key-pressing muscle. It so happened that each of these occurred with a frequency of about 600 per hour, or about once every 6 seconds, with their emission completely independent of each other. To demonstrate that the thumb-twitch was coming to serve as a discriminative stimulus for the incipient key-press, the latter had to follow the former within a stipulated time with significantly increasing frequency. This, of course, is what did take place. Interestingly, however, the overall number of responses, either in the thumb or the key-pressing muscle, did not increase in the course of the experiment. The training effect consisted of a bunching of occurrences of the small response in the key-pressing muscle right after occurrences of the thumb-twitch. You get the twitches occurring at various levels, and you also get twitches in the key-pressing muscles at intervals. So what one has to do is determine the operant level for both and then one can work with a change in how they are timed and a change in frequency. In this way it is possible to determine that the response is occurring as a result of a proprioceptive stimulus, rather than simply reflecting the operant level. Interestingly enough in this situation we did get a grouping of the responses, so that they came closer together, but the overall number of responses, either in the thumb or the key-pressing muscles, was not increased during the experiment. It was simply a re-grouping before they occurred.

BRUNER: Generally when we speak about skill there are two properties to it which are very important. One of them is that basically a set of discrete, small reactions are put into a larger pattern. Secondly, that larger pattern is somehow related to an objective in the environment, approach to which, or recession from which, provides different signals that make possible a basis for correction. Now in these experiments what you do basically is to detach a specific part of a larger reaction pattern. You have something similar, I think, to a fractionation procedure; you are picking out small responses which are usually part of larger patterns, and the response is divorced from an object or from some form of environmental dependent with which it is in contact. Now, in what way does this relate to skill? It seems that it has to do with skill inasmuch as you would have to get control of this very fine-grained response in order to adjust the requirements, for example, that are involved in things like threading a needle. You have to get control of things like the adductor response. Yet in this situation there is a relationship between the response and some object in the environment. You are trying to get a thread through a hole. Basically this has to do with emitting a response, which I think is the abiding trouble with all kinds of motor theories that do not specify anything about the relationship between a movement and the environment. It suspends an organism in some kind of an indifferent environment, and gives you not really responses but movements. This is my dilemma, I wonder if you could clarify how you see the relationship of this to the problem of skill regulation.

HEFFERLINE: I certainly agree with you that many of the things psychologists have their subjects do are rather arbitrary and artificial, but so, you might argue, are many of the things that the child is taught to do in the very process of socialization. But I don't believe it is at all appropriate to speak of responses being fractionated in the studies I have described. The responses are simply very small, too small to have any direct effect upon the external environment, including the experimenter's eyes, but they can be made to have very large effects through the mediation of amplification and display.

In our studies of these small responses there was always some environmental consequence which was made contingent on their occurrence, such as the elimination of an environmental noise or the sight of a numerical increase on an illuminated scoreboard. This is a clear indication of the trainability of such responses in their own right and not simply as components of a larger or more complex response. However, one of the potential applications of this technique is that in terms of your own hierarchical notion of skills it may well provide a way of building up the constituent parts of a complex skill by effectively welding together the underlying substrata of behaviour. The approach may be particularly useful in cases of mal-development or delayed development where you are able to give a child, for instance, external indications of internal happenings.

Basmajian is using such an approach in treating children with residual motor weaknesses. One of the big problems in such conditions is to motivate the children to work, since ordinarily there is so little to show for their effort. The amplified display on the other hand, gives clear cut evidence of work performed and improvement accomplished. Seeing one's muscle potentials or hearing them is tremendously reinforcing to young and old alike. If you give instructions on what is a desirable change to have appear on the oscilloscope, individuals will work and work to bring this about.

Later a subject may be able to produce the effect without the external feedback. If you urge him to tell you how he manages to do this, he is likely to say something like, "Well, I just have to get into exactly the position I was in when I did it before." Or some may say, "I just think how it looked on the 'scope the last time I saw it, and then lo and behold there it is."

KAY: This has been very enlightening for me. Annett (1959, *Quart. J. exp. Psychol.*, **11**, 3) published some experiments which were similar to the kind of things which you have been describing. These were training studies in which he was trying to teach subjects to exert a particular pressure on a rigid bar. The subject could see what he was doing by watching a display of his response on an oscilloscope. When given visual feedback the subject learned to make the response accurately and quickly, but when visual feedback was withdrawn the response promptly deteriorated.

HEFFERLINE: What were the instructions?

KAY: Subjects were asked to learn to exert a precise pressure on the handle of a plunger. Under certain trial conditions this meant that the spot on the oscilloscope moved to a particular target area and the subject could see it as he exerted the pressure. Learning was poor under these conditions and better when visual feedback was given *after* making the response.

HEFFERLINE: You may get quick deterioration such as this in teaching pigeons a complex discrimination. But you can get them to hold their gains if you use the right technique.

CONNOLLY: Are you referring to a carefully designed fading programme here?

HEFFERLINE: Yes, that's right.

BRUNER: It seems to me that the crucial point which came out strongly in Hefferline's report is the fantastic amount of potential signalling from which we could select. Probably we don't know the range of channels it could be tuned into, principally because we are trying to get rid of information rather than utilize the information which is available. We have the overload problem. What you have shown here is that there is a new range of combinations and new signals which can be used.

CONNOLLY: In the case of Annett's experiment, it is important to appreciate exactly what he was requiring the subject to do. He was asking subjects to "make a pressure". When they have visual feedback one can only expect them to use it since it is a very powerful form of feedback. It does not seem surprising to me therefore that once you take the visual feedback away the response deteriorates. The subject tries to perform the task as well as he can and of course uses the most effective form of feedback which is available to him. He does not pay any attention to less veridical forms of information feedback or less readily accessible forms of feedback. It seems to me that this is just where operant techniques come in again because one can make use of them, in principle at least, to shift control from one modality to another. That is, to shift control from visual feedback to proprioceptive feedback.

PRECHTL: It is very important to differentiate between posture and movement, when you press something constantly this is posture. Not long ago I tried to find out how fast I could fire a single motor unit, having an EMG-needle in the anterior tibial muscle. The anterior tibial muscle makes more gross movements than fine movements and in voluntary contractions I was nowhere able to fire one single unit faster than ten per second. As soon as the frequency came above this another unit came in. I did the same with a thumb adductor and was able to go to twelve per second. Then I thought, if I use pressure so that I have tactile feedback as well, then I can speed up my single motor unit activity. That was wrong. The other thing is that, when you flex your elbow at a certain speed the movement is completely smooth. When the movement is fast you get a ballistic line. As soon as you want to move slowly then the movement becomes discontinuous and the line is wavy (Fig. 9). In fact, you can never make this slow movement really smooth (Fortuyn and Gramsbergen, *Europ. Neurol.* in press).

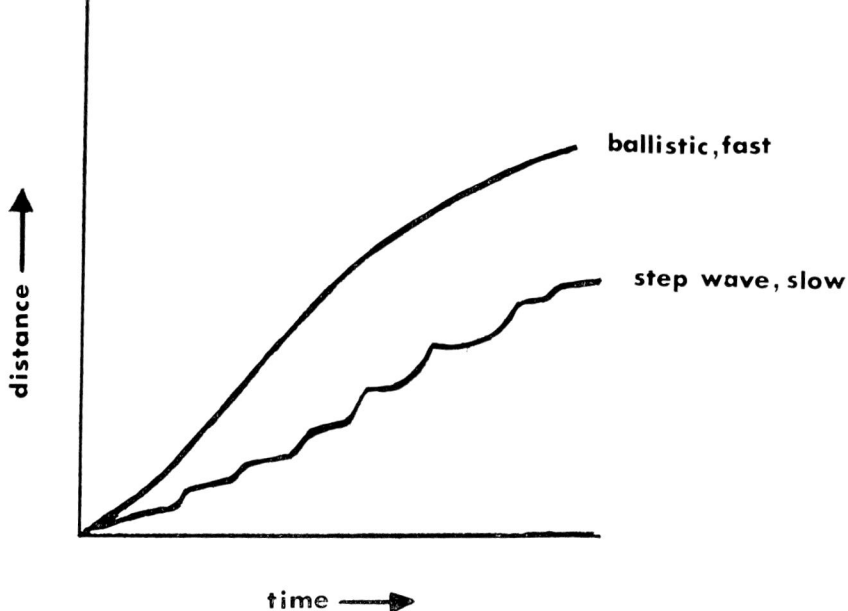

FIG. 9. The nature of fast and slow movements.

CONNOLLY: Did you put the needle electrode right into the muscle?
PRECHTL: This is a concentric bipolar needle electrode; in the muscle—yes.
BRUNER: You get exactly the same thing in the turning of the head, if you turn your head slowly you come up with a step wave.
PRECHTL: Yes, you do the same with the eyes.
HEFFERLINE: The twitches occur apart from simply "wanting to make a slow movement". They occur in subjects who, so far as they know, are doing nothing at all, in fact, even when they are asleep.
TWITCHELL: Can I just get myself clear about these twitches? They were twitches on the oscilloscope—right?
HEFFERLINE: Yes, the twitch is invisible to the subject but we make it visible ourselves by amplifying it on an oscilloscope.
LEFFORD: I have always been fascinated by people who can separate their small finger or their middle fingers apart, who can waggle their ears, and who can levate their nostrils. I trained myself to do two of these, but I cannot waggle my ears. I wonder if there is some sort of heightened awareness about feeling certain parts of the body.
HEFFERLINE: If you want to waggle your ears, come around to my lab

when we get back to New York and for a small fee we will train you.
LEFFORD: If I had visual feedback I am sure it could be done. It seems to me that the critical thing is getting in contact with the appropriate proprioceptors.
HEFFERLINE: It doesn't have to be conscious though, you simply have to have feedback, auditory, visual or some such.
CONNOLLY: I taught myself to waggle my ears by looking in the mirror when I was a small boy.
BRUNER: Do you recall how you did it?
CONNOLLY: Not really, originally I think it involved moving the whole of my scalp, and then eventually refining it down until I was just moving my ears. I suppose it was some kind of shaping procedure that I was doing.

Animal Studies

The Development of Bird Song

ROBERT A. HINDE

University of Cambridge

SOME OF THE most interesting work on the development of motor skills in animals has come from the study of bird song. Although it may be regarded as a special case in that it lacks orientation to the environment, bird song involves a motor output which, though often complex, is readily subject to analysis by sound spectrographic techniques. In addition, its development can be studied under relatively well-controlled conditions. For the most part I have myself been associated only indirectly with the study of bird song: this paper will review the work of a number of investigators—particularly Thorpe, Marler and their colleagues.

While in some cases the species-characteristic song develops in birds raised under conditions of auditory isolation, in others exposure to the specific song is necessary for normal song development. One of the most intensively studied species is the chaffinch (*Fringilla coelebs*), and it is convenient first to review briefly the findings on this species (Thorpe, 1961):

(i) The characteristic song lasts about 2·5 seconds, ranges from 2 to 6 kHz, and consists of three phrases usually of successively lower frequency, each consisting of several notes, followed by a terminal flourish. Each individual has a repertoire of several songs, differing in their details (Fig. 1a).

(ii) The song develops from a rambling subsong of indefinite length by progressive omission of extreme frequencies and approximation towards the normal pattern (Fig. 2).

(iii) Individuals hand-reared in isolation from other individuals develop only a single form of the song which is not divided into phrases (Fig. 1b).

(iv) Chaffinches hand-reared in groups, but isolated from normal

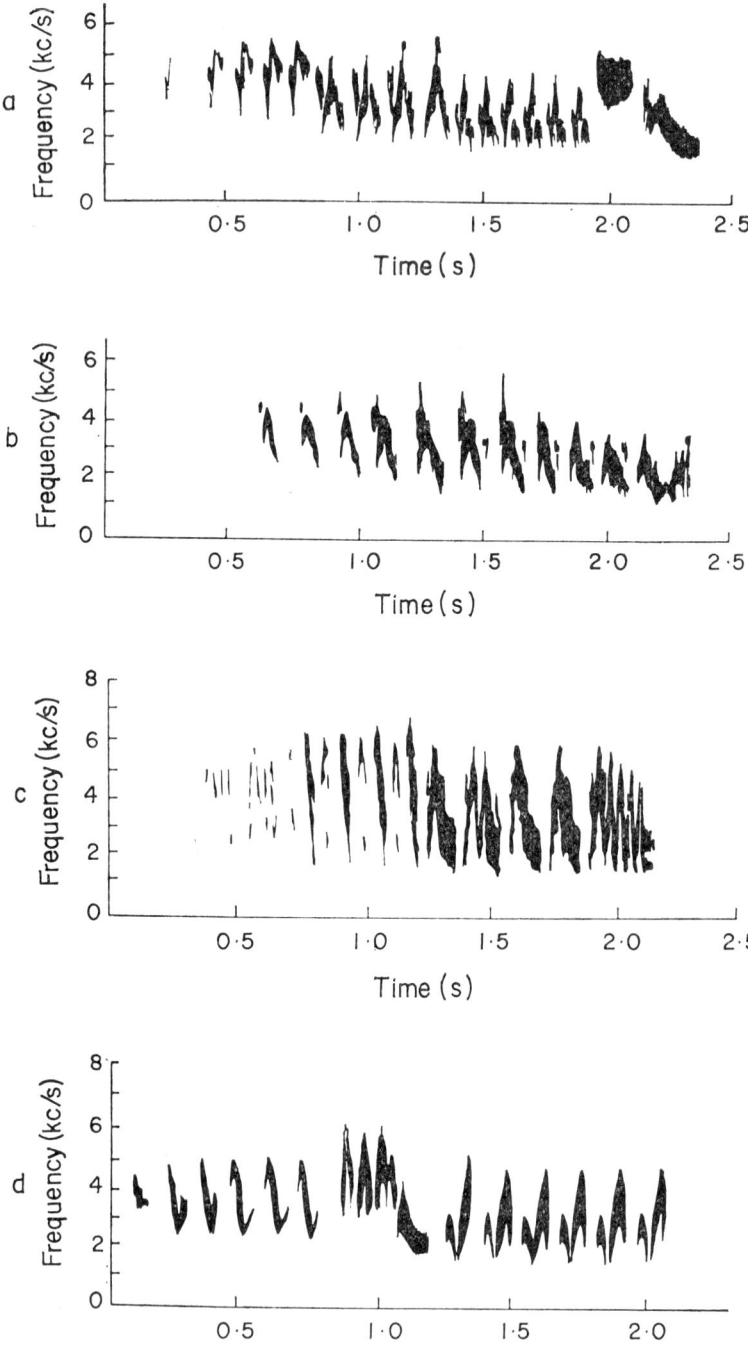

FIG. 1. (a) Characteristic normal song; (b) song of an individual reared in isolation; (c) song of an individual from a group reared in isolation; (d) song produced by a bird reared in isolation after tutoring with a disarticulated chaffinch song with the ending in the middle. (After Thorpe. 1961. Reprinted with permission of the Cambridge University Press, London.)

THE DEVELOPMENT OF BIRD SONG 289

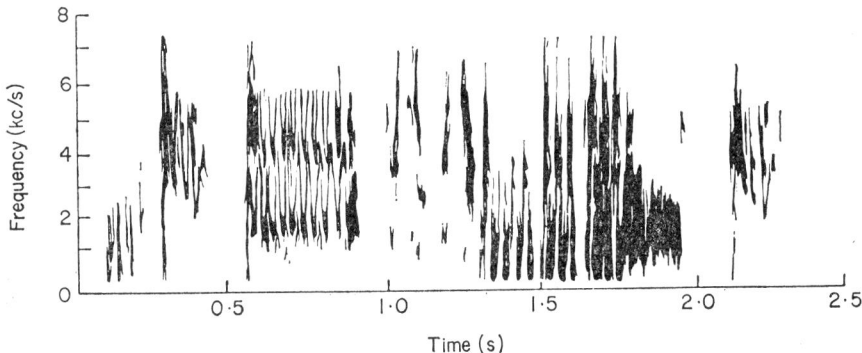

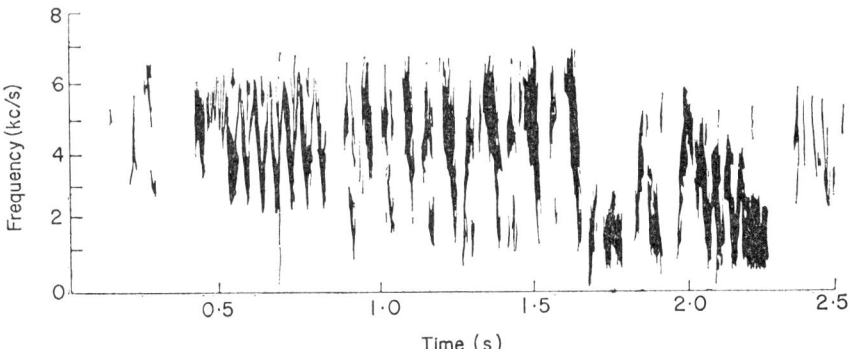

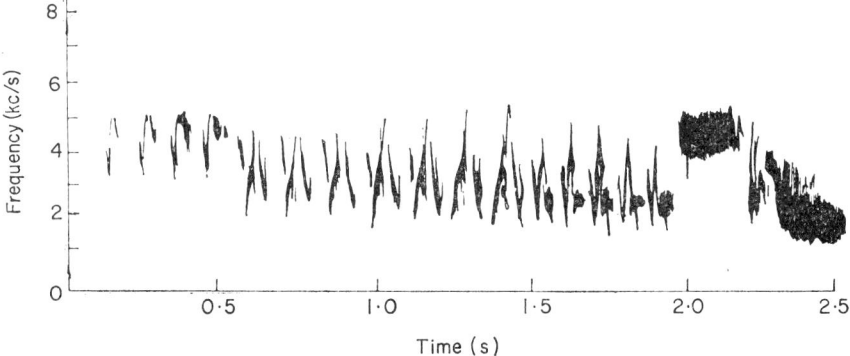

FIG. 2. Three successive stages in the development of full-song from sub-song in the chaffinch. (After Thorpe, 1961. Reprinted with permission of the Cambridge University Press, London.)

song, develop songs more elaborate than those of individuals reared in isolation. The songs are similar within groups, but differ between groups: the indication is that learning occurs within each group (Fig. 1c).

(v) Individuals trapped in their first autumn and kept in isolation thereafter develop songs more or less within the normal range. The difference between these birds and those hand-reared from an early age, (iii) above, indicates an effect of experience during the first few months of life, long before the birds themselves begin to sing.

(vi) Chaffinches caught in their first autumn and kept subsequently in groups develop group songs just like those of wild birds. The difference between these birds and the autumn-caught isolates, (v) above, indicates the importance of experience during the period of song development: this probably occurs in the course of countersinging.

(vii) Hand-reared isolates, exposed to tape recordings of chaffinch song during their first autumn and winter, subsequently produce near-normal songs. Such birds will not learn anything which is played to them. A chaffinch song played backwards, or with the end in the middle (Fig. 1d), is imitated, but an artificial chaffinch song with notes of pure tonal quality is not. The wider range of sounds in the subsong shows that the restriction in what they will learn is not a matter of the range of sounds which the bird's own syrinx can produce; Thorpe suggested that the criterion may be a resemblance in note-structure to normal chaffinch song.

(viii) Chaffinches isolated from their first autumn are more restricted in what they will learn when tutored in this way. They will not learn reversed or re-articulated song, but are affected by hearing normal chaffinch song. The greater selectivity of these birds, as compared with the hand-reared isolates, must be due to experience before they themselves started to sing.

(ix) Once a chaffinch has acquired its repertoire of songs in its first breeding season, little further change takes place.

These results indicate that song development depends on experience at two periods of the life history—early on, before the bird itself has started to sing; and in the first spring, in the course of countersinging with other individuals. One possibility is that the effect of early experience is to increase the reinforcing effectiveness of song. On this view, the development of full song from subsong would be due to the reinforcing value to the bird of hearing itself sing the full song. Two predictions would follow from this:

(i) Deafening the bird after it had experienced song, but before it started to sing itself, would make it impossible for the bird to monitor its own output and thus would nullify the effects of the early experience.

(ii) Since reinforcers are usually effective for a wide variety of responses, any reinforcing effects of hearing song on singing should also operate for other responses.

Both of these predictions have been confirmed. We may consider first the effect of deafening (Konishi and Nottebohm, 1969). Chaffinches which have already developed their songs before deafening maintain them subsequently, relatively unaltered. The effects of deafening before song has fully developed depend on the time of the operation: the earlier the stage of song development, the greater its effects. Individuals deafened at about 100 days of age, who had heard no chaffinch calls other than their own nestling, fledgling and perhaps juvenile calls, subsequently produced only very unstructured and rudimentary songs. Birds deafened in their first winter, with some previous experience of subsong, produced songs with syllables more like those of wild birds, but of considerable simplicity. Birds deafened during full song development produced songs much nearer the wild type; but even if the operation was performed after several days of practising the full song—though before it had reached its final stereotyped form—the song subsequently underwent considerable deterioration which was not reversed by testosterone therapy (Nottebohm, 1967).

These experiments thus showed that the effects of deafening depend on the stage of vocal development at which the operation occurs; there was also strong evidence that sound patterns developed before the loss of hearing may be incorporated, perhaps in a modified form, into the full song. Song development is thus a gradual integrative process, intimately bound up with the development of other vocalizations (Nottebohm, 1967).

We may now turn to the second prediction—that song should serve as a reinforcer for other responses. Stevenson (1969) tested this with chaffinches left in cages containing three transverse perches. The two end-perches operated microswitches, which in turn operated counters: in addition, that end-perch which had been the less preferred during preceding preliminary observations could operate a tape-loop which played a single chaffinch song. Distribution of perching between the two end-perches during stimulus conditions in which every fifth or sixth response to one of the end-perches did produce song, was compared with that during control conditions when perching was simply recorded. A reinforcing effect of song would be indicated by an increase in the proportion of responses to the active perch during the stimulus conditions.

As shown in Fig. 3, song was found to be a reinforcer for autumn-caught chaffinches treated with testosterone. A burst of white noise of similar duration and intensity did not show reinforcing properties. Furthermore, none of the eight chaffinches hand-reared in isolation from chaffinch song and tested without testosterone treatment, behaved as though song were a reinforcer. Hand-reared, testosterone-treated and autumn-caught, non-injected groups showed intermediate results. Thus two of the conditions upon which normal song development depends—experience of song and testosterone—also appear to affect the reinforcing effectiveness of song.

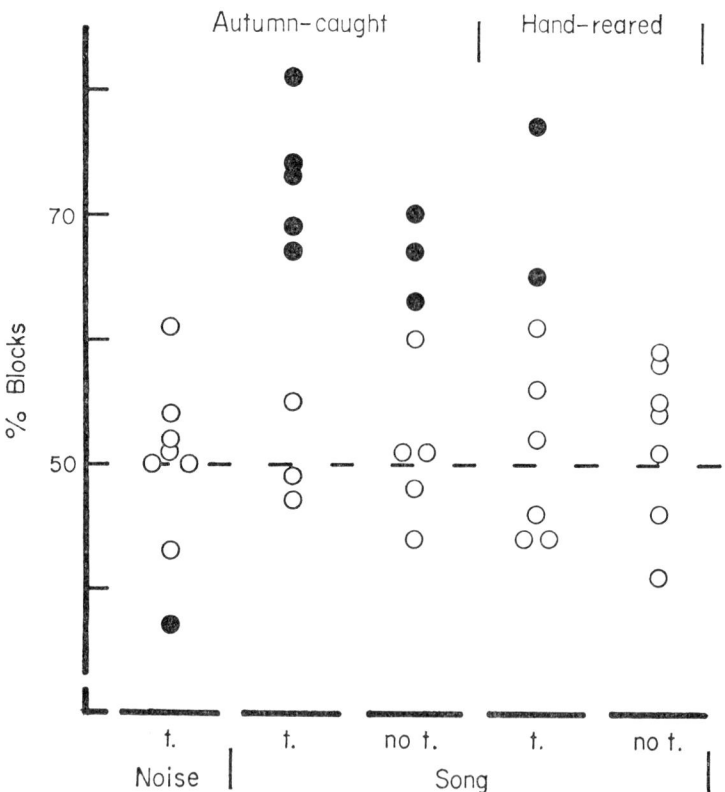

FIG. 3. Measures of the reinforcing effect of white noise or normal song for individual first-year male chaffinches. Ordinate: percentage of blocks of control and reinforcement conditions in which a reinforcing effect was shown. Filled circles indicate a significant effect (Sign test, two-tailed, $p < 0.05$), in either the positive or negative direction. Abscissa: t, testosterone-injected; *no-t*, in winter condition and not injected (from Stevenson, 1969. Reprinted with permission of the Cambridge University Press, London).

One way of relating all these findings is to suppose that song development involves a "model" or "template" which is influenced by experience—particularly experience of the species-characteristic vocalizations. Sounds which approximate to this model are reinforcing. Of course the postulation of a model is merely a device for tying together the experimental data: the corresponding physiological reality is quite another issue. However, it also permits us to relate song development to certain data concerning the elicitation of song in the adult: that song-type which is most frequent in each individual's repertoire is also the most effective in eliciting song from that individual. This suggests that sound patterns which approximate to the model are both reinforcing and effective in eliciting song (Hinde, 1958).

Studies of other passerine species have shown that song-learning occurs in a basically similar way in a number of other species, though in each the process has its own peculiarities. This literature has recently been reviewed by Konishi and Nottebohm (1969) and by Immelmann (1969): here a few points of special interest will be selected.

(i) *Restrictions on learning.* In the chaffinch the restriction on the sounds which will be imitated and incorporated into the full song seems to depend on their resemblance to normal chaffinch sounds. In other species there is a strong tendency to learn the song which the father sings. Bullfinches (*Pyrrhula pyrrhula*) reared by canaries develop a canary-like song and ignore the song of adult bullfinches kept in the same room (Nicolai, 1959). In the zebra finch there are preferences both for the father's song and for songs of the right tonal quality: if the two do not coincide, the former tends to predominate (Immelmann, 1969). In other species, a very wide range of sounds may be imitated (e.g. the meadow lark, *Sturnella magna* and *S. neglecta*; Lanyon, 1957).

(ii) *Sensitive period.* In the chaffinch, song learning is limited to a sensitive period which normally comes to an end when full song develops in the first breeding season. A bird not allowed to sing at that time by castration, did so later under the influence of testosterone therapy: thus the end of the sensitive period is not age-dependent, but depends on song development itself.

In other species, the sensitive period ends before the onset of full song. For instance the white-crowned sparrow (*Zonotrichia leucophrys*) has rather distinctive local dialects. Birds taken from the nest and reared in the laboratory develop song patterns which lack the characteristics of the local dialect. If they are brought in a few weeks later, their song develops normally and they develop the characteristics of the dialect of their own locality. In tutoring experiments, birds exposed to recordings of a particular dialect during the first weeks of life subsequently reproduce it, but birds brought into the laboratory after about 3 months of age cannot be taught a fresh dialect (Marler, 1967). Since the sensitive period during which white-crowned sparrows can learn a fresh dialect ends before they themselves start to sing, it cannot be ascribed to motor fixation, as in the chaffinch. Konishi and Nottebohm suggest that there are two sensitive periods, one for acquisition of the template and one for the motor learning; in the chaffinch the two coincide, but in other species they do not. In the zebra finch, which in this respect resembles the white-crowned sparrow, the different characteristics of the song can be affected at different ages. In this species singing starts at 35 to 40 days, and full song appears at 9 to 11 weeks. Tutoring before singing starts can affect the elements of the song, but the length and sequence of song elements and the rhythm can be affected between the fortieth and eightieth days of life.

(iii) *Effects of group-rearing.* Grouping of hand-raised chaffinches leads to the production of more elaborate song patterns than are produced by isolated individuals. No such effect occurs in white-crowned sparrows (Marler and Tamura, 1964), but group-reared Arizona juncos (*Junco phaenotus*) produce more complex syllables and larger repertoires than isolates. Such data suggest that stimulation received in the course of counter-singing in the group situation leads to greater "improvization". However, comparative evidence emphasizes the need for caution here: the Oregon junco (*Junco oreganus*), which in nature has a simpler song than the Arizona junco, produces more complex songs if reared in isolation than it does in nature. Individuals reared in isolated groups are more likely to produce near-normal songs than are the isolates: mutual stimulation thus serves to bring the course of development back to a normal pathway, rather than to produce further elaboration (Marler, 1967).

(iv) *Effects of deafening.* All passerine birds so far studied produce abnormal songs if deafened before the completion of song development. Particularly interesting results were obtained with white-crowned sparrows, where song development consists of two stages separated in time (see above). Normal song development depends on the young bird being exposed to the species song during part of its first 3 months of life; but during the period of motor development the bird does not have to hear the species song from any external source. Deafening after the sensitive period but before the onset of singing annuls the effect of the earlier experience (Konishi and Nottebohm, 1969).

(v) *Nature of the learning involved.* The first phase of song-learning fits neither the paradigm of classical conditioning, which involves the attachment of a response to a new stimulus, nor that of operant conditioning, which involves a change in response frequency as a consequence of reinforcement. In that it does not involve the response by which its occurrence is subsequently revealed, parallels can be found in studies of perceptual learning (e.g. Gibson, Walk and Tighe, 1959), discrimination learning (e.g. Sutherland, 1959; Mackintosh, 1964) and latent learning (e.g. MacCorquodale and Meehl, 1954; Thistlethwaite, 1951).

It will be apparent that the comparative study of song development provides material pertinent for a number of basic problems in developmental psychology.

REFERENCES

GIBSON, E. J., WALK, R. D., and TIGHE, T. J. 1959. Enhancement and deprivation of visual stimulation during rearing as factors in visual discrimination learning. *J. comp. physiol. Psychol.* **52**, 74–81.

HINDE, R. A. 1958. Alternative motor patterns in chaffinch song. *Anim. Behav.* **6**, 211–218.

HINDE, R. A. 1969. (Ed.), *Bird vocalisations in relation to current problems in biology and psychology*. Cambridge University Press.

IMMELMANN, K. 1969. Song development in the zebra finch and other estrildid finches. In R. A. Hinde (Ed.), *Bird vocalisation in relation to current problems in biology and psychology*. Cambridge University Press.

KONISHI, M. and NOTTEBOHM, F. 1969. Experimental studies in the ontogeny of avian vocalisations. In R. A. Hinde (Ed.), *Bird vocalisation in relation to current problems in biology and psychology*. Cambridge University Press.

LANYON, W. E. 1957. The comparative biology of the meadowlarks (*Sturnella*). *Wisconsin. Pub. Nuttal. Ornith. Club. No. 1*. Cambridge, Mass.

MACCORQUODALE, K. and MEEHL, P. E. 1954. Edward C. Tolman. In Estes *et al.* (Eds.), *Modern learning theory*. Appleton-Century-Crofts, New York.

MACKINTOSH, N. J. 1964. Selective attention in animal discrimination learning. *Psychol. Bull.* **64**, 124–150.

MARLER, P. 1967. Comparative study of song development in sparrows. *Proc. 14th Int. Ornith. Cong. Oxford*, 231–244.

MARLER, P. and TAMURA, M. 1964. Culturally transmitted patterns of vocal behavior in sparrows. *Science*, **146**, 1483–1486.

NICOLAI, J. 1959. Familientradition in der Gesangsentwicklung des Gimpels (*Pyrrhula pyrrhula L*). *J. Ornith.* **100**, 39–46.

NOTTEBOHM, F. 1967. The role of sensory feedback in the development of avian vocalizations. *Proc. 14th Int. Ornith. Cong. Oxford*. 265–280.

STEVENSON, J. G. 1969. Song as a reinforcer. In R. A. Hinde (Ed.), *Bird vocalization in relation to current problems in biology and psychology*. Cambridge University Press.

SUTHERLAND, N. S. 1959. Stimulus analysing mechanisms. In *Proc. sym. mechanization of thought processes*. Her Majesty's Stationery Office, London. 575–609.

THISTLETHWAITE, D. 1951. A critical review of latent learning and related experiments. *Psychol. Bull.* **48**, 97–129.
THORPE, W. H. 1961. *Bird song*. Cambridge University Press.

Discussion

INGRAM: I am interested in the imitations of different species and so on and I couldn't help wondering whether any efforts had been made to discriminate between the types of noise which affected the birds. You have rhythm, intonation, and combinations of rhythm and intonation, and so on. I should very much like to see the effects of reinforcing rhythmic patterns in birds which have been hand-reared for a period of time. Is anything known about this?
HINDE: There are two approaches to this. The first is to establish that not just any sound is a reinforcer, and this was done by finding a reinforcing effect of song, but not of white noise. The next stage is to explore what parameters of full song are reinforcing though in a sense I find this a bit dull. One would find that the important factor is the rhythm or the tonal structure or something.
INGRAM: I find it anything but dull. In children we knew the intonational and rhythmic patterns, certainly in the first 6 or 8 months of life, are far more important than the word sound-patterns.
BRUNER: How do you know that?
INGRAM: We know this by the reactions of the child to statements made by parents.
BRUNER: Yes, at that particular point, but what about later on? It may well be that you could produce retardation or failure to develop a phonology if you are not exposed to the linguistic community of words.
INGRAM: Yes, this tends to happen in children of deaf and dumb parents, doesn't it? Such children are certainly retarded unless they are put into nurseries early or circulate with other children.
CONNOLLY: Physiological responses can be more easily elicited in the human neonate with complex sounds than they can with pure tones.
INGRAM: Exactly. I should be very interested to know what the reinforcer is, whether it is tone or rhythm, or even volume. One is dealing with such a large number of variables. I don't think song exists; I think song comprises a large number of different variables. I would like now to study these variables.
HINDE: May I just say one other thing which is relevant to what you are saying? Falls (1969. In R. A. Hinde (Ed.), *Bird vocalisations in*

relation to current problems in biology and psychology. Cambridge University Press) in Canada has been doing this, not in the reinforcing situation, but in seeing what song a wild, territorial bird would respond to. He worked with birds whose songs could be relatively easily doctored on tape, and he played back to them songs doctored in different ways to see whether they responded. I don't remember all the details of this, but he found that there were certain characteristics of the song which were necessary to produce a response at all. In addition he found that there were other characteristics which were responsible for individual recognition of one bird by another. In these experiments he was of course asking about the eliciting effectiveness rather than the reinforcing effectiveness.

WHITE: What is the life span of the chaffinch?

HINDE: The expectation of life under natural conditions is probably about 18 months to 2 years. In captivity you can keep them alive for 8, 9, or even 10 years.

WHITE: It seems to be a very large chunk of the entire life span that we are talking about.

INGRAM: You mean all the birds are suffering from senile dementia?

WHITE: No, I mean I have been very impressed by the suddenness with which so many other things seem to develop, for example, the imprinting phenomenon.

HINDE: Yes, but this is normally a seasonally breeding bird. You can, by injecting them with testosterone, make them learn their songs in the autumn, whereas otherwise they would not sing until their first spring.

WHITE: In the wild, is there any difference in the rate at which they acquire their song? You have said that this can be altered to some extent by using testosterone. From what you said I am left with the impression that in the wild it takes quite a time, and there is a good deal of opportunity for variation. You see this long period seems to me to be in marked contrast to the acquisition of other skilled behaviours by animals. For example, in Held and Hein's (1963, *J. com. physiol. Psychol.* **56**, 872) work with kittens I think a brief period in the order of 12 minutes is enough to show some recovery of visually directed responding.

HINDE: The only experiment which gives a time, so far as I know, was that cited by Riesen (1961, *J. nerv. ment. Dis.* **132**, 21) where kittens showed visual placing after 5 hours of continuous practice of visuomotor co-ordination. In the zebra finch, which is a desert bird, and can breed when it is 80 days old, the total amount of time spent listening to song probably doesn't amount to more than 5 hours.

WHITE: Well I suppose Held has not published anywhere these findings on how long it takes the kitten to acquire ordinary co-ordination. And I suppose eye/paw co-ordination is a little more common to the natural repertoire of the kitten. But it is extraordinarily fast.

TWITCHELL: I thought it was a period of several hours. The kitten in the gondola, I do recall, recovered the reactions fairly rapidly, that is, in a few hours.

BRUNER: Was this the kitten fitted with a ruff around its neck?

TWITCHELL: In the case of that kitten it was about 12 hours for the guided response. You can get visually elicited extension however, almost immediately after the ruff has been removed.

BRUNER: It seems to me that what you are looking for basically is: is there a deep structure and a surface structure to bird song, such that they will respond to some fundamental aspect of it? The other point is variation. In this case you may look for some parallels in terms of how they learn. Do they learn some sort of deep internal structure first then learn variations on it? It certainly doesn't sound that way from the results that Hinde presented.

CONNOLLY: You said you could extend the sensitive period of song learning by injecting testosterone. Can you push it at the other end too, by various kinds of exposure perhaps to complex song patterns?

HINDE: The sensitive period has been extended by preventing the bird from coming into brooding condition in its first Spring. (Konish, M. and Nottebohm, F. 1969. In R. A. Hinde (Ed.), *Bird vocalisations in relation to current problems in biology and psychology*. Cambridge University Press).

CONNOLLY: Yes. You can do this in an imprinting experiment, it is possible to extend the sensitive period by isolating the bird and to shorten it by group-rearing. The sensitive period can also be manipulated by other variables.

HINDE: I don't think this is the case with respect to bird song. The clearest experiment is that with the white crown sparrows.

CONNOLLY: Following that sort of thing, what I was thinking of was what would happen if you presented these birds with something that was more complex. Off-hand I am not sure exactly what, but something which is both complex and has a structure to it. White noise, for example, would not fit what I have in mind. I am trying to get away from the reinforcement pattern here.

INGRAM: I was thinking the other way. I wonder what would happen if you presented them with something more simple, without the tonal variations, but with the rhythmic patterns. Or alternatively with the

tonal variation and without quite the same rhythmic pattern. You are asking the same question but in a different way I think.
CONNOLLY: I don't think I am. I am not quite so interested in what the components of song are, but whether or not one could produce a super-song.
HINDE: Why do you want to get away from the reinforcement?
CONNOLLY: Suppose one suggested that, for the bird, the problem is essentially one of utilizing its experiences to form some kind of cognitive structure. This structuring, which is presumably reflected by changes in the organization of the central nervous system in some way, will of course be a function of the experience which the bird has. There will be differences dependent upon whether the animal experiences a rich or an impoverished environment. Perhaps the optimal experience is its own, species characteristic, song. This is why I wonder whether or not there is a super-optimal one. Can one devise a sort of "prosthetic" song?
HINDE: There is a possibility here. There is a species of chaffinch, which lives on the Canary Islands, called the blue chaffinch. The adults of this species produce a song which is rather like the isolate song of the European chaffinch. This would be a very interesting species to play the European chaffinch song to: it may for them be a super song in your sense.
CONNOLLY: You can do this quite easily in imprinting experiments. If in addition to presenting a visual stimulus you also link it with an auditory one, or perhaps vary the temperature in certain ways, you produce a much more potent stimulus. No doubt this is very complex but what you can say about this is that you are providing a stimulus which is maximizing the information input. If what is happening is some kind of structuring, some kind of initial organization in the nervous system, then the basic thing is to produce a form of super stimulus.
HINDE: But you see, maximizing the information input you could do by giving, let us say, the song of another species, but that is not learnt. You cannot just put it into simple quantitative terms because its qualitatively different.
BRUNER: Considering the qualitative aspect, and to pursue Connolly's point for a moment, suppose you decompose the elements of this song by looking at the things that drop out. For example, at one point the terminal warble may be a part that should not be in. If it drops out, it could also be maximized. So you look at it and find out whether it has a structure that can be sharpened. You take the noise out of the terminal warble and you play it as a simple warble and in this way build the thing up. I am really thinking, in the back of my mind, about the model of

Jakobson and Halle (*Fundamentals of Language*. 'S-Gravenhage: Mouten, 1956). They were analysing language in terms of guessing which features might be central to it. Having done this they were "pumping them up" in the same way that Connolly is suggesting, getting them noise-free, extended, and sharpening possible amplitude differences. I wonder whether a super-stimulus of this kind would lead to a super-response, I must confess I never thought about a super-response before!

WHITE: In one of my investigations we put red and white striped mitts on babies. This did affect the age at which they discovered their hands and peered at them. Although we haven't done the next study, I have a very strong suspicion that providing palpable objects which interfere with the spontaneous disposition of the fist, along with the striped mitts, would probably be the most effective way of getting the child to attend to his hand earlier. In the home-reared infant, for example, the hand is discovered anywhere from 70 to about 100 days of age. We have had them finding their hands well before 40 days of age by these experimental techniques. The mitted-fist does appear to be a kind of super-stimulus.

KAY: Are we not discussing this as if we wanted to produce a bunch of prima donnas? I was struck by the fact that the range was narrower in certain species if they were reared under their natural conditions. What I am puzzled about is, is this just a question of identification? I mean, is it in fact that it started off with one species making a little tweet, and another one just having a single note, and so on? And, that due to increasing complexity of their environment, they have had to go into longer and longer identification notes of this kind. What is the general logic of the whole exercise? If we go on to rear more birds in isolation, are we going eventually to get more variability?

HINDE: I can answer you in functional terms if that would help at all. Its function is that it has to be recognizable as a song of this species and, in addition, it has to be recognizable as the song of a particular individual within the species. A certain stereotypy is therefore necessary so that it will be distinguished from other species, but within this individuals have to be recognized themselves.

KAY: Thank you, I hadn't quite got this point of how much individuality there was within the species group.

BRUNER: Eventually we shall come back to the general point that you raised, about the conditions which in effect have a high price for precocity, in the sense of cutting down variability.

HEFFERLINE: Something which may be relevant to this is the claim made by some about the babblings of small babies. The claim is that the human child in tribes throughout the world makes all of the sounds of every known or possible human language. But then gradually through selection there comes to be a particular range of phonemes of a particular language. Then later, when the individual maybe has the job of learning a foreign language, he does not have his German sounds or his French sounds which did occur spontaneously to start with.

BRUNER: Unfortunately that is not true.

HEFFERLINE: I was struck by the first spectrogram that Hinde showed us, where there is a lot of randomness at first. I was also curious as to whether, when the species' typical song comes out, it comes out in a fragmentary fashion, phrase by phrase, or it emerges as a unitary pattern.

HINDE: The sub-song rambles on and on. You suddenly hear within it phrases that are recognisably of full song type. They become more and more recognizably full song, finally you hear a full song in the middle of all this.

BRUNER: From work on the early development of language in human children, it appears that the parental role is to modulate the way in which the particular contrast develops. Thus early on there is a warping in the direction of the speech community of the native speaker, towards the language of the parents. In this way there is a shaping which is very reminiscent of the kind of thing which Hinde talked about.

I do hope we have an opportunity to talk more specifically about the differences between the acquisition of motor response patterns in speech, the acquisition of phonology if you will, and the acquisition of other motor skills. One thing which is certainly not coming from the literature is that these are parallel in any way.

HINDE: May I ask a question which I think bears on this? One of the things that has struck me in the past as a casual observer of children is that when a child pulls himself up and stands on his feet for the first time, or nearly the first time, it looks as though it is a tremendously rewarding performance for the child. Similarly, in the case of Held's monkey who saw his hand for the first time, I got the impression that this was quite a fascinating experience for the animal. How much do people who work on the development of skills in children look at the question of why they develop as opposed to how they develop? Has anyone ever tried to see whether standing up is reinforcing to a child, for example by rotating his carry cot so that he gets into the vertical position, or by giving it any of the appropriate leg feedback when it was in the prone position? Or any of these sorts of experimental manipulation which I should have thought would have been quite possible. I raise this point because I think that the relevance of the work on the reinforcing aspect of bird song to this group has little to do with language, it just happens that sounds are involved. I think the relevance of bird song to the development of skills is this question of the model or template, or the reinforcing effectiveness or whatever you like to call it. It seems to me that there is an implication of this reinforcing effect in the case of a child first standing up. That is, approximation to a given pattern of feedback is of itself reinforcing. It may be along these lines that there is a parallel.

CONNOLLY: When a child reaches a certain point in an activity there appears something which looks very much like satisfaction, he smiles or he seeks to repeat the thing. Are you saying: is there something about having achieved an upright posture which may be rather like having issued forth with a song? It seems to me that if a child reaches that point, all things associated with it become stabilized and form part of an organization, at that time in the child's life.

WHITE: How far do you have to extend that kind of thing?

CONNOLLY: I don't know, what I was trying to do was really to clarify things rather than propose hypotheses.

HINDE: This is precisely what I meant, and if this is the case one should be able to analyse what it is about standing up that is reinforcing. It could be a change in visual input, it could be a change in proprioceptive feedback, or any similar thing.

BRUNER: I can tell an anecdote about this which I think is very much to the point. Papousek and I this past summer tried to repeat some of his Prague experiments with head-turning. We were working of course with American babies—things turned out to be very interesting. We got the babies into the apparatus and they were lying supine, and lo and behold the moment you put them in a supine position they are so swamped by this new position that the head-turning doesn't show. It is unusual for our babies to be put in a supine position; our paediatricians tell American parents that their babies are supposed to lie in the prone position.

CONNOLLY: How old were the babies?

BRUNER: Three months, and you can imagine by 3 months they are not put on their backs any more, so you tilt them up a little, about 30° and under these circumstances everything is fine. We have hit upon a rather interesting cultural difference here I think. To be sure, Prague babies don't have any different genes from Cambridge, Massachusetts babies. Apparently, some kind of position is modal and the achievement of that position signals that all is O.K. to the baby.

CONNOLLY: On this question of preferred posture, I was very struck when nursing my young daughter just how much she preferred to be held in the upright position. When held in the nursing position she often became very upset but was fine as soon as she was put upright again.

PRECHTL: I think the upright position should be right from the beginning because there is a tremendous righting effect even in the newborn.

BRUNER: What we are saying is that at every stage there is some postural thing which the child takes to be natural, and if you take the child off this you are going to get all kinds of efforts to regain it. Whether this is a version of the righting reflex or not I don't know. Perhaps a child cannot scan properly when in other than a vertical suspension.

HINDE: Let me say this for a third time and then perhaps someone will take some notice of it; surely the experiment to do is to see whether this is reinforcing by seeing whether it will increase the frequency of some other response.

BRUNER: No, no, no! That is a kind of odd way of saying "Does it have an effect on an arbitrarily associated stimulus?" and that isn't necessarily what is going to tell us the story. This is the notion that somehow if something is reinforcing it can be used in a kind of Pavlovian situation.

HINDE: Not a Pavlovian situation, a Skinnerian situation.

INGRAM: There is another situation which doesn't seem to involve posture, and which children seem to enjoy greatly, and which I am sure everyone has seen. This is when the child learns to release his grasp. Outside any supermarket or grocer's shop you see this, the child dropping everying out of the pram.

WHITE: It amazes me that the notion of schema disequilibrium in a Piagetian sense has not been brought up before this.

INGRAM: Exactly, this is what Piaget says isn't it? The child will practise anything that he has learned.

WHITE: No, the child will practise what he is in the process of acquiring in that particular area. Once he has acquired it he doesn't practise it.

BRUNER: I am worried about taking something out of context and saying that it would be reinforcing for other events. It may very well be the contextualization of standing up and the expenditure of effort to stand up.

HINDE: Yes, it may be, sure. But if you were to get further understanding, one method is to see whether you could find out what it is about standing up that is reinforcing. And that is all I am saying. It is possible that none of the experiments which I am suggesting would work, and negative results wouldn't tell you very much. But positive results would. What you said about Piaget, that is nothing more than a description, it doesn't tell you anything at all.

Sensory-Motor Integration

Learning to Draw

M. L. J. ABERCROMBIE

University College London

I. INTRODUCTION

DRAWING MOVEMENTS RESEMBLE many other skilled movements that are made under visual control, and differ from them only in that they produce a permanent visible record of themselves. I shall be dealing mainly with the copying of very simple line figures, not with drawing from memory or from imagination, when the subject has to decide what his picture should look like; in copying this decision is already made for him. In perceiving the figure the subject relies on schemata or engrams of similar figures he has seen in the past, and in copying it he sets into action a series of movements whose results he has predicted. These are usually, of course, movements of the hand but there are artists who draw with the foot or the mouth.

Some apes, as is well known, have enjoyed drawing, and it is natural to me, as a biologist, when in difficulty about any aspects of human behaviour, to turn for guidance to those surviving representatives of our evolutionary past. Morris (1962) reports that it was not movement alone that made drawing such an absorbing occupation for his apes, but the visual stimulus that resulted from their own movement. They were not enthused by the effects of using a stick that left no trace; and if with surfeit of excitement their interest should flag, it could be revived by giving them a different colour to paint with. They liked making their mark, and they did this in various ways, with simple scratching or finger painting movements, or with several different ways of grasping a brush.

It was not, however, drawing as a source of aesthetic pleasure that stimulated my early interest in the development of this skill, but the importance of drawing for representing objects veridically, and thereby stimulating accurate observation. The art of apes does not help us much here. Apes may revel in colour; they may be sensitive to the sizes and shapes and positions of blobs on paper; they may appreciate symmetry or balance, or prefer complexity to simplicity, but (as Morris and others have shown) apparently no sub-human has ever been known to attempt to represent anything. I am disappointed in apes, who care only about aesthetics, and turn to normal and brain injured children for help in understanding, for scientific purposes, the difficulties of drawing.

Young children and mentally deficient people have drawing difficulties, i.e. drawing ability is a function of mental age; the peculiar thing about the drawing difficulties of brain-injured children is that in some cases they may be *specific*, i.e. unexpectedly bad compared with their mental age. The drawing difficulties of brain-injured children are one aspect of their visuomotor or constructive disorders, such as are exemplified when they are asked to copy two- or three-dimensional shapes or construct them on request. A convenient measure of these specific difficulties is got by comparing the score on the WISC performance scale with the verbal score (more specifically, scores on the Object Assembly and the Block Design sub-tests with the verbal score). Or, if the Stanford Binet test is used, by comparing the mental age on the drawing items with that on verbal items. It is interesting to note that a similar discrepancy between Verbal and Performance IQ, and difficulties in copying figures, is shown by some women with Turner's syndrome (sexual infantilism and gonadal dysgenesis with chromosomal anomalies, usually absence of an X chromesome; Alexander *et al.*, 1966).

The kinds of difficulties that spastic children may have is illustrated in their drawings of a man or a diamond. A drawing of a man by a spastic diplegic girl, 15 years old, whose verbal mental age was about 13 years, shows extreme simplification. It is equivalent to that of a $4\frac{1}{2}$-year-old child, and contrasts markedly with that by an athetoid girl aged 14, Performance IQ 61, or by a non-brain-damaged boy, aged, 9, WISC verbal IQ 84, Performance IQ 74 (Abercrombie, 1964). It is his kind of drawing which people regard as exhibiting a body-image disorder. But the same girl's drawings or ordinary line figures show the same kind of backwardness (Abercrombie and Tyson, 1966). She could copy a circle, a square, and an upright cross, but she had great difficulty with oblique lines as seen in her copy of a diamond, an oblique cross, or the Union Jack. In the Bender-Gestalt items in which there are two figures touching each other, she drew these separately. She can be given a mental age on these drawings of say 4 or 5 years, which is very similar to that on her drawing of a man. Similar tendencies of simplification of figures and fragmentation of them can be seen in the drawings of young children, mentally deficient people, some adults with brain injury, and those with Turner's syndrome.

II. DRAWING DIFFICULTIES

I shall discuss these drawing difficulties under two headings (the influence of Piaget's and Werner's theories of perceptual development will be apparent): first that they seem to be signs of a more primitive or simple level of perception and of representation, and secondly, that there seem to be more specific difficulties of hand-eye co-ordination. The first seems to be related to generally inadequate experience of skilled movement, and the second to more specific disorders of co-ordination of movement, possibly due to conflicting instructions to the muscles.

Specific drawing difficulties are not restricted to children with motor disorders, of course; they are found in children with minimal brain damage who have very slight signs of motor disorder, amounting only to clumsiness (Gubbay et al., 1965). And they are not found in children with physical handicap which prevents their exploration of space to the same extent as the motor disorders of cerebral palsy do, but who do not have brain damage (Abercrombie et al., 1964a). Among cerebral palsied children, the athetoids do not show these disorders to marked extent, whereas the spastics do. This is not to say that these children with disorders of movement do not have a delay in perceptual development, as distinct from visuomotor development. Indeed one would expect that they would be backward in, for instance, recognizing or matching shapes and in general mental development (Abercrombie, 1968a). The work of Held (1965) and others (see discussion by Connolly, 1969) underlines the great importance of active bodily movement for visual perceptual development. Kittens do not learn to see as well if they are pushed around instead of walking around, while being exposed to the same visual environment, and men do not compensate very well for the effects of distorting spectacles if they do not move actively while wearing them.

More specifically, it is to be expected that any disorder of eye movement would affect perceptual development, and more general mental development, because it would reduce the input of relevant information (Abercrombie, 1968b). Yarbus's (1967) studies of the eye movements used in looking at a picture, "The Unexpected Visitor", illustrate that the patterns of eye movements used when the subject is just looking at the picture, or when given a variety of specific instructions, are very different. If the subject is asked to make a guess how long the unexpected visitor has been absent, his eyes flash backwards and forwards between the children's and adults' faces. If he is asked to remember the people and furniture in the room, they make more comprehensive exploring movements. In the normal subjects swift and accurate eye movements are used to bring significant parts of the visual display on to the fovea, and other parts of it may be perceived only by the peripheral part of the retina, whose visual acuity is much lower.

Studies of children's eye movements show that at the age of 6 they have less control than at 10, and brain-injured children have very much less control over their eye movements than normal children (Abercrombie et al., 1963). Pursuit movements were recorded by asking a child to watch a train moving backwards and forwards, and wait for it to come from behind the screen; a normal child gives a smooth line, showing that the eyes were on target most of the time, whereas a cerebral palsied child has extremely irregular movements, a great deal of the time spent off target. Similarly, saccadic movements were recorded by asking a child to look at a row of dots as though he were reading words. Again, a normal child following instructions fixes his eyes on the dot and then makes a sharp movement to the next dot, and so on, a long backward movement to begin the line again. The cerebral palsied child is not able to command his eyes in this way. Not only does the latter wobble about on a dot, but he hops irregularly backwards and forwards along the line. The cerebral palsied child is working on noisy channels; half the time he is getting information from other parts of the visual field than his targets. One would expect this to show in slower general mental development, in lowered IQ. Abercrombie et al. (1963) found that accuracy of eye movements was more closely related to mental age than to chronological age.

III. THE "GLOBAL" RESPONSE

There is a rather more particular way in which disordered eye movements might affect learning; many psychologists, notably Hebb and Piaget, have argued that eye movements are important in learning to perceive shapes. This would require that some record of the eye movements is made in the central nervous system, but this possibility has been questioned because of the controversy about feedback from the eye muscles. It is known that proprioceptive input from the eye muscles is poor (Howard and Templeton, 1966). The recent work of Festinger and Cannon (1965), however, shows that the outflow of impulses to the eye muscles in saccadic movements, though not in pursuit movements, is recorded. Knowledge of saccadic movements of the eyeball is not, therefore, dependent on proprioception.

Studies of the eye movements of children looking at a shape beautifully illustrate the relation of movements to perceptual development (Zinchenko and Ruzskaya, cited by Zaporozhets, 1965). At the age of 3 to 4, a child tends to fixate in the middle of the shape and to make only a few excursions to the contour; at 5 years old, the number of excursions is increased and at 5 to 6, there is a much greater tendency for the outline of the shape to be scanned by the eyes. The ability to perceive differences between similar shapes develops parallel with this habit of outlining the contour. Similarly, if a young child is given a cut-out shape to hold, it will clasp it in its fist, but an older child makes more deliberate finger movements around the contour, differentiating the shape more clearly.

The ability to represent differences in shapes by drawing lags behind the ability to perceive differences. Children will represent a circle, a square, a triangle and a diamond, all with a rough circle, when they can actually distinguish these shapes (Piaget and Inhelder, 1956). Indeed, the little twigs they may put on the circle representing the corners of a square show that they do perceive the differences between a circle and a square but cannot represent them adequately, or perhaps do not see the need to do so.

Zaporozhets (1965) reports some interesting work by Boguslavskaya in which children learned how to draw through being trained in analysing shapes, not by drawing them. She shows a drawing made by a $3\frac{1}{2}$-year-old child, of a cup and a shovel, which is just a scribble, and a recognizable cup and a house drawn by the same child after he had been taught how to analyse the shapes by modelling with sticks. The child's attention was directed towards the contours of the pattern which, as we saw previously, he does not trace spontaneously with his eyes until the age of 5 or 6.

If the figure is so complicated that the child cannot analyse it properly, and the representing task is therefore too difficult, he falls back on a simpler, global sort of statement, as the too young child falls back on the circle in attempting to draw a square. In the Frostig test (Frostig *et al.*, 1961) a child is asked to copy a line figure on a grid of dots on to an empty grid of dots. The first figure is a bar across the middle of three rows of dots (Fig. 1a). Too young a child will draw the line anywhere on the grid (Fig. 1b). Successive figures increase in complexity; a child who can accurately reproduce the early ones may get a general impression of a more complex one but not draw it in relation to the grid of dots

(Fig. 1c and 1d). A boy who found a more complex one too difficult said, "Oh, it's a sort of eight", and drew a little eight starting on the wrong dot, and much too small (Abercrombie, 1964). He did not refer back to the model to see if it was right, but looked up at the tester for

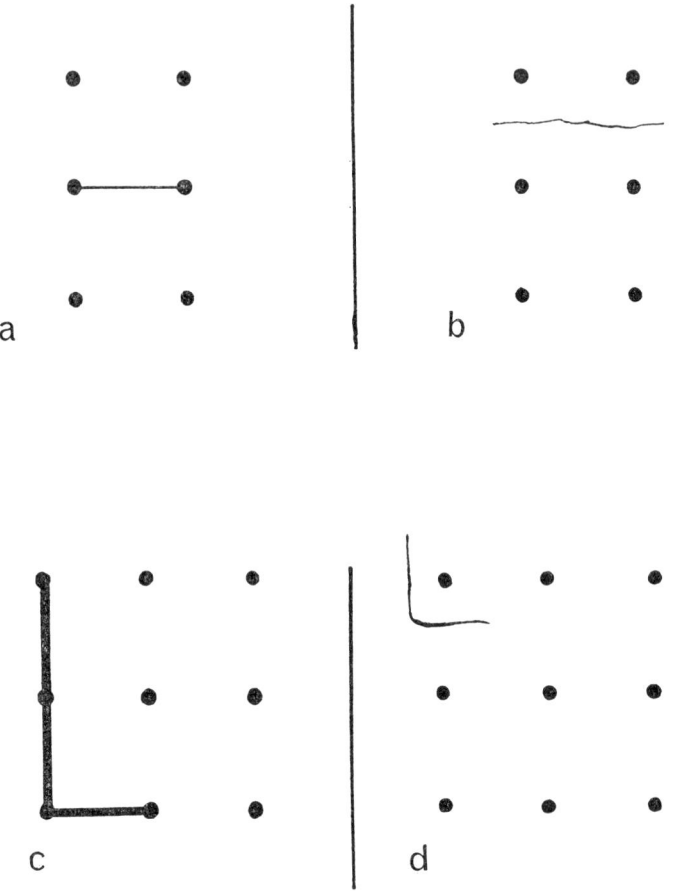

FIG. 1. Items from the Frostig test (a, b) and attempts of children to copy them (c, d) (from Frostig, Lefever and Whittlesey, 1961. Reprinted with permission of the author and publisher).

approval. Another boy of the same age made a more determined attempt to copy the figure instead of the schema in his head, by moving to and fro, from the model to his own drawing. He counted along the row of dots and started on the right one, made the first line at the right slope and the right length, but then he got lost. He analysed the model and tried to copy it bit by bit, using the finger of his left hand to help locate the dots, instead of representing a global "idea" of it. It may be that the need to analyse too difficult a figure by eye or hand movements, in order to represent it, explains why it is easier for a child to draw a figure if he watches someone draw it, than if he is presented with a static model to copy; the other person's movements are analysing it for him.

The more difficult the task for any particular person, the more likely he is to regress to a "global" approach for its execution. It is common for an architect to make a rough sketch of a building he is thinking of designing, which is recognizably the embryo "idea" of the building which, often years later, materializes. Such a sketch by Gibberd of Liverpool Cathedral has the same sort of relationship to the actual building as the boy's "eight" has to the model figure. My colleague John Weeks has made an interesting point about the role that style plays in the design of predominantly functional buildings or complexes of buildings. The design of schools or hospitals or airports has to be preceded by a considerable amount of research, of gathering information about needs, materials, costs, and all sorts of other constraints, and a sketch on the back of an envelope may seem irrelevant to this analysis. However, Weeks regards style as a design tool; it restricts the number of decisions which have to be made to manageable proportions, and provides an overall "idea" which makes a coherent, easily comprehended whole. Students who have been trained to collect all the necessary information first in an attempt to meet the demands of functionalism (i.e. to analyse intensively without, at the same time, attempting to synthesize) sometimes have great difficulty in designing at all.

IV. THE "CONFLICT" RESPONSE

A characteristic of the global way of representing a percept is that it seems to be done quickly and surely, without much doubt or questioning. I am not suggesting that the child does not see that his copy does not match the model, but only that he is not unduly concerned about the mismatch; he accepts that his copy is good enough. There is a quite different kind of behaviour shown by some brain-injured children, when they seem tormented by indecision. They will make attempt after attempt to copy a figure, often without improving. This behaviour can be more easily seen when the child is constructing a pattern with sticks or blocks, rather than when leaving a permanent record with a pencil in drawing. He assembles and reassembles the pieces, and may repeatedly destroy a pattern which is approximating the copy, instead of improving it. It is often reported that a child will say something like "I can see it, but my hand won't do it" or, "why can't my hand do what my eye sees?" or, "I'd better by careful or it'll turn into a square". Luria *et al.* (1963) report a brain-injured adult as saying "I can visualize it well, but my hands don't move properly". This behaviour seems to belong to a later stage than the global one; unsuccessful attempts at construction after analysis are now being made, and the hand seems to be receiving conflicting instructions.

I have no personal experience of brain-injured adults and it may be presumptuous of me to venture an interpretation of some of the published descriptions of them. However, I am tempted to do so, because of the considerable interest that has been aroused by the differences in drawing disorders of adults with unilateral lesions of the left and right hemispheres. I suggest that the differences are comparable with the two stages of development of skill in drawing described above, the global and the analytical. McFie and Zangwill (1960) report that left-sided cases (all of whom had moderate or marked degree of general intellectual impairment) showed in their drawings a reduction of the parts represented, and simplification. In copying a four-pointed star with matchsticks they often arrived at a simplified figure which is coherent but no longer a star; the figure shows one effort as a circle. In copying a Koh's block design, they preserved the square outline, even if they did not get the pattern right. By contrast right-sided cases moved the matches about a great deal, but had difficulty in representing any coherent structure, and in copying a block design might even lose the square outline of the design. Piercy *et al.* (1960) also noted that severe incapacity in left-sided cases tended to result in simplicity in copying e.g. a cube, whereas in right-sided cases the drawings, although disorganized, were comparable in complexity to the model. The mean number of lines used by the left-lesion cases in making unrecognizable cubes was significantly smaller than that used by the right-sided cases. They conclude that constructional apraxia associated with right hemisphere lesions involves greater impairment of perceptual functions than is the case with left hemisphere lesions. Warrington *et al.* (1966) also noted that left-sided cases showed less tendency to build up complex figures systematically from their parts, and included fewer details. They comment that the left-sided cases seem to experience difficulty in planning the drawing process leading to simplified versions of the model, while the right-sided cases have difficulty in incorporating spatial information into their drawings, leading to disproportion and faulty articulation of parts. An alternative way of describing the phenomena,

I suggest, is that the left hemisphere cases have regressed to an earlier, global stage of development than have the right-sided cases.

In attempting to understand this second sort of difficulty in learning to draw, I shall concentrate on the difficulties of drawing oblique lines; the average child can copy a vertical line at the age of $1\frac{1}{2}$ to 2, a horizontal line at the age of 2 to $2\frac{1}{2}$, but an oblique line, not until 5 or 6; or 4 if he watches someone else doing it. He can copy a circle at 3, a square at 5 and a diamond at 7. The difficulties of copying oblique lines are illustrated in Fig. 2 which gives a selection of diamonds taken from some recordings, made by Dr. Tyson, of drawings by a hundred 6-year-olds in ordinary schools (Abercrombie, 1965). Three-quarters of the children produced recognizable diamonds; these are the worst ones, and they resemble the products of much older brain-injured children.

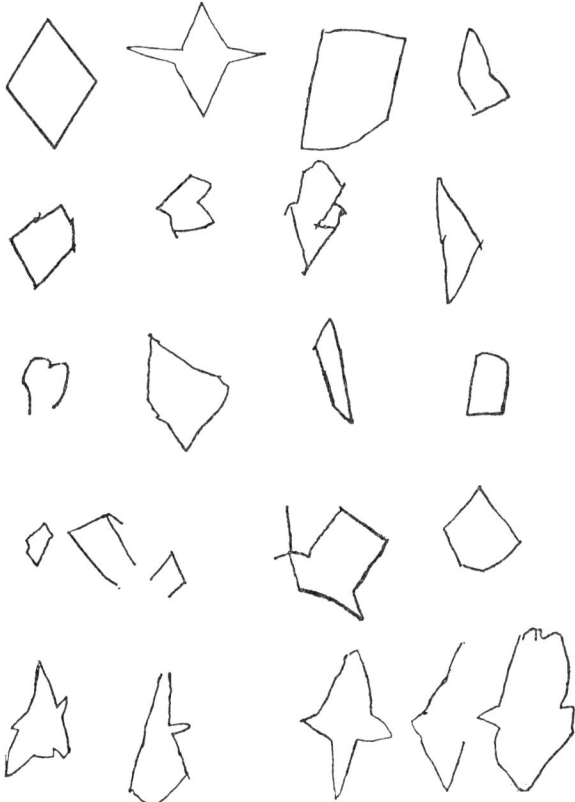

FIG. 2. Diamonds drawn by 6-year-old children; the model is in the top left hand corner (after Tyson).

Yarbus (1967) shows that oblique lines are outlined by different eye movements from those used for vertical and horizontal lines. The latter are scanned with straight saccades whereas oblique lines are scanned with curved ones. He believes that this is due to non-simultaneous movements of the eye muscles being made in following an oblique. It is conceivable that the greater complexity of such movements may contribute to some of the difficulty of seeing oblique lines. When the perceptual task is too difficult relative to present competence, gross movements of the whole or parts of the body may be called into use. A young child, or an older spastic child, will run his finger along a line, or turn his head and shoulders to align with it, as though attempting to imitate it and incorporate it with bodily movements. Vereecken (1961) has described how difficult it is even for adults to copy oblique lines in certain positions. If a subject is given an oblique line on a piece of paper which is askew on the table and is asked to copy this on to another piece of paper which is askew in a different direction, without moving the paper and without moving his head, he gets a pain in the eyes, as though from frustrated attempts to "copy" the line by bodily orientation. It is common for people to reorientate a sheet of paper on which they are drawing an oblique line in order that the line, and consequently their movement may be vertical or horizontal, instead of the edges of the paper being so, as is normally the case. Piercy *et al.* (1960) noted that adults with right-sided brain lesions, unlike those with left-sided ones, often orientate their copies of a cube or a house diagonally on the paper. Their special difficulty in representing three-dimensional objects on a two-dimensional surface may be related to the difficulty in drawing obliques. Perception of the relationships of lines is also easier if they are preponderantly vertical and horizontal rather than oblique. A tutor's spontaneous reaction to a student's plan for a group of old people's dwellings was to call it chaotic; then he said that a great improvement in design had been made later when the student had redrawn the plan with little change, though differently oriented on the paper.

Landmark's (1962) report of a 15-year-old spastic girl of normal intelligence who could not draw the 12-year Binet figure of a diamond enclosing two others (Fig. 3a) is of great interest in helping to analyse drawing difficulties. The girl was shown the figure for 10 seconds, it was then removed and she was asked to draw it. Her effort is shown in Fig. 3b. She could visualize it quite well and describe it verbally, but could not draw it. However, using a ruler, she drew Fig. 3c; she moved the ruler around until she could see that it was in the right position. When drawing freehand, she did not know how the stroke she thought

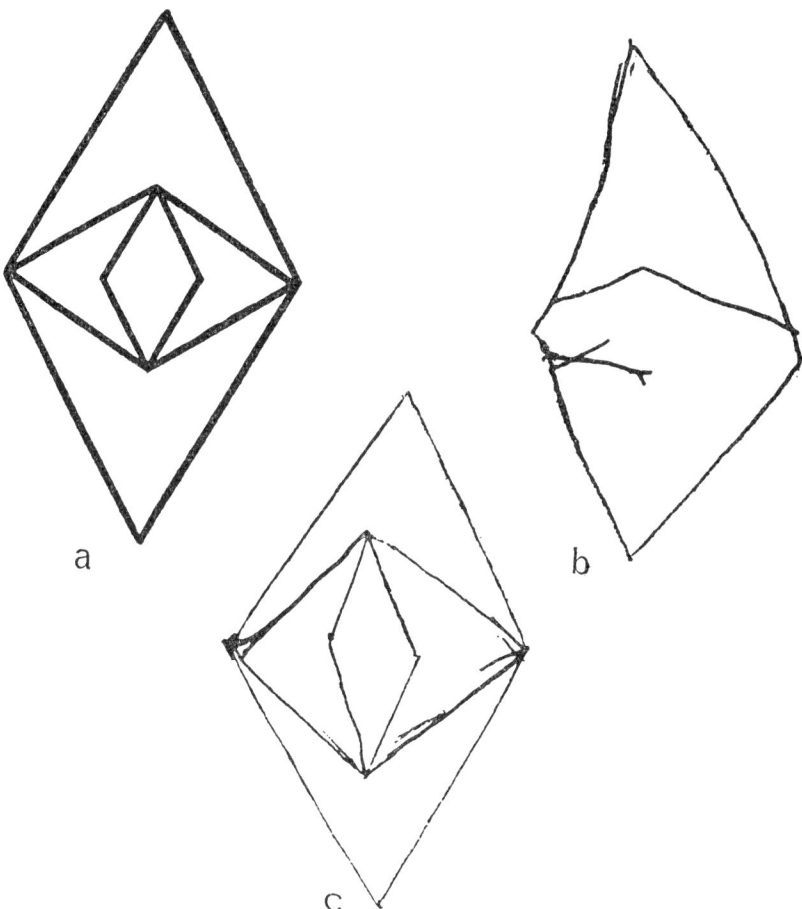

FIG. 3. The Stanford-Binet complex diamond (a) and attempts of a spastic girl to copy it, (b) free hand, (c) with the aid of a ruler (from Landmark, 1962. Reprinted with permission of S.I.M.P. and Heinemann, London).

of drawing was going to look. It was of no help to her to know that a particular stroke was wrong, because she did not know in what direction the new stroke ought to go. One might explain Landmark's observation in temporal terms: the use of the ruler makes the task easier because the child can match the line (with the model if she is copying, or with her schema if she is drawing it from memory) instead of having to project it. Over and Over (1967) have made a useful distinction between detection and recognition which is relevant here. It has often been reported that young children and some animals do not discriminate between mirror-image oblique lines. Over and Over asked children either to say whether two shapes were the same or not (detection), or which of the two was "right" (recognition). They were better at detection than recognition, and the authors suggest that the difficulty of recognition is due to deficiencies of memory of spatial information.

V. CONTRALATERAL ASSOCIATED MOVEMENTS

Since one seems to perceive the direction of oblique lines so much by bodily movement, I wondered whether associated contralateral movements might possibly contribute to the difficulty in distinguishing the slope of lines and copying them. The persistence of these movements in brain-injured and mentally defective children is well known (Abercrombie *et al.*, 1964b) and Cernacek (1961) found that in normal subjects during simple voluntary movement of the hand, inapparent contralateral motor irradiation to the symmetrical muscle was detectable by electromyography. If, when a child intends to move one hand along an oblique line, there is a natural tendency for mirror-image associated movements to occur in the other hand, then it is possible that there would be a conflict between the information received from the right and left hands, as to the direction of the line.

We have studied the hand movements of children copying figures when their hands are screened from their view (Abercrombie *et al.*, 1968). I shall only refer to the circle, and horizontal, vertical and oblique lines. Each was copied first with the right hand and then with the left, and then two of each of the same figures were presented side by side, one to be copied with each hand at the same time.

In normal children, when drawing a circle, there was a strong tendency for the hands when moving singly, to move anti-clockwise. Fifty-one per cent of the children showed this; 7 per cent of them moved each hand clockwise, and the other 42 per cent moved the hands in opposite directions, one hand anti-clockwise and the other clockwise. But when they were drawing two circles simultaneously, 91 per cent of the children moved the hands in opposite directions. Similarly, in drawing a horizontal line, when the hands were used separately, 63 per cent of the children moved both hands dextrad, from left to right, 4 per cent moved both sinistrad, and 33 per cent in opposite directions. But when both hands were being used simultaneously, 91 per cent of them moved in opposite directions, either towards each other or away from each other, and only 9 per cent of the children drew with both hands dextrad or with both hands sinistrad. In drawing a vertical line, both hands, whether used separately or together, tended to go vertically downwards (towards the child on a horizontal surface). Thus for the vertical component of a movement, the two hands tend to move in the same direction whether moving singly or simultaneously. For the horizontal component, when moving simultaneously they have an overwhelmingly greater tendency to move in opposite directions, than when moving singly.

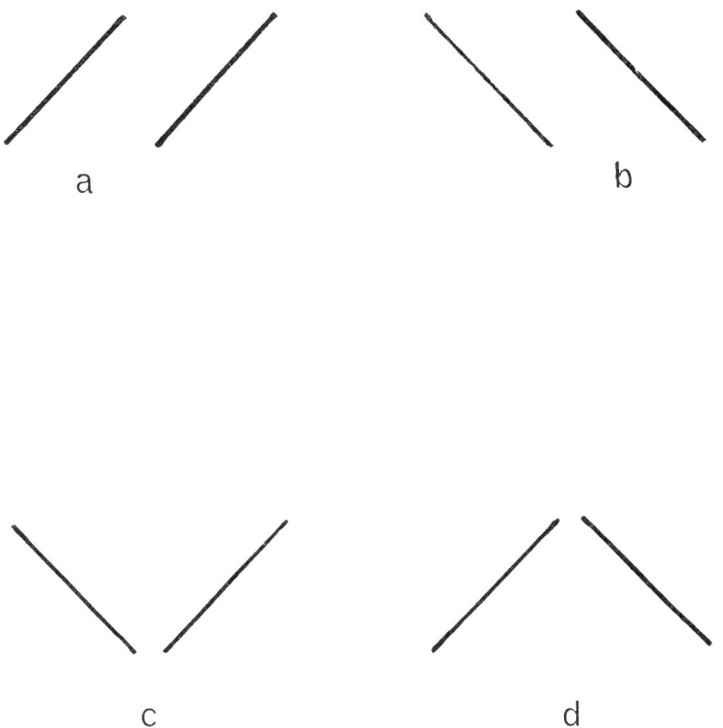

FIG. 4. Pairs of oblique lines, (a, b) parallel obliques, (c, d) opposite obliques.

In drawing oblique lines, there was a tendency to move downwards, but it was not so strong as with the vertical lines, and the tendency to move downwards was stronger when both hands were being used together. In drawing the single oblique, there were only two errors of direction out of 180 possibilities. There were four pairs of obliques, two parallel and two converging, Fig. 4. In copying the parallel obliques (Fig. 4a and 4b) there were ten errors and these were of such a kind that the hands made converging or diverging movements. The two pairs of opposite obliques (Fig. 4c and 4d) which might seem perceptually more difficult than the parallel ones, produced only two errors, the lines being drawn parallel. Of the total of 12 errors made in the double obliques, ten were spontaneously corrected, so that these were not errors of either visual or kinaesthetic perception: the children knew that the movement of their hands had not imitated the direction of the lines that they were looking at. It could be that they were responding to the tendency to make movements in opposite directions in the horizontal component, as when both hands are used simultaneously in drawing the circle or horizontal line. Brain-damaged children showed the same tendency as normal children, to produce a high frequency of opposite movements when they were drawing the pairs of horizontal lines or the pairs of circles. There was a difference between them and normal children in making the single movements, their single movements resembled the normal simultaneous movements. With the single horizontal line there was a significantly greater preponderance of opposite movements than in the normal children, and there was a similar tendency for an excess of opposite movements in drawing the circle, though the differences were not statistically significant. In drawing the oblique lines there were, of course, more errors than in the normal children, especially in copying the parallel obliques. We suggest that the condition in the brain-damaged children who have a comparative weakness of lateralization is a more primitive state; the pattern for single movements resembling that for simultaneous movements, with less effect of dominance of one hand. It is interesting that Maki in 1928 reported a case of a brain-damaged adult who, when copying simple line figures in the air, was unable to make other than left to right movements with the right hand, and right to left with the left, whether he was copying with one hand or with both simultaneously. The disturbing, confused feeling that comes with ambiguity of perception of which hand is which is beautifully evoked by M. C. Escher's (1968) print of "Drawing hands".

VI. VISUAL AND PROPRIOCEPTIVE INPUT

Another possible source of difficulty is conflicting attention to visual and proprioceptive input. Recent work has shown that when there is a conflict between the two inputs, the eyes win in normal people (Over, 1966; Rock and Harris, 1967). There are a few cases reported by Witkin *et al.* (1954) in the tilting-chair/tilting-rod experiments which recall the condition of brain-injured children when they show such indecision and confusion in drawing or in making stick patterns. The subjects sat in a tilting chair in a darkened room and were asked to judge when a tilted luminous rod was set to vertical. The rod was seen against a luminous rectangular frame, which was tilted. Some people caused the rod to be set to align with their own body, whether the chair they were seated in was vertical or tilted, others set it to align with the axis of the frame. That is, some relied mostly on postural clues in judging the vertical and referred to their own body as a standard in setting the rod, while others were so strongly influenced by the visual field of the frame that they could not set the rod vertical. Although many people did not hesitate in making their judgement and felt quite happy about the result even if the rod was by no means vertical, there were some who found the task extremely difficult. They could not achieve certainty, and in some extreme cases had to give up; one after 50 minutes of trying. The rod might appear to them to be vertical when in a variety of positions, and they sometimes made paradoxical statements—that the frame was tilted when it was at 28°, but that the rod which was aligned with it, also at 28°, was vertical. They seemed to be orienting the rod by the frame, and the frame by their own body, and did not see the contradiction that resulted. In a few extreme cases, the rod was put wildly out of vertical because the subject suddenly switched whichever side of the square frame he saw as the top, turning it through 90° as it were. These troubled subjects might become quite ill with dizziness, excessive sweating, headache and nausea.

This description reminds one of extreme cases of difficilty of performing constructional tasks which some cerebral palsied children have; in doing the stick or block test they may assemble the pieces over and over again, getting quite near to the required pattern, and then undoing the whole thing in a confused and disoriented way. One gets the impression that they suffer from being torn in different directions, as though they are attempting to conform alternatively to two different frames of reference. Another print of Escher's, "Relativity", evokes the sense of unease that this sort of behaviour may cause.

Consideration of some work by Wober (1966) on the responses of Nigerians to the rod-and-frame and other tests takes us away from drawing difficulties in particular, but is relevant to the problems of individual differences in the development of skills in general. Wober found that performance on the rod-and-frame test in his Nigerian subjects (unlike Witkin's Americans), did not show significant correlations with two other tests of field independence (the embedded figure test and Koh's blocks), nor with Raven's matrices, nor with degree of formal education. All of the latter are indices of analytic ability in the visual field (Western education in the English language involves literacy and familiarity with diagrams and figures), and the correlations between them are significant. Performance on the rod-and-frame test, however, correlated with job efficiency, whereas the measures of visual analytic ability did not. Wober relates his findings to others, suggesting that people develop different patterns of relative importance of the different senses (or "sensotypes") not only in response to sensory loss (e.g. blindness) but through different cultural experiences; African cultures, for instance, differ from American and European cultures in being more proprioceptive and auditory than visual.

Drawing has always played a large part in the education of architects (and of other designers) and continues to be an important design tool, as well as the main medium of communication between members of the building and planning team. Difficulties of space visualization seem to be a major obstacle to learning to design big buildings and urban spaces. Could this be connected with different ways of storing and of integrating the experience of small-scale movements (eye and hand) and of large-scale movements and translocations of the whole body? Certainly our literate habits encourage the development of eye-movement skills in reading and of the co-ordination of these with hand movements in writing, while we get much less practice in co-ordinating the experiences of locomotion with eye-hand movements. Birch and Lefford (1963) showed that, while at 5 years old children can readily relate visual and haptic experiences of geometric shapes, they cannot so well relate either of them with kinaesthetic input until they are several years older. It may be that the integration of information about bodily orientation in space is even slower, and some of us seem to have missed out on it almost entirely.

The notion that each of us has a potential array of talents which are unused because we did not happen to start paying attention to them at the right time is not new, but the possibility that it is never too late, that by taking thought a perceptual habit can be broken and things can be felt that were not experienced before, opens exciting possibilities for the extension of human skills. Jacobson (1929) helped people to become aware, as they had not been, of muscle tension, as distinct from cutaneous and other sensations accompanying muscle contraction. Having been taught how to stop getting a pain in the neck, or rather, how to stop putting it there (Barlow 1964), I have a deep personal interest in this aspect of learning better how to manage one's own cerebral processes. It has potentialities far beyond the obvious ones of helping to control some psychosomatic disorders. It may help to develop further our spatial abilities, which tend to get neglected in our literacy-oriented culture

(Macfarlane Smith, 1964). Some of us let lie dormant the kinaesthetic senses which are concerned with the orientation of the body in space and with its use as a standard for the appreciation and manipulation of extra-corporeal space. The work of Hefferline (1958) gives the subject amazingly increased control over his own muscular contractions by making his proprioceptive impulses visible to him. This boosting of sensory acuity does for proprioception what the telescope and microscope do for vision. It opens up new possibilities for the extension and elaboration of human experience and skill.

VII. SUMMARY

To summarize, I am suggesting that two components can be distinguished in the causation of drawing difficulties in brain-injured children: one is the persistence of immature, global, generalized ways of perceiving and representing a figure, and the other may be the result of conflicting orders given to the hand in the attempt to reconstruct it after analysis. The first kind of execution is not necessarily experienced by the child as a mismatch, but the second is; he is tormented by his failure to represent what he can see. The more difficult the task, the greater the tendency to recruit more and more patterns of movement which add complexity to complexity because of reafference. It is a great pity that he cannot just enjoy himself as the apes do, pleasing themselves that the movements of their hand leave a mark that their eyes can see; but then the apes are making no attempt to represent anything. The origins of our more scientific endeavours, like the apes' purely hedonistic ones, are rooted in the pleasure of making our mark and seeing it, and seeing that it fits harmoniously into its context. But the attempt to *represent* the world depends on the perception of an endless series of self-generated mismatches, and the attempt to correct them is necessarily attended by conflict and frustration.

REFERENCES

ABERCROMBIE, M. L. J. 1964. *Perceptual and visuomotor disorders in cerebral palsy: a review of the literature*. Spastics Society, Heinemann, London.

ABERCROMBIE, M. L. J. 1965. On drawing a diamond. In S. A. Barnett and A. McLaren (Eds.), *Penguin science survey B*. Penguin Books, Harmondsworth. 36–54.

ABERCROMBIE, M. L. J. 1968. Some notes on spatial disability: Movement, intelligence quotient and attentiveness. *Develop. Med. Child Neurol.* **10**, 206–213.

ABERCROMBIE, M. L. J. 1969. Eye movements and perceptual development. In P. Gardiner, R. MacKeith and V. Smith (Eds.), *Aspects of paediatric and developmental ophthalmology*. S.I.M.P., Heinemann, London.

ABERCROMBIE, M. L. J., DAVIS, J. R. and SHACKEL, B. 1963. Pilot study of version movements of eyes in cerebral palsied and other children. *Vision Research*, **3**, 135–153.

ABERCROMBIE, M. L. J., GARDINER, P. A. G., HANSEN, E., JONCKHERE, J., LINDON, R. L., SOLOMON, G. and TYSON, M. C. 1964a. Visual, perceptual and visuomotor impairments in physically handicapped children. *Percept. mot. Skills Monogr. Suppl.* **18**, 561–625.

ABERCROMBIE, M. L. J., LINDON, R. L. and TYSON, M. C. 1964b. Associated movements in normal and physically handicapped children. *Develop. Med. Child Neurol.* **6**, 573–580.

ABERCROMBIE, M. L. J., LINDON, R. L. and TYSON, M. C. 1968. Direction of drawing movements. *Develop. Med. Child. Neurol.* **10**, 93–97.

ABERCROMBIE, M. L. J. and TYSON, M. C. 1966. Body image and draw-a-man test in cerebral palsy. *Develop. Med. Child Neurol.* **8**, 9–15.

ALEXANDER, D., EHRHARDT, A. A. and MONEY, J. 1966. Defective figure drawing, geometric and human, in Turner's syndrome. *J. nerv. ment. Dis.* **142**, 161–167.

BARLOW, W. 1964. Rest and pain. *Proc. IV Internat. Cong. Phys. Med.*, Paris, 494–498.

BIRCH, H. G. and LEFFORD, A. 1963. Intersensory development in children. *Monog. Soc. Res. Child Develop.* **28**, 5.

CERNACEK, J. 1961. Contralateral motor irradiation—cerebral dominant. *Arch. Neurol.* **4**, 165–172.

CONNOLLY, K. 1969. Sensory-motor co-ordination: Mechanisms and Plans. In P. M. Wolff and R. MacKeith (Eds.), *Planning for better learning*. S.I.M.P., Heinemann, London.

ESCHER, M. C. 1968. *The graphic work of M. C. Escher*. Oldbourne, London.

FESTINGER, L. and CANNON, L. K. 1965. Information about spatial location based on knowledge about efference. *Psychol. Rev.* **72**, 373–384.

FROSTIG, M., LEFEVER, D. W., and WHITTLESEY, J. R. B. 1961. A developmental test of visual perception for evaluating normal and neurologically handicapped children. *Percept. mot. Skills* **12**, 383–384.

GUBBAY, S. S., ELLIS, E., WALTON, J. N., COURT, S. D. M. 1965. Clumsy children: a study of apraxic and agnosic defects in 21 children. *Brain* **88**, 295–312.

HEFFERLINE, R. F. 1958. The role of proprioception in the control of behavior. *Trans. N.Y. Acad. Sci.*, **20**, 739.

HELD, R. 1965. Plasticity in sensory-motor systems. *Sci. Amer.* Nov, 84–94.

HOWARD, I. P. and TEMPLETON, W. B. 1966. *Human spatial orientation*. Wiley, New York.

JACOBSON, E. 1929. *Progressive relaxation*. University of Chicago Press.

LANDMARK, M., 1962. Visual perception and the capacity for form construction. *Develop. Med. Child Neurol.* **4**, 387–392.

LURIA, A. R. PRAVDINA-VINARSKAYA, E. N., YARBUS, A. L. 1963. Disorders of ocular movement in a case of simultanagnosia. *Brain*, **86**, 219–228.

MACFARLANE SMITH, I., 1964. *Spatial ability*. University of London Press.

MCFIE, J. and ZANGWILL, O. L. 1960. Visual-constructive disabilities associated with lesions of the left cerebral hemisphere. *Brain* **83**, 243–260.

MAKI, N. 1928. Natürliche Bewegungstendenzen der rechten und der linken Hand und ihr Einfluss auf das Zeichnen und den Erkennungs-vorgang. *Psychologische Forschung* **10**, 1–19.

MORRIS, D. 1962. *The biology of art.* Methuen, London.

OVER, R. 1966. An experimentally induced conflict between vision and proprioception. *Brit. J. Psychol.* **57**, 335–341.

OVER, R. and OVER, J. 1967. Kinaesthetic judgements of the direction of line by young children. *Q. J. Exper. Psychol* **19**, 337–340.

PIAGET, J. and INHELDER, B. 1956. *The child's conception of space.* Routledge, London.

PIERCY, M., HECAEN, H., and DE AJURIAGUERRA, J. 1960. Constructional apraxia associated with unilateral cerebral lesions—left and right sided cases compared. *Brain* **83**, 225–242.

ROCK, I. and HARRIS, C. S. 1967. Vision and touch. *Sci. Amer.* **216**, 96–104.

VEREECKEN, P. 1961. *Spatial development: constructive praxia from birth to the age of seven.* Wolters, Groningen.

WARRINGTON, E. K., JAMES, M., and KINSBOURNE, M. 1966. Drawing disability in relation to laterality of cerebral lesion. *Brain* **89**, 53–82.

WITKIN, H. A., LEWIS, H. B., HERTZMANN, M., MACHOVER, K., MEISSNER, P. B., and WAPNER, S. 1954. *Personality though perception.* Harper, New York.

WOBER, M. 1966. Sensotypes. *J. soc. Psychol* **70**, 181–189.

YARBUS, A. L. 1967. *Eye movements and vision.* Plenum Press, New York.

ZAPOROZHETS, A. V. 1965. The development of perception in the pre-school child. In P. H. Mussen (Ed.), *European Research in cognitive development. Monog. Soc. Res. Child Develop.* **30**, 82–101.

Discussion

HOWARD: I was interested in the finding that the child is easily able to copy the inclusion of the triangle in a circle. This reminded me of Piaget's topological stage which he claims precedes the precise shape discrimination stage. Gross topology of shape is a prerequisite for the later development, these results would fit with this, wouldn't they?

ABERCROMBIE: Yes.

HOWARD: The other thing is the diamond. In one of the diamonds which you used the angles at the top and the bottom were acute and the angles at the sides were obtuse. The difficulty here, compared with the square, is due not only to the difficulty of oblique lines, as opposed to verticals and horizontals, but the difficulty that children have with obtuse angles as compared with acute angles. When a child has to draw an obtuse angle he has much more difficulty than when he has to draw an acute angle. With the acute angle there is a definite change in direction, there is a contrast principle at work here I think. It is easier to discriminate on the basis of movement (a) from (b) in Fig. 5; (b) is less discriminable both sensorially and motorically.

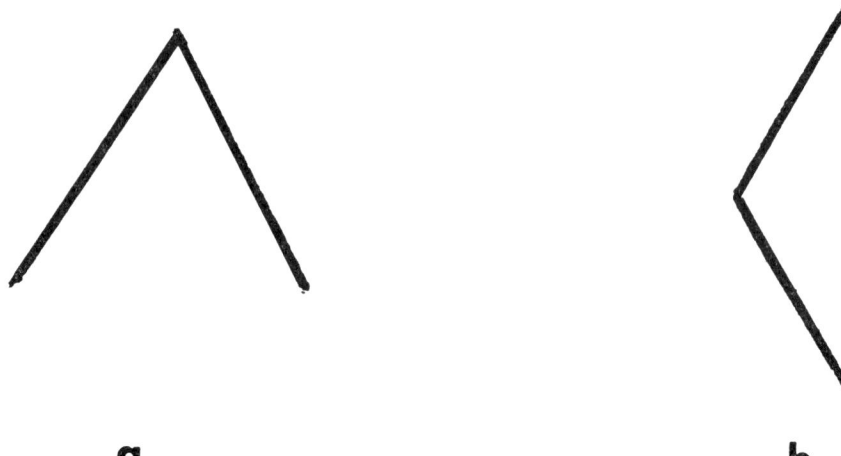
FIG. 5. Acute and obtuse angles involved in drawing a diamond.

INGRAM: An interesting example here is the child who can draw a square but not a diamond, if you ask such a child to put a square on its point quite a lot of children will, in fact, produce a good diamond.

HOWARD: I think there are other factors involved in comparing squares with diamonds. Discriminating horizontal from vertical lines is easy compared with discriminating oblique lines and by the same token drawing oblique lines is more difficult. The discrimination of the horizontal from the vertical is easier because of our body symmetry; one runs along the principle axis of the body, the other across it. Oblique lines do not have any such associated contrast. It is well known that in discrimination tasks, quite apart from drawing, children are relatively poor at discriminating obliques from each other (Fig. 6a) but they are good at discriminating verticals from horizontals (Fig. 6b), I think the octopus shows similar properties.

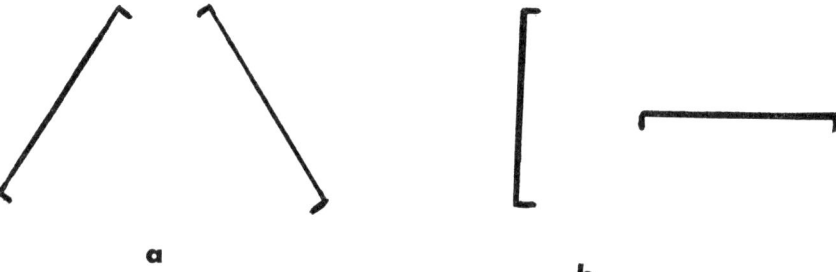
FIG. 6. Discrimination problems, (a) obliques, (b) horizontal from vertical.

CONNOLLY: I think you could test this hypothesis by making a diamond of the usual long thin form and turning it through 90° so that the obtuse angle is at the top and the acute angles are at the sides.
HOWARD: Is this the difficulty of acute versus obtuse?
CONNOLLY: Yes.
HOWARD: It is well known that when children are observed drawing acute and obtuse angles that the acute angle presents no problem but the obtuse angle is produced in a very precarious fashion.
ABERCROMBIE: There is another difficulty which is that children apparently find it easier to do the top rather than the bottom, so this is a very complicated thing. However, I have heard a child say, "I had better be careful or it will turn into a square", that is to say, that both of the angles turn into right angles.
BRUNER: May I ask a general question? My point may be naïve and if so I apologize for it. I should like to raise the issue, "What is involved psychologically in the process of representing something in graphic form?" Let me expose my own confusion. If I ask myself about drawing as a skilled activity, the first thing I have to ask is, "What is the objective?" The old notion that what I am doing is creating a match between my experiences and what is on the piece of paper clearly is not a good enough answer to this. We find, as I think someone has already pointed out, that for the representation of something by graphic means there is usually a well developed set of conventions which are in effect the constituents which we use. These conventions were slow to develop, if you look, for example, at the representation of drawn parallax going back to the 16th century. There are of course cultural differences in terms of the conventions which are used in graphic representations. A. C. Mundy-Castle dealt with some aspects of this in his work in Ghana.

One can recognize that there are local variants like local dialects. Things produced by young children give one the impression that they are working away trying to re-invent the conventions. They don't have a convention, they are trying to construct a language almost for representing things to themselves and along the way one is struck by the fact of their inventiveness. I keep coming back to what it is that one is trying to do when one draws and I find myself going back to Lefford's paper. There we had the question of when a child can go from his hand to a representation of his hand. I will put it that way round so that everything is topographically, not topologically isomorphic; so that in a sense when you draw something what you are doing is drawing the hand that you are going to point to afterwards. It is necessary therefore to have control of a whole set of things, like orientation, number of elements, and so on. It is almost as if the abstraction process were more compelling in drawing than in fact it is in language, because in language you get early phonological shaping. There appear to be certain innate capacities. For example, it seems to be the case that the first whole phrase is broken into pivot and open class, and it differentiates from here. In the case of drawing we don't have the innate, though I am not entirely sure of this, perhaps vertical/horizontal distinctions are innate. In effect it seems to me that what you have opened up here is this very powerful question of what in the world do we mean by drawing? What is representing by graphic means?

CONNOLLY: I think I see what you are driving at: but how do you apply conventions to the problem? A very important feature in Abercrombie's material is what is required of the child is objectively defined; it is something which matches the model against certain criteria which are set.

BRUNER: Against certain criteria which are highly selective.

CONNOLLY: Yes, and in the case of the child who puts little twigs on a circle, and that then is a diamond, I agree this is very interesting. How does he become so inventive and where do these notions come from? But the question remains, why can he not produce what is there in front of him?

INGRAM: If you ask him if his representation is correct he will very often tell you that it is wrong.

BRUNER: Oh yes, he will recognize that he has not got it exactly, but he does seem unable to make the necessary correction.

LEFFORD: I think I can illustrate children's inventiveness. We showed the children a model of a diamond. Assuming that it would be helpful, we gave them guiding points, as architects and artists use. What we found was that the children drew the diamond and put the dots indicating the points afterwards. If that isn't inventiveness then I don't know what is.

INGRAM: I wonder if you will agree that it is possible to teach young children to draw a diamond?

CONNOLLY: I have tried this with one of my students. We devised two different training programmes and took two groups of pre-school children (age 3 to 5 years) through these programmes. I don't think there was any single case where we did not get some measurable improvement, and in many cases it was quite clear that children who could not apparently draw a diamond when we first asked them could do so with ease and confidence at the end of the training programme.

LEFFORD: We were surprised to find that what we thought would be helpful in fact turned out to be confusing. The child was apparently confronted with a task of analysing two figures, then co-ordinating them and so on. For the child it was an entirely different task than for the adult.

CONNOLLY: An experiment which we did in our lab a couple of years ago may be of interest in this context (Connolly, 1968, *Aspects of Education* **7,** 82). We devised a set of about nine straight line figures similar to those shown in Fig. 7. We wanted to find out whether the

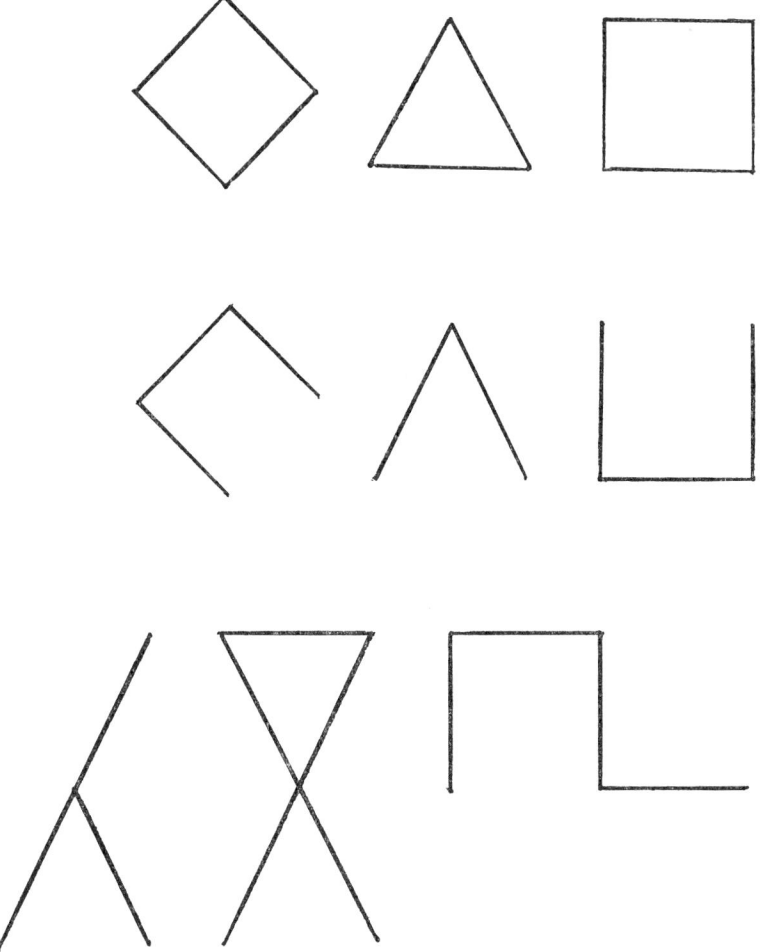

FIG. 7. Various straight line figures used in copying experiment.

difficulty which young children are reputed to experience in copying such figures was a function of perceptual difficulties, or of motor difficulties, or whether it was some integrative problem. The experiment was done with three groups of children aged 4, 5, and 6 years. The first part of the experiment was a simple matching-to-sample test in order to ensure that the children were able to discriminate and identify all the figures. None of the children had any problems in doing this, even those who had only been at school for 10 days. We then asked them to draw some lines, and they drew lines, all but about three children produced vertical, horizontal and oblique lines. When we asked those few children who did not produce oblique lines to draw them they did so without any apparent difficulty. The children were then asked to make paper and pencil copies of all these shapes. Following this they were given a pile of coloured match sticks and asked to make models of them. In both these cases the child was given a card with a drawing of the figure on it, so they had before them the model the whole time. We analysed these drawings by use of some of the criteria which Loretta Bender (1938, *A visual motor gestalt test and its clinical use*. Monog. 3. Am. Orthopsychiat. Assoc.) described. The results of the two copying tasks are shown in Fig. 8. There were no differences in the 4-year-old group between their pencil copies and their match stick models. At 5 there was a significant difference, and by 6 it had disappeared again. The point I want to bring out here (because Abercrombie said something in her paper which triggered it off) is the difference between the two types of copying in the 5-year-old. They were very much better with the match sticks. At the time I thought about these results in terms of Birch and Lefford's (1967, *Monog. Soc. Res. Child Develop.* **32**) work, in terms of the integration between different sensory modalities. There is, however, another point which I think is very important. If the child is positioning three or four match sticks to produce one of those figures, then he may readjust them as he goes. He can check his position against the model and if it does not correspond in a suitable way he can move the sticks; this I think makes the task a lot easier. This is one important variable in the situation, there is another, which is the fact that there is a much higher stimulus-response compatibility where the subject is fitting together a whole figure. For example, if I am to draw a diamond I must first put my pencil on the paper and then I have got to decide in which direction I must make my pencil go. I begin to produce a line and I have to decide if it is correct, I then have to decide where I should change direction and in which direction any subsequent line should go. With the match sticks this problem is not so difficult. The results we

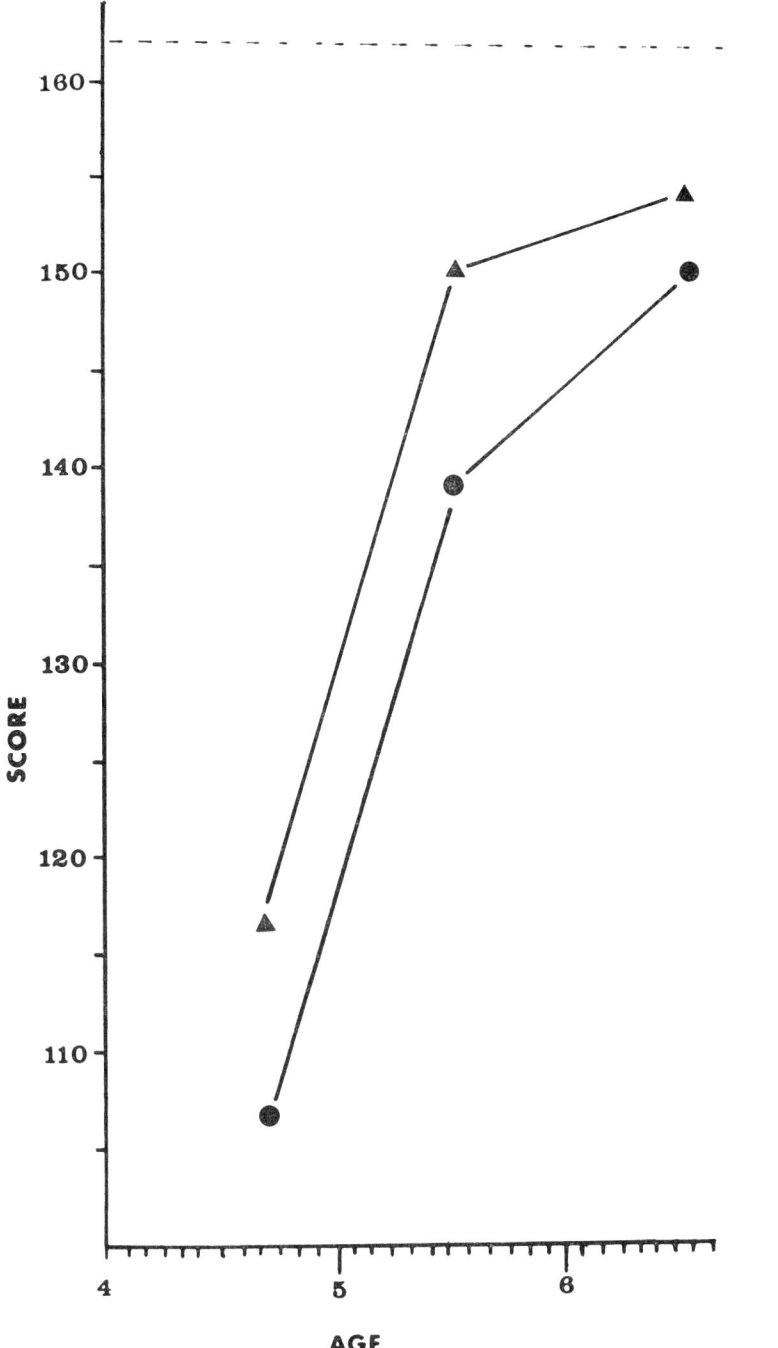

FIG. 8. Results from copying experiment at various ages, triangles represent scores on matchstick models, circles scores on paper and pencil copies.

obtained from this experiment remind me very much of Landmark's (1962, *Develop. Med. Child Neurol.* **4,** 387) findings with a spastic girl who could not draw a diamond. When given a ruler, however, this child used it in order to determine the orientation of the lines which she must draw to produce the diamond.

LEFFORD: I believe that the child can visually discriminate and differentiate the parts of a figure. I would suggest that it is in the kinaesthetic modality that the child does not "know" that particular angle. I am, of course, coming back to the notion of reafference and motor feedback which may be basic to an ability to draw.

HEFFERLINE: I should like to take up what Lefford was saying about the kinaesthetic angle that the child may or may not have. This reminded me of a method of art education that was invented about 20 years ago in Ohio State University. An art teacher by the name of Sherman wrote about drawing by seeing. (H. L. Sherman, 1947, *Drawing by seeing.* Hinds, Hayden & Eldredge, New York). It was a curious, essentially tachistoscopic way of getting art students to draw what they saw. The stimulus was flashed at them whilst they were standing at drawing desks listening to background music being played, they were supposed to stay very relaxed and sketch out with quick strokes what they saw. I think the idea behind this is rather similar to what you were talking about when you spoke of children having to regress in order to get rid of a lot of corrections, reafferences and conventions. This technique was not designed to teach draftmanship but to get the flow and some kind of artistic individuality into drawing.

BRUNER: Could I add something to this? It is what I thought was a brilliant analysis of Jakobson's, about the difference between representing something linguistically and representing something graphically. The distinction is something like this. In language, what you have are sets of conventions concerning the segments that are going to make up the message, and you have, moreover, the form of a sentence which has slots in it. These are form classes and they require that you know what you have to drop in. There is no set segmentation possible in drawing (until you start getting things a little more stylized, but forget about the conventions for the moment), so that what you have got to do basically each time is to work up a segment of your own. Now the main thing about segments, in anything which has this quality of symmetry when representing something, is that you have to have a means of analysing it in terms of the overall sentence. This is given in the nature of language. Connolly mentioned the fact that the child has great difficulty in knowing that the line he has begun to draw is relevant to the overall diamond

which he has been set. This task requires that the child keep in mind the orientation of the total diamond all the way through the task. I think in that extraordinary book which Sherman wrote a number of years ago that this is what he is getting at. By giving a person a brief flash of 50 milliseconds or so you are demanding that he should break it down into segments which can be copied more easily. They have to simplify and this aids them in extracting the important features from the display. Perhaps we can get a little bit closer to this by talking of the constructive nature of the perception itself, the taking of elements and building them up into a whole. I wonder if the child can already make these elements?
LEFFORD: A young child can't.
ABERCROMBIE: I think there is something in this because children can much more easily copy a person drawing than they can copy a static thing. So what the person's drawing movements are doing is presumably analysing the segments for them.
KAY: I think Burner may have got us stuck on this word "segment". At some point we are going to get back to the old one of ballistic and graded responses. One might think of it in this way: that the child has not yet got the graded responses in a skilled task such as drawing. The problem therefore for drawing is not that he canot set off the ballistic responses, it is that he has not got the target orientation. The error of discrepancy is at the end of the task and the beauty of Connolly's stick experiment is that it allows the child to manipulate as he proceeds to the solution of the problem. In addition the discrepancy can be measured and the child can see the extent of any errors.
INGRAM: One of the things I find interesting about situations such as this, is that there does seem to be some transfer between making a diamond with sticks and copying a diamond in a paper and pencil task. Our experience in Edinburgh would suggest that the child who has made diamonds with sticks learns more quickly to draw them; but this was not from a controlled study.
CONNOLLY: How old are the children in this Edinburgh study? I should be surprised if you found this in the 6-year-old, unfortunately in our experiment the children did not draw the diamonds after having made the models.
INGRAM: The children we worked with were of superior intelligence and aged about 5; I think their average IQ was about 125.
PRECHTL: Yes, but will it help them if you do it the other way round, that is, make the model having attempted to draw the diamond? In the example which Hefferline mentioned certainly kinaesthetic learning comes in a great deal. I am very impressed by how fast one can improve

one's own kinaesthetic and tactile perception. Perhaps I can illustrate what I mean by an anecdote. Some years ago I felt tempted to build a violin, so I did. When you do the carving from a block of wood it has to be thick in the middle and become thinner towards the edges, also it has to be very smooth. There are instruments to measure the exact thickness. To begin with, by tactile assessment I was able to pick up differences of half a millimetre. Two weeks later I was able to do this down to one tenth of a millimetre, by repeating it again and again.

TWITCHELL: I am interested in Ingram's studies concerning the way in which he trained children to draw diamonds. Occasionally I run into a number of 4-year-old children who can do all these geometric drawings quite perfectly. These children, as I recall, all happened to have older siblings who liked to do lots of drawings, so there were many attempts to copy what the older siblings were doing. What I wonder is, whether this is the natural course of things or whether these children were all exceptional?

ABERCROMBIE: I would have thought that these were all very bright children.

TWITCHELL: I think it would be true to say that these children have all been making attempts at drawing for 2 or 3 years.

INGRAM: The sample I am talking about is a very selective one, Edinburgh middle class, social class 1 and 2 that is, with an average IQ well above 120. These children were selected as a control group for other children with slow speech development. They may therefore be a very atypical group, and it may be much easier to teach such children. I wouldn't put any stress on this work at all except to say that the children who cannot draw a diamond one week can draw it the next when we have shown them how to do it using sticks.

CONNOLLY: The student of mine who took on the task of trying to teach young children to draw diamonds used my own daughters as guinea-pigs. We were concerned to try out some of the programmes which we had devised in order to see which of them had most promise as a teaching aid; we were trying the effects of tracing over diamonds and going through a procedure not unlike Lefford's of connecting up dots. One afternoon she tried these with my 3-year-old daughter who produced rather poor tracings. However, about halfway through one of the programmes she produced a perfect diamond quite spontaneously. This was a great surprise and needless to say it posed something of a problem; should one hold it there or go on? Well, we went on. At the next stage the reproduction was relatively poor again. Now the good diamond she produced was really a very good one, this is what is so difficult about doing experiments on training, it really is a great problem to know when one has effectively come to an end. How does one account for these apparently perfect responses? I don't find an explanation in terms of chance very convincing for a task as complex as drawing a diamond.

The Adaptability of the Visual–Motor System

I. P. HOWARD

York University, Toronto

In recent years many experimental studies have been done on the adaptation of visual–motor behaviour to displaced vision. Several models and theories have been proposed to account for the processes underlying such adaptation and although practically all the experiments have been done on adults, the results have been assumed to have implications for understanding visual–motor development. This paper will present a general scheme of the hand–eye control system and its functional properties, and show that current models and theories are arbitrary subsets of the elements of this scheme.

I. COMPONENTS OF THE VISUAL–MOTOR SYSTEM

Consider the task in which a subject is asked to place a forefinger on a visual target when no part of his hand or arm is in view. The structural components of this task are: the target, the eye, the head, the upper part of the body, and the arm.

Each component is optically or mechanically linked to the next component in the loop at what may be called "artiulations". The points of articulation are: the nodal point of the eye, the centre of rotation of the head, the centre of rotation of the eye and the centre of rotation of the elbow joint. Each of these points of articulation will be discussed, together with a brief summary of the ways in which spatial information is coded at each.

A. *Image Motions*

The nodal point of the eye may be considered to be the point of articulation lines of sight for the stationary eye. The projections of lines of sight into a distal frontal plane may be specified by the international perimetric system. The proximal projection of lines of sight defines the corresponding retinal oculocentric space values. Lines of sight for the two eyes may be considered to have a common point of articulation in a single cyclopian eye or egocentre at a point midway between the eyes (Hering, 1942).

The relative locations of images on each retina are topologically preserved as far as the visual cortex, and it is this anatomical topology which codes the oculocentric position of visible objects. The eye has a unique central spatial landmark—the fovea. No other sensory surface has such a spatial "Kernpunkt". Usually when we wish to judge the egocentric direction of an object, that is, its direction relative to the head, we fixate it by bringing its image on to the fovea. This is done with great accuracy and consistency. Thus a judgment of the egocentric position of a visible object is reduced to the task of knowing the direction of gaze; the oculocentric (retinal) direction of the object is always the same. Simple as this point is, we shall see later that it seems to have been overlooked in discussions about the relative lability of oculocentric spatial judgments. Outside the fovea, three things happen: (1) the ability to discriminate oculocentric directions (acuity) declines rapidly; (2) spatial judgments become progressively more and more anisotropic, that is, lacking an exact geometrical correspondence with the relative positions of distal stimuli; and (3) spatial judgments become increasingly labile, that is, subject to modification by training. This latter point is a prediction rather than a statement of fact, but it will be seen later that there is evidence to support it.

B. Eye Movements

The centre of rotation of the eye is the point of articulation for movements of the eye. The conventional polar co-ordinate system here is Listing's system. It is unfortunate that this system has a different meridional zero from the perimetric system. For binocular viewing a common cyclopian eye may be assumed, and the eyes can be assumed to have a common point of fixation.

All the evidence suggests that there are no proprioceptors indicating the position of the eyes in the head. What muscle spindles there are in the extraocular eye muscles apparently do not serve this function (Merton, 1964), and there are no joint receptors in the eye socket. Eye position is apparently coded as follows: by virtue of the springiness of the extraocular muscles, the eyes have a tendency to return to a "position of rest". It has recently been shown that the degree of tension in any one muscle is a linear function of the length of that muscle (Robinson et al., 1969). If the eye is to be held in one position each agonist must match the tension in its antagonist; thus each eye position is associated with a unique pattern of innervations. The eye, unlike a limb, never has to work against externally imposed loads, even gravity has little effect because the eye rotates approximately about its centre of gravity. The pattern of innervation of the eye muscles or its corollary discharge is thus ideally suited to serve the sense of eye position. It is conceivable that the velocity signal in the corollary discharge could serve to compensate for the retinal image motion, so as to produce stability of the visual world during eye movements. This so called "cancellation theory" of visual stability seems to have become generally accepted (Gregory, 1958). It is most unlikely to be true, however, for two reasons: in the first place, velocity during a saccade is not a constant function of innervation because of variations in tension with position; in the second place, there is no evidence that the visual world is stable during saccadic eye movements. Vision is somewhat suppressed during saccades (Volkmann et al., 1968), and we probably pay no attention to what we see at such times (Stoper, 1967).

Eye-position sense seems therefore to be based upon the corollary discharge of patterns of tonic innervation in addition of course to purely visual factors, such as the position of a fixated object in the field of view as bounded by the visible parts of the nose and orbital ridges.

C. Head Movements

The centre of rotation of the atlas joint in the neck may be considered to be the point of articulation of the head. Its position is probably coded in terms of inputs from joint receptors and utricles. Motor outflow is probably of minor importance because there is no unique relationship between motor innervation and head position.

D. Arm Movements

The centre of rotation of the ball-and-socket joint of the shoulder is the point of articulation of the shoulder joint. The elbow and wrist joints will be ignored and the spine is outside the control loop we are considering. All the evidence suggests that the sense of position at skeletal joints is provided by inputs from joint receptors and not by muscle spindles, nor by corollary discharge. This is what one would expect, because a limb has to work against variable external loads, and hence muscle-spindle activity and the motor outflow will not be uniquely related to limb position. In any case, limbs are not "springy" as eyes are and hence there is no invariant relationship between innervation and position for limbs as there is for eyes.

If the eyes and the arms are considered to have cyclopian points of articulation, it is a noteworthy fact that all points of articulation lie very close to a common vertical axis. Perhaps this is no accident, there is a distinct behavioural advantage in having all spatial judgments referred to a common origin.

II. BASIC PERFORMANCE OF THE VISUAL–MOTOR SYSTEM

Let us now take a look at the performance of this visual–motor system. A person is normally able to point with unseen hand consistently to within approximately one degree of a visible target at arm's length. Consider first the situation where one arm is aiming at a target, seen with one eye. In this situation there is no feedback of pointing error and the control system is said to be in the "open-loop" mode. Furthermore, all the articulations are in series. In any such open-loop series, linear system the following relationships should hold: (1) the variance (consistency or precision) of performance of the whole system is the sum of the variances of the separate articulations round the loop; (2) the constant error (bias or accuracy) of the whole system equals the albebraic sum of the constant errors of the separate articulations round the loop.

Whether or not these additive properties are true in practice, it is certainly true that, in the first place, the variance of the whole performance can be no better than the variance of the performance of the articulation with the largest variance, and in the second place, the constant error of the total performance is not limited by the constant error of any one separate articulation. These latter statements are seen to be true when one considers that variances are not signed and therefore cannot cancel, but that constant errors are signed and those with opposite sign will tend to cancel out.

The only systematic experimental approach to these questions was a study by Howarth and Fisher (reviewed in Howard and Templeton, 1966). The results of this study were equivocal and further work is needed.

III. GROWTH AND ADAPTABILITY OF THE VISUAL-MOTOR SYSTEM

What can we predict about the development of such a system? As the body of the child grows the limbs get longer and the shoulders further apart, the eyes also grow further apart. It is to be expected that the neural control centres would need to be adaptable in order to compensate for constant errors which such growth changes would otherwise introduce.

Nobody has made a systematic study of the ontogenetic growth of accuracy and precision in such a task. However, in recent years there has been renewed interest in how adults learn to point to a target which is prismatically displaced. As in so many other things, Helmholtz was the first to study the adaptation of pointing behaviour towards prismatically displaced targets, but interest in this problem has only recently been revived. Somewhere in the system, as a result of feedback during training, information regarding the space values at one or more of the points of articulation must become "recalibrated" in order that the motor command may bring the arm back into "registration" with the target. This is the process with which I am concerned.

There are two main questions which have been studied, one concerns the necessary conditions for visual–motor adaptation and the other the site of the adaptive change. These will be dealt with in turn.

IV. CONDITIONS FOR VISUAL–MOTOR ADAPTATION

An important hypothesis about the conditions necessary for the adaptation of visual–motor behaviour to prismatic displacement has been put forward by Held. The essentials of the hypothesized mechanism are represented in Fig. 1 (taken from Held, 1961). Except for the addition of the "correlation store", it is the same as the model which von Holst developed in connection with his work on visual–motor

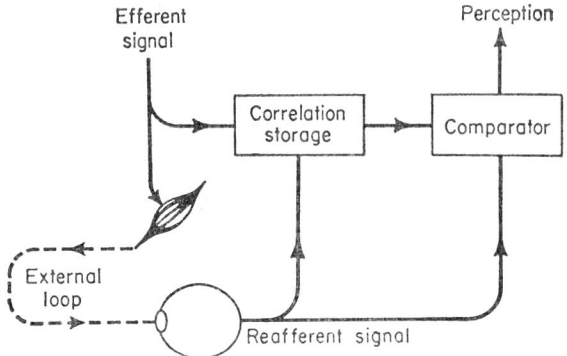

FIG. 1. Schematized process assumed by Held to underlie the adaptability of the visual–motor system (from Held, 1961. Copyright by Williams and Wilkins, Baltimore).

co-ordination in animals. In Held's words, "the reafferent visual signal is compared (in the Comparator) with a signal selected from the Correlation Storage by the monitored efferent signal. The Correlation Storage acts as a kind of memory which retains traces of previous combinations of concurrent efferent and reafferent signals. The currently monitored efferent signal is presumed to select the trace combination containing the identical efferent part and to activate the reafferent trace combined with it. The resulting revived reafferent signal is sent to the Comparator for comparison with the current reafferent signal. The outcome of this comparison determines further performance" (Held, 1961, p. 30).

The model predicts that a self-produced efferent signal is required for the building-up of stored traces upon which are based further modifications of the system.

The evidence which Held produced to demonstrate the necessity of reafference is now well-known and may be summarized as follows. The subject's ability to aim at a visual target with an unseen hand was first established; the subject then viewed his hand for a few minutes through prisms which shifted its apparent position by 2·2 inches to one side. During this time the hand was waved from side to side, either actively by the subject, or passively by the experimenter. Only after the active condition did subjects show evidence of having adapted to the prisms when they were tested after training in an aiming test.

Held concluded that self-produced movement coupled to visual reafferent stimulation is necessary for a change of visual–motor co-ordination. However, if Held's exposure or training procedure is examined it can be seen that his model is not appropriate to account for his results (Templeton, 1969). The motor outflow determines only the *amplitude of the arm movement during the exposure condition*, and the *amplitude of movement was not affected by the prisms*. In other words, the prisms did not alter the correlation between corollary discharge and the visual reafference.

In Held's training condition the arm is, and appears to be, moving through the same amplitude as the motor outflow commands. Furthermore, the motor outflow required to hold the arm in a given position is very little affected, if at all, by a change of 2·2 inches and in any case all evidence suggests that motor innervation does not serve position sense in a limb (Howard and Templeton, 1966). The only discordance in Held's experiment was between the visual position of the arm and its position as detected by joint receptors. But Held's model makes no mention of visual-joint-sense correlation, and it is therefore inappropriate for this situation.

It is surprising that there was no adaptation in Held's passive condition; for the discordance between vision and the joint sense should have been just as great in the passive condition as in the active condition. There are four possible reasons for this lack of passively induced adaptation.

The first is that the type of prism which Held used does not displace the visual scene evenly. The displacement is greater on the prism-base side than on the other side, so that the scene is compressed from one side to the other. This means that the seen excursion of the hand may have been minified or magnified depending on its position in the field of view. Such an effect would disturb the correlation between corollary discharge and visual reafference and may therefore be expected to produce differential effects between active and passive movement. However, it is not clear in Held's account where the hand was in the visual field and hence it is not possible to assess the effect of this factor, which in any case must have been very small.

Had Held explicitly studied the effects of visual minification or magnification on visual–motor adaptation he may have found some support for his model, at least it would have been appropriate. But in any case, a model which accounts for only one selected set of experimental conditions has little generality.

The second factor which may have produced adaptation under only the active-movement condition is that there was probably a difference in the degree of visual or motor asymmetry between the active and passive conditions. There is some evidence that asymmetry alone can induce a change in visual–motor behaviour (Harris *et al.*, 1966; Howard, 1967).

The third possible reason for Held's results is that his test procedure involved active movement and hence was more like the active training than the passive training procedure. This gives an unfair advantage to the active condition. It has been shown that a passive training procedure produces a change in a passive test (Pick and Hay, 1965) and even in an active test (Templeton *et al.*, 1966).

Finally, Held's active exposure condition may have caused the subject to pay more attention to what he was doing, and this may have potentiated the adaptive process. Held has produced other evidence for his reafference model, notably the now famous experiment in which it was found that only those kittens which had moved actively in relation to their visual surroundings developed visual–motor behaviour. However, these experiments were biased in favour of the active kitten, for the passively moved kitten was provided with virtually no information regarding the relationship between body movement and vision (see Howard and Templeton, 1966, p. 394).

In more recent experiments, Held and his associates have demonstrated the adverse effects on the visual–motor behaviour of kittens and monkeys produced by rearing them with occluding neck ruffs (Hein and Held, 1967; Held and Bauer, 1967). These experiments seem to provide evidence for Held's reafference model. However, it is not clear from these results whether it was the absence of the sight of the actively moving limb which was crucial or merely the absence of the sight of the limb, whether moving or not.

In any case, deprivation studies such as these, although interesting, are always open to the criticism that the procedures cause the degeneration of structures and functions, rather than merely remove the conditions necessary for their growth.

In summary therefore, I am saying that Held's early theory based on the idea of mismatch between motor outflow and visual reafference was inappropriate for his own data and in any case it has been shown that voluntary movements are not essential for adaptation. What are the alternative theories of the conditions for adaptation? Harris's theory, that adaptation involves a change in the felt position of a part of the body, is a theory about the site of the adaptive change and not about the conditions for its occurrence. I should like to propose what may be called "discordance theory" (Howard, 1966). According to this theory visual–motor adaptation will occur whenever there is discordance as defined by one of the following conditions.

(a) Intersensory discordance involving the unusual spatial association of stimuli in different modalities. This leads to judgemental shifts as in ventriloquism or visual capture, as well as to sensorimotor adaptation. An example of the way in which intersensory discordance may lead to sensorimotor adaptation is provided by an experiment by Howard, Craske and Templeton (1965). In this experiment a rod seen through mirrors so as to be apparently displaced to one side was moved towards the subject and touched his face. The tactile and visual sensations were discordant and tests given immediately after exposure showed that the subject displaced his aims at a visual target in a direction which compensated for the optical displacement of the rod.

(b) Sensory-motor discordance involving the unusual association between motor innervation and consequent sensory inputs (reafference). The reafferent signal may result from a movement of the sense organ or of a part of the body being sensed. Discordance of any kind is very disturbing; motion sickness, for instance, is the result of conflicting action signals from vestibular and visual stimulation. Held's theory is seen to involve a special type of sensory motor discordance, that between the voluntary motor command and reafferent visual signals. Held apparently no longer insists that self produced movement is necessary and insists only that this type of discordance is more effective in producing adaptation than other types of discordance. In this he may be right, but the essential factor inducing modification of sensory motor behaviour is discordance of spatial information.

So much for theories about the necessary conditions for adaptation. I shall consider now the second general issue in this area.

V. SITE OF THE ADAPTIVE CHANGE IN VISUAL–MOTOR ADAPTATION TO DISCORDANCE

There are two related methods for studying this question: one may be called the "transfer-of-training" method, the other the "component analysis" method. The logic underlying the transfer-of-training method is that, if the change is in the visual system, the effects of training with one arm and with one eye open will *not* transfer when the subject is tested with the other eye, or another sense organ, but *will* transfer when he is tested with the other hand. But if the change is in the arm–body joint then training *will* transfer from one eye to the other, and to other modalities, but *not* from one arm to the other. Interocular and intersensory transfer has generally been found to occur, but there is conflicting evidence on interlimb transfer: some investigators have found some degree of transfer, others have found none.

Several attempts have been made recently to discover the conditions under which intermanual transfer occurs, in the hope of resolving the contradictions in the literature. However, whenever differences have been found to be associated with a certain factor, it has not been made clear why this is so (Hamilton, 1964; Freedman *et al.*, 1965).

The inspiration for an experiment I did recently was the thought that recalibration may occur at that articulation which shifts its mean position during training. It is usually the arm which has to shift its mean position in order to hit the displaced target; however, it is possible to arrange things so that the retinal image, eye, head or arm articulation changes its position. If the articulation which adjusts to the displaced target determines the articulation where a recalibration occurs, it should be possible to reveal the fact by the interlimb test. Specifically, if the position-shift and recalibration occur at the neck or above, there will be intermanual transfer because these articulations are common to both arms, but if the shift and recalibration involve the arm joint, interlimb transfer should not occur.

In the training task the subject had to point to a small target light in otherwise dark surroundings. The target was at eye level and its position could be varied along a horizontal arc at arm's length. The subject viewed the target binocularly through variable prisms which displaced the apparent position of the target up to 15° to left or right of straight ahead. At the beginning of training the prisms were set at zero displacement and were increased by approximately $\frac{1}{4}°$ steps between each pointing response up to a maximum of 16°. A further 40 pointings were made with the prisms at full displacement. The increase at each step was less than the mean variation of normal pointing, so that the subject remained unaware that a displacement was being introduced. This gradual "shaping" procedure ensures that any intermanual transfer that might occur is not merely the result of a conscious attempt by the subject to allow for displacement. During training, the subject's finger tip came into view at the termination of each aiming movement and he was instructed to attempt to hit the target as accurately as possible. During pre-training and post-training test-trials the finger did not come into view. The subject was asked to rest his arm between pointings on a horizontal padded surface and to avoid contact between the two hands. Ten pre-tests and ten post-tests were given for each hand before and after training, with the prism in its fully deflected condition. The difference between the mean pre- and post-test scores for the trained hand as compared with the untrained hand was taken as the measure of intermanual transfer.

The following training conditions were used:

(a) *Arm-shift condition*. In this condition the target was coupled to the prism-drive mechanism in such a way that it moved through the same angle as the prisms but in the opposite direction. In this way the target light was kept in the straight-ahead position of the subject. I shall refer to this as a "compensated target". The subject's retinal image, eyes, head and body therefore remained in the same position during training, but the arm had to aim more and more to one side in order to hit the target.

(b) *Body-shift condition*. Here the target was compensated (kept in the optical straight-ahead position), and the body was rotated by rotating the chair upon which the subject sat. Now the image, eye and arm articulations remained fixed and the neck became more and more deviated.

(c) *Eye-shift condition*. Here the target remained in the same actual position and the subject was asked to fixate it. The subject's retinal image, head and body remained in the same position, but the eyes became more and more eccentric.

(d) *Image-shift condition.* Here the subject was asked to fixate a second light which remained optically straight ahead, but to point to a stationary target light which appeared to become eccentric. Now the eyes, head and body remained in the same position, but the retinal image of the target became more and more eccentric.

A set of controls was run in which the effects of asymmetry were the same as in the experimental conditions, but in which there was no discordance between vision and reaching.

The variance of the data was disappointingly large, and although there was a tendency for intermanual transfer to occur in each condition, the only condition producing a significant degree of transfer was the image-shift condition. (A previous report that transfer occurred in all conditions was based on an inappropriate analysis.) This result suggests that the site of recalibration was largely, if not wholly, at the arm joint, irrespective of which motor articulation was involved in the realignment of limb and target, but that when the target was in the periphery of the visual field the recalibration was visual (retinal) at least in part. In other words, the arm joint is the most labile member of the control loop when the target is imaged on the fovea but the retina accounts for some of the lability when the target is imaged on the periphery.

It must be stressed that all pre- and post-tests were given with the prism at full deflection. This means that the visual target in the "image-shift" condition was in the periphery of vision during testing. When I talk of lability of retinal space values I refer only to the retinal periphery; the space value of the fovea would surely have remained unaltered.

We are always certain, to within a fraction of a degree, which part of the field of view we are fixated upon and the sensory features of foveal stimulation are so distinctive that training with prisms is most unlikely to alter its oculocentric space value. However, when a subject is trained to point to a displaced visual target imaged on the periphery of the retina, one might expect a change in peripheral retinal spatial values. Indeed, the retinal periphery would seem to be more labile than any other sensory component in the loop.

When I looked in the literature for evidence bearing on this question, I came across an experiment by Cohen (1966). He found that training transfers from foveal fixation to peripheral fixation, but not from periphery to fovea. This is just what one would expect on the assumption that the space value of the fovea is fixed and that the space values of the periphery are labile. When training involves peripheral fixation, recalibration is of the labile retinal space values of the periphery and is therefore specific to that location.

All other investigators of visual–motor adjustment to prismatic displacement, from Helmholtz onward, have used foveal fixation, the very part of the retina where the oculocentric space value will not shift. It is hardly surprising therefore that evidence of visual recalibration has not been found. It is unfortunate that it has been generally concluded that visual recalibration never occurs.

Harris (1965) has maintained, as the cornerstone of his theory of recalibration, that recalibration always involves a change in the "felt position" of the limb, head or eye. Harris defines "felt position" as being determined by all relevant sensory inputs, such as those from joints and tendons, as well as the corollary discharge (efference copy). With "felt position" defined as broadly as this, it is apparent that the only change which Harris claims does not occur is a change in the oculocentric space values of the retina, for these are the only elements in the system which are not subsumed under the term "felt position". It seems therefore that Harris's theory boils down to the statement that the recalibration of the visual–motor system to discordant information never involves a shift in the oculocentric space values. If I have interpreted Cohen's and my data correctly, then the theory is wrong because it is possible to shift oculocentric space values outside the fovea.

Incidentally, if this is the correct interpretation of Harris's theory, the differences between this theory and Held's theory of remapped potential orientations are only apparent. "A change in a felt position" and a "remapping of orientations" are apparently only different ways of talking about recalibration of space values of articulations. Held's description has the advantage of being objective. A detailed examination of the evidence Held has put forward to support his theory as against Harris's theory (e.g. Efstathiou, Bauer, Greene, and Held, 1966), reveals that both theories can accommodate the evidence equally well.

The second factor which has been overlooked in discussions of interocular transfer of prismatic training concerns the motor innervation to the eyes. The eyes do not have a passive position sense, and therefore what position sense they possess must arise from the efferent command signal or what Helmholtz called "sensations of innervation". Now according to Hering's law of equal innervations, one eye never moves unless the other eye moves through the same angle. The two eyes are yoked together and always move as a pair. Therefore, even if spatial recalibration of the efferent signal to the eye muscles were to occur, it is unlikely that it could be confined to the command to the muscles of one eye. Recent evidence (McLaughlin and Webster, 1967) suggests that recalibration of eye position does occur.

What I am saying then is that in the first place it was futile to look for a recalibration of the spatial value of the fovea, and in the second place, the presence of interocular transfer cannot be used as evidence for the absence of a recalibration of eye position because such a recalibration would not be confined to one eye anyway. It may also be argued that the presence of interlimb transfer cannot be used as evidence for the absence of a recalibration of the limb joint, for the two arms may be to some extent yoked together.

What I have stated about the use of evidence from transfer of recalibration from limb to limb or eye to eye leads to the following conclusion. It is not legitimate to argue from the presence of transfer that recalibration is not confined to a particular level in the system. However, it is probably legitimate to argue that, if the effects of training do *not* transfer, the recalibration *is* confined to one articulation.

Finally, there is a dimension to the problem of the site of visual–motor adaptation, which has been very much neglected. In almost all the studies done in the area, the arm has been used as the organ actively engaged in training. It may be that *recalibration occurs at that joint which is actively engaged during training, whether or not that is the joint which modifies its mean position during training*. Even though it has been shown that recalibration can occur in the absence of motor innervation, it is generally agreed that it is more complete when training involves self-produced movement (corollary discharge). It is reasonable to hypothesize therefore that recalibration will mainly involve the joint which is "active" during training. If we were required to "aim" our heads or our eyes to a target then perhaps these joints would be just as labile as the arm joint when the arm is doing the aiming. The only evidence I could find on this question was the results of an experiment by Craske (1967). It was shown that subjects who inspected immobile parts of their own body through prisms, subsequently pointed incorrectly towards visual targets with both hands, i.e. they behaved as if the eye position sense had been recalibrated. It was further shown that the eye position sense had indeed been changed by the predicted amount.

REFERENCES

COHEN, H. B. 1966. Some critical factors in prism adaptation. *Amer. J. Psychol.* **79,** 285–290.

CRASKE, B. 1967. Adaptation to prisms: change in internally registered eye-position. *Brit. J. Psychol.* **58**, 329–335.

EFSTATHIOU, A., BAUER, J., GREENE, M., and HELD, R. 1967. Altered reaching following adaptation to optical displacement of the hand. *J. exp. Psychol.* **73**, 113–120.

FREEDMAN, S. J., HALL, S. B., and REKOSH, J. H. 1965. Effects on hand-eye co-ordination of two different arm motions during adaptation to displaced vision. *Percept. mot. Skills* **20**, 1054–1056.

GREGORY, R. L. 1958. Eye movements and the stability of the visual world. *Nature, London* **182**, 1214–1216.

HAMILTON, C. R. 1964. Intermanual transfer of adaptation to prisms. *Amer. J. Psychol.* **77**, 457–462.

HARRIS, C. S. 1965. Perceptual adaptation to inverted, reversed and displaced vision. *Psychol. Rev.* **92**, 419–444.

HARRIS, C. S., HARRIS, J. R., and KARSCH, C. S. 1966. Shifts in pointing "straight ahead" after adaptation to sideways-displacing prisms. Paper read at Eastern Psychological Association, New York, April, 1966.

HEIN, A. and HELD, R. 1967. Dissociation of the visual placing response into elicited and guided components. *Science* **158**, 390–392.

HELD, R. 1961. Exposure-history as a factor in maintaining stability of perception and co-ordination. *J. nerv. ment. Dis.* **132**, 26–32.

HELD, R. and BAUER, J. 1967. Visually guided reaching in infant monkeys after restricted rearing. *Science* **155**, 718–720.

HERING, E. 1942. *Spatial sense and movements of the eye.* Amer. Acad. Optom, Baltimore.

HOWARD, I. P. 1966. Displacing the optical array. In S. J. Freedman (Ed.), *The neuropsychology of spatially oriented behavor.* Dorsey, Homewood.

HOWARD, I. P. 1967. Response shaping to visual–motor discordance. Paper presented to the Psychonomics Society, Chicago.

HOWARD, I. P., CRASKE, B., and TEMPLETON, W. B. 1965. Visuo-motor adaptation to discordant ex-afferent stimulation. *J. exp. Psychol.* **70**, 189–191.

HOWARD, I. P. and TEMPLETON, W. B. 1966. *Human spatial orientation.* Wiley, New York.

MCLAUGHLIN, S. C. and WEBSTER, R. G. 1967. Changes in straight-ahead eye position during adaptation to wedge prisms. *Percept. Psychophys.* **2**, 37–44.

MERTON, P. A. 1964. Absence of conscious position sense in the human eyes. In M. B. Bender (Ed.), *The oculomotor system.* Harper & Row, New York.

PICK, H. L. and HAY, J. C. 1965. A passive test of the Held reafference hypothesis. *Percept. mot. Skills* **20**, 1070–1072.

ROBINSON, D. A. O'MEARA, D. M., SCOTT, A. B., and COLLINS, C. C. 1969. Mechanical components of human eye movements. *J. Appl. Physiol.* **26**, 548–553.

STOPER, A. E. 1967. Vision during pursuit movement: the role of oculomotor information. Ph.D. Thesis, Brandeis University, U.S.A.

TEMPLETON, W. B. 1969. The effects of abnormal stimulation on the judgement of visual direction. Ph.D. Thesis, Durham University.

TEMPLETON, W. B., HOWARD, I. P., and LOWMAN, A. E. 1966. Passively generated adaptation to prismatic distortion. *Percept. mot. Skills*, **22**, 104–142.

VOLKMANN, F., SCHICK, C., AMY, M., and RIGGS, L. 1968. Time course of visual inhibition during voluntary saccades. *J. Opt. Soc. Amer.* **58**, 562–569.

Discussion

KAY: Can it be said that the adult subject accepts the brief half-hour experience which he receives in your experiment against a lifetime of normal experience? The interesting question is how quickly can a person accept this new information, does he really accept this new tactile, kinaesthetic-proprioceptive information as normally related to what he sees?

HOWARD: Yes, that is exactly what happens in all these experiments.

KAY: Would the effect, in fact, show when visual displacing prisms are removed.

HOWARD: Exactly, that is what always happens. He has to readjust his pointing back to normal.

WHITE: This is a well known after-effect.

HOWARD: The effect I end up with, with gradual shaping, is no different from what other people get, with their training procedures. In the initial stages of the procedures used by others the discordance between sight and movement is apparent, but after practice the subject ceases to be aware and the apparent discrepancy is removed. Subsequent pointing behaviour is affected and shows an after-effect with both types of procedures, showing that the effect is "deep" in the system. If the subject remained aware of the discordance, the change in his visual-motor system would be trivial and not reflect a real recalibration of his habits. No one in the field who has worked with prisms denies that there is a deep shift, a real recalibration.

WHITE: The beauty of these alterations here is that by introducing the displacement by gradual stages, the subject has been deliberately "conned".

HOWARD: Yes, even that initial conscious discordance has gone. The other techniques get to where I get in the end, but there is always the possibility of a conscious remembrance of that discordance, which could effect the subject's subsequent behaviour.

WHITE: I think the thing that is so exciting about Held's conceptualization in relation to these studies is that you do not need conventional feedback in the sense that you are aware of the error. You get the feedback of the information in this automatic way. Held showed that all you have to do to produce adaptation is to watch the hand moving in the visual field, but with no target and no error. There are problems about understanding what induces the adaptation in the absence of conscious error, but both your study and Held's show that any conventional notion that one has to have a conscious error when reaching for a target just does not apply.

HOWARD: I call Held's procedure "no target training". It does not work anything like as effectively as training with a target even though conscious error correction is not necessarily involved in either.

WHITE: Was it Wallach who said that the best way to do it is to tell the subject how far off they are. But the matter is still apparently in dispute.

Intersensory Integration and Motor Impairment

GENERAL DISCUSSION

Motor Impairment, Sensory Integration and Training

CONNOLLY: During the early stages of acquiring a new skill an adult tends to monitor his performance primarily through vision. As skilled performance is acquired the monitoring function is gradually transferred to kinaesthesis. I think a similar transition takes place over a rather longer time scale during development. The work of Held and his colleagues on reafference, and in particular their work on the sensory-motor development of immature organisms, lends support to this view. Lefford's paper and the monographs which he has published in collaboration with Birch (1963, 1967, *Monog. Soc. Res. Child Develop.* **28, 32**) indicate that the development of voluntary motor control and the emergence of skill are linked with the ability to use and interrelate information from several sense modalities. This work can be subsumed under the general title of integration. Twitchell (1959, *J. nerv. ment. Dis.* **129**, 105) has suggested that the motor deficit in cerebral palsy is related to a defect in sensory-motor integration and it is possible that further ideas about inter-sensory integration and its relationship to the development of skill may emerge from a consideration of the motor handicap suffered by children with certain neurological abnormalities.

One of our primary interests in Sheffield is in the motor problems of cerebral palsied children and I should like to describe briefly some of the work which we have done in this field. We set ourselves the task of seeing to what extent we could improve the performance of a child whose motor responses are uncoordinated, inaccurate and slow. Is there in the nervous system of these children any remaining plasticity or is the damage such that performance is irremediably impaired; given a child whose motor control is poor can we, by carefully programming his behaviour, bring about any lasting and substantial improvement?

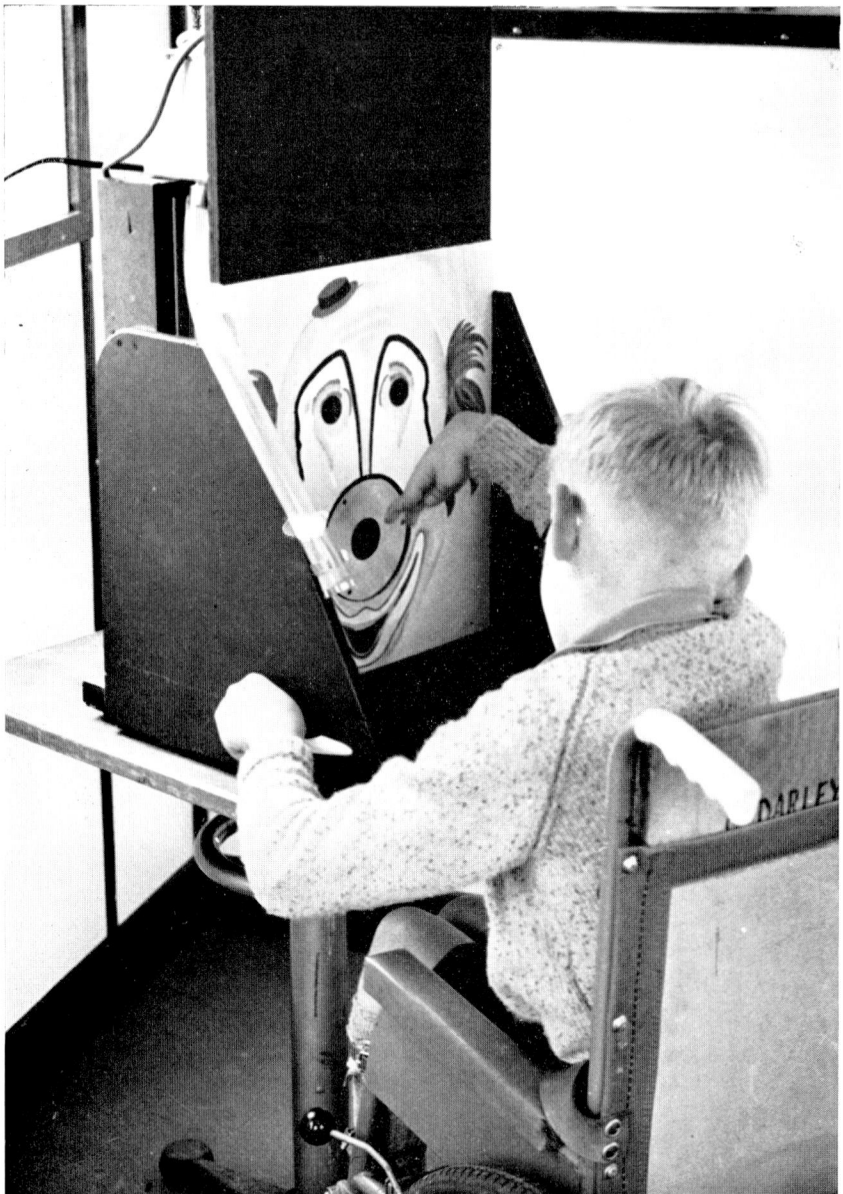

FIG. 1. Hemiplegic child operating clown apparatus.

We began our work by concentrating on a simple target response where a child is required to move from a specified position in space to a target, on command. Since our experimental programme necessitated that the children undergo extensive practice, and since motivation is important the apparatus which we developed took the form of a toy, Fig. 1. From the child's aspect he is confronted by a clown's face mounted in a frame. On the base board about 9 inches in front of the clown is a start button, painted bright red to contrast with the black frame, about 1·5 inches in diameter. The child is asked to put his finger, fingers, fist or whatever he can control in at least a rudimentary fashion, on this button. When the clown's nose lights up his task is to turn the light out as quickly as he can by hitting the nose with the hand which was resting on the button. A number of reinforcers are used to maintain the child's interest in the task; when a correct response is made, the nose light goes out, the eyes flash, the clown says "well done" or sings a snatch of a song, it also dispenses Smarties (M & M's). An incorrect response, not hitting the illuminated nose, results in the clown emitting a 2,000 Hz pure tone for 3 seconds, this is a signal of failure, and of course the nose light remains on. The positive reinforcers, apart from the nose light going off are put onto various schedules as the training progresses. The nose light and the negative 2,000 Hz pure tone provide immediate knowledge of results and are always available. Details of the equipment have been published elsewhere (Connolly, 1968, *Develop. Med. Child Neurol.* **10**, 697).

Two time measures are taken; reaction time, the time between the nose light going on and the child releasing the microswitch mounted under the start button, and flight time, the time between leaving the home button and arriving at the target. The pattern of errors under the various experimental conditions is also recorded automatically. We have been interested to discover how far it is possible to shape an initially crude response in terms of the time required to execute the movement and the size of target which could reliably be hit. At the beginning of training our subjects, who were mostly hemiplegics showing varying severity of impairment, were given a large target (approximately 16 square inches) and unlimited time in which to make the movement. Once a response to a large target was established the target size was reduced by small incremental steps. This was accomplished by fitting annulus rings (see Fig. 1) over the nose and so gradually reducing its effective size. The final target size is quite small, approximately 1·5 square inches. A similar temporal shaping is also achieved by progressively decreasing the time allowed for the execution of the response, this is defined operationally for the subject by withholding reinforcers for responses which are not completed within the allocated time.

The child shown in Fig. 1, as can be seen from the exaggerated posture of his right arm as he carries out the movement, is a hemiplegic. When we began work with him he was able, only with the greatest difficulty, to hit the largest target and the movement required about 2·7 seconds. After a few weeks of training he was able to hit, with relatively few errors, the smallest target and he could hit a medium sized target within about 700 milliseconds. The results of our initial experiments convinced us that it was possible to improve simple skills of this kind in cerebral palsied children. Many problems remain however. One of my students, Sandy Cohen, is looking into questions of generalization and the stability of performance once training is discontinued. The results which he has obtained so far are most encouraging though of course there are wide individual differences between the subjects. Following training, the subject's performance on a range of motor tasks shows improvement and this improvement is on the whole maintained after 6 weeks with no practice. There is some suggestion therefore of generalization and some indication that improvements following training are stable.

The clown apparatus indicates the feasibility of bringing the motor responses of neurologically impaired children under stimulus control. However, as a teaching, as distinct from measuring device it may be of limited value. Kinaesthetic feedback is necessary for the fine control of motor responses and it does not seem unreasonable to postulate that one of the problems confronting the cerebral palsied child is inadequate kinaesthetic feedback. The problem then becomes one of devising ways of augmenting feedback, such that the child can learn to discriminate signal from noise. If motor responses can be brought under control by amplifying feedback in another modality (visual) then it might be possible to shift the control to kinaesthetic/proprioceptive systems by suitable training procedures. Hefferline's work suggests that this should be possible (Hefferline, 1958, *Trans. N.Y. Acad. Sci.* **20,** 739; Hefferline and Perera, 1963, *Science* **139,** 834). In the case of the cerebral palsied child the proprioceptive feedback signals from his own movements may be so attenuated by noise in the neuromuscular system as to render the feedback signals almost useless. If we hypothesize that this is one of the major difficulties which the brain injured child has to face in learning to control his movements then our problem becomes one of devising ways of training the child to extract the signal from the noise. This is where questions of intersensory integration come in because I am suggesting that one modality be used to train another.

Hefferline's work has shown that it is possible to bring a single motor unit under voluntary control providing that appropriate experimental techniques are used. The subject may not be able to verbalize about it but the fact remains that he can do it, though whether a neurologically impaired patient can do this remains an open question. In the course of our discussions it has been suggested that this is a long way from the skilled responses which psychologists are usually concerned with, a whole complex set of movements and muscle responses which are integrated and put together in a variety of serial orders, but this may only reflect the level of analysis which we are used to dealing with.

Our pilot studies have made use of a joystick arrangement which the subject is required to move in a graded fashion. The movement of the joystick is transduced, via potentiometers, and displayed on an oscilloscope so that a spot of light is under the subject's control. In the early stages of training mechanical or electronic damping may be used to reduce the effects of tremor and any jerky or athetoid movements. A target is displayed on the screen and the subject's task is to move his spot of light to the target. A range of criteria may be used to measure the response; time taken, track of subject's spot, overshooting, under shooting etc. Once an acceptable response is established under these conditions of high grade visual feedback we have to devise means of transferring control from vision to proprioception. The technique which we have experimented with consisted in making the subject's spot disappear just before it reached the target so that the last fraction of the movement must be performed without visual feedback. The extent of this "blind band" is then gradually increased by very small steps. If control can be maintained over a graded response by using such a fading technique the response must be monitored by internal signals and the subject must therefore be able to discriminate some kinaesthetic signals from other activity in the neuromuscular system. No doubt the training will be difficult and some kind of adaptive system, perhaps by on-line control of the display, would be desirable. This work is very much in its early stages and I cannot present to you the results of any controlled experiments but I should be interested to have your views on the feasibility of educating one sensory modality by another.

ABERCROMBIE: I wonder if I could go back to your point about manual skill being primarily under visual control. We are of course talking about skills which are directed to a visual goal. Quite obviously this does not apply to Hinde's birds or to athletics. I am not sure that this presumed predominance of the visual system is justified from an evolutionary point of view.

I should like to make another point about the idea of environmental enrichment and the brain injured child. I think you are implying that what is of primary importance for the brain injured child is that his perceptual experiences be structured and carefully linked together. Now, whilst I do not deny this, it is becoming increasingly clear to me that it is not so much difficulties in the selection of sensory input that the brain injured children suffer from, so much as the lack of selection of the output. With the increasing difficulty of tasks set by too complicated a sensory input, the child's response makes the matter very much worse. The greater the child's effort, the greater the number of associated movements. The cerebral palsied, and in particular the athetoid child, is producing all sorts of unwanted movements. The central nervous system is being bombarded with all this reafferent rubbish, and, if I am right in thinking that the contralateral mirror image movements are important, what is even worse is the *non-random* opposite stimulation. If on top of this there is a recording of efference, then the whole system is being terribly overloaded. I do not want to deny the importance of intersensory association and integration but I think it is important to remember that far too much is being done on the motor side, more than the child can cope with; it is being swamped by reafference and possibly efference.

CONNOLLY: I take your point about "motor overload", and I quite agree that this is probably a basic problem however input synchrony is also fundamental.

ABERCROMBIE: May I just add that I think Hefferline's approach provides an answer to this, that is in terms of helping the child to inhibit all the other, irrelevant, movements. His experiments so far have been designed to show that people can produce these minute responses but the technique may be used equally well to *inhibit* unwanted movements.

CONNOLLY: Let me say again that my ideas are hypothetical, I postulated that one of the severe problems facing the cerebral palsied child was inadequate kinaesthetic feedback and that this arose from an unfavourable signal to noise ratio in the neuromuscular system. I am not suggesting that the somaesthetic senses are completely degenerated in those subjects nor am I suggesting that vision is completely dominant in the normal child. What I have in mind bears some similarity to the experimental paradigm which Held called decorrelation—where one set of inputs is not related to another set. He demonstrated the consequences of this by quite a simple arrangement of having the subject view his hand through a pair of prisms which were revolving in opposite directions. When the subject moved his hand the felt movements were not correlated with the visually perceived movements. I think this experimental situation might provide an analogue of the problem which I am suggesting faces the cerebral palsied child.

BRUNER: Is there not a great deal of this integrative function already built in? A very young baby for instance will orient its eyes in the direction of a source of sound. I think apparent movement can go from one modality to another; this is something which interests me greatly and we are in the process of investigating it. Certainly different senses can stand for each other in terms of marking off time limits, so that in space and time there appear to be certain relationships between sensory modes. I do not doubt that there is a tremendous amount of integration to begin with and that this gets elaborated by certain kinds of experience. What bothers me a little is that we have been talking thus far as if association is what ties together the senses. What we know about the structuring of responses both serially and spatially tells us that they are not linked together simply by being next to each other.

INGRAM: I am rather worried by this notion of the nervous system of the cerebral palsied child being bombarded by impulses. Surely one of the characteristics of a great many cerebral palsied children is a lack of stimulation. Take for an example a child with a congenital hemiplegia, he will have very little experience of movement and you cannot say he is being bombarded by an excess of confusing sensations.

CONNOLLY: Perhaps not, but what sensations he does have may be disordered or in terms of my hypothesis decorrelated. The brain dysfunction may be largely a deficit in the integration of different sensory and motor systems.

INGRAM: The sensations may be totally disordered, is it not therefore the lack of movement experience that is likely to be important. I would have thought that poverty of movement in infancy is likely to be far more important than any excess of confusing stimulation.

The Concept of Noise

HINDE: May I ask for a point of information? In all this talk about noise I really have no conception yet as to what the dependent variable is, or what it is that these conjectures are based upon.

CONNOLLY: There is a wealth of evidence in the literature indicating that in order to perform skilled operations it is necessary that a person should have feedback from his own movements. This implies that internal signals of some kind are involved. In order to monitor his performance therefore, the individual has to select the relevant cues from the total ongoing activity in the neuromuscular system. My hypothesis is that cerebral palsied children are unable, or have great difficulty, in picking out the relevant cues from all the other signalling going on: the relevant and important cues are in fact lost amongst all the other activity of the neuromuscular system, which I have called noise.

HINDE: I think this is a different and more circumscribed use of the term noise than the one which we discussed yesterday. It seems to me that, whereas this may be a useful concept within particular limits, there is nevertheless a danger in extending the concept of noise from the restricted use which you have just described to some sort of broad "motor noise".

PRECHTL: If you consider eye movements then the optimal sort of eye movements could be thought of as a signal. As soon as this is defined as a signal every deviation from that can be considered as noise.

HINDE: This is very different from what was said a little while ago about too little noise: this is quite a different sort of concept.

CONNOLLY: I think Ingram was talking about too little stimulation and too little experience, not too little noise.

INGRAM: Yes, I was referring to a lack of stimulation; a lack of experience and in particular a lack of movement experience. I am worried about this concept of noise from a different point of view, because presumably it is coming from within the nervous system rather from without.

BRUNER: I should like to point out a mathematical reason for caution in the use of this notion. The concept has some very sharp restraints on it; when one talks about noise level it is necessary to make the assumption that noise is additive. Secondly whenever a model of information theory is used in this context it assumes that you can specify something about the nature of the information transmitted which means that you have full knowledge of the number of alternatives from the set in which the signal is embedded.

CONNOLLY: I accept what you say, I am using the term primarily for heuristic reasons. I should be just as happy to talk about the message which is required to produce a particular response, and the difficulty of extracting this from all the other activity which is going on. An analogy would be to consider the difficulties involved in transmitting a message on a very bad telephone connection, the interference makes this difficult and the message is in danger of becoming garbled. If I am given a cue however, such as the general topic of the message I can reduce the number of alternatives.

PRECHTL: A good example to which the mathematics have been

applied in detail is Stark's (1968, *Neurological control systems*. Plenum Press, New York) analysis of the pupillary response in humans. The pupils are never quiet, they are continually moving though when the retina is stimulated by an increase in light intensity they constrict. Constriction can be regarded as the signal and this is superimposed on the whole system which is continually undergoing change. What makes sense in this context is to have a clear definition of the signal itself and the rest then is noise.

HINDE: I think Prechtl may be over-interpreting what I said. I am not disputing the usefulness of the concept, all I am saying is that we must not use it in many different senses at the same time.

Neurological Considerations

INGRAM: From a neurological standpoint most of our information about the integration of sensory activities is in a way negative, it comes from evidence of brain lesions in adults. Luria (1966, *Human brain and psychological processes*. Harper & Row, London) provides many examples but I do not think one can argue very much about the developing child from what happens in the brain injured adult.

TWITCHELL: I think some of the work done by Hubel and Wiesel (1965, *J. Neurophysiol.* **28,** 1029) is important in this context because it shows up many of the difficulties which underlie this problem. If a kitten is deprived of vision from birth for a number of months and then that eye is stimulated subsequently, we find that most of the binocular cells in the occipital cortex which are fired by that eye have been knocked out. However, if both eyes are blindfolded and the experiment repeated then we find that the effect does not occur, most of the binocular cells are still effective. This I think brings us to the real problem of dysfunction. Performance is certainly related to efferent brain injury but it seems to me that it is also related to the undamaged parts of the brain which remain. Some of the defects which we have talked about may well be related to what some have called perceptual rivalry, but there is also rivalry of various motor systems. Part of the defect of motor function in the hemiplegic for example, is not only the loss of contributions from the injured hemisphere but also some effect from the intact hemisphere; this of course complicates the issue very considerably. A similar situation arises if one limb of a monkey is de-afferented then it is virtually useless, however, if both limbs are de-afferented then the loss of function is less than when only one limb is de-afferented.

BRUNER: The notion of plasticity is almost one of the working criteria for a skill. When we say that a skill has been achieved we mean basically that a person can perform the task under a range of conditions—he can climb a small tree or a large tree.

INGRAM: I think a neurologist would understand plasticity to mean the ability of other parts of the brain to take over the functions of a damaged part.

TWITCHELL: Which does not happen.

BRUNER: That is rather discouraging.

INGRAM: I wonder if that is really true? What about children who sustain damage to the dominant hemisphere in the first 3 or 4 years of life, their speech development continues. They do not become dysphasic as would adults who sustained the same damage.

TWITCHELL: Well that may be because both left and right hemispheres can serve language function for the first 3 or 4 years.

HINDE: Let's go back to this question of intersensory integration. I should like to press Twitchell a little further on what he meant about the importance of the Hubel and Wiesel work. It seems to me that he was making a point as to the difficulty of interpreting these observations and I am not quite sure just what he was driving at.

TWITCHELL: Consider again cerebral hemispherectomy in the monkey which produces a profound hemiparesis. The motor deficit surely is related in large part to the loss of contact placing and grasping reactions and concomitant enhancement of avoiding reactions. But neglect of the contralateral limbs is also a feature. Vocalization following nociceptive stimulation of these limbs is depressed. Following ablation of the intact motor cortex, a more natural balance between groping and avoiding responses appears; motor function improves and even a more natural reaction to nociceptive stimulation of those limbs returns. I think, in a sense, the same may be true with the Hubel and Wiesel study. Perhaps the marked binocular depression which results from "blinding" one eye may not be so much the result of "blinding", but that something is coming from the intact side to intefere with it or to rival it. I am suggesting that those parts which are left intact contribute to the deficit in a very important way.

HINDE: That is exactly what I was getting at. Perhaps the best experiment is not the lesion experiment but the artificial squint experiment (Hubel and Wiesel, 1965, *J. Neurophysiol.* **28,** 1041) which decreases the number of striate cortical cells driven from both eyes.

TWITCHELL: I would think this is another demonstration of the effect of a disequilibrated afferent input.

LEFFORD: I should like to call attention to observations made on the congenitally blind. In the case of those people whose sight was restored surgically there was no visual recognition of objects which they could appreciate tactually. One might expect that there would be some kind of recognition if there were integration at an earlier level.

Our own work has been with relatively complicated perceptual stimulation. One of our experiments in the intersensory field is concerned to discover whether a child can recognize numbers in different modalities. Can the child count six coins? Can he count six taps? Can he also count six touches on a finger? If this ability appears in one modality is it already available in another? One feature that does seem fairly clear to me is that education appears to occur within a modality. First the pattern within two different modalities must be learned within each modality before they can be related. Now as I understand Connolly's experiment he was using vision to educate the somaesthetic modality: once the child can make the correct movement then there will be some sort of stimulation of the somaesthetic modality and in consequence there will be some learning. This brought to mind an experience which I once had in examining a patient. We showed the patient a noise maker such as is used on New Year's Eve. He looked at it with a most perplexed expression on his face and clearly did not know what to do with it. However, if we said "New Year" he would whirl it around appropriately and make the correct noise and the correct action. apparently by using a different input line we could trigger off his recognition of the object. I was very impressed by this. Apparently one can lose "intelligence" in one modality whilst retaining it in another.

TWITCHELL: Connolly's cases point to a problem with respect to the sensory factors involved in motor function. When I discussed the development of the reflex substrata for voluntary prehension in the infant a few days ago, I noted the importance of the instinctive groping and avoiding reactions and of the grasp reflex, the latter as a facilitator of finger flexion. All of these reactions require contact as an adequate stimulus, and when their mechanisms are intact, extremely adroit orientation of the hand can occur without visual direction. Note that this does not imply any conscious perception of the contact. Now the motor cortex is intimately concerned with the function of these reactions—the instinctive reactions are abolished by ablation of the motor cortex and the grasp reflex seriously impaired. In such instances, vision is required to direct the residual movement.

In this regard, it is instructive to follow the course of recovery from hemiplegia in man after a stroke (Twitchell, 1951, *Brain* **74,** 443). At a stage prior to recovery of the grasp reflex some voluntary finger movement may be accomplished under visual control—blindfold the patient, however, and he is no longer able to perform that movement even though there is no defect in any modality of perceived sensation including cortical discriminating sensation. If the grasp reflex returns during the course of recovery, he is able to perform these movements without the aid of vision.

Monkeys with lesions in the motor cortex can reach out and pick up peanuts and sometimes these animals have been observed to groom themselves. If you prick one of these monkeys with a pin, it will reach out and brush the examiner's hand away. If the animal is blindfolded he is no longer able to do this. There is no loss of perceived sensation: prick him and he will vocalize. Histological examination reveals no damage in the primary sensory receiving areas; yet without vision and in the absence of this very important cortical contact facilitator the animal is unable to execute a movement.

The importance of the exteroceptors in the skin for the control of highly co-ordinated motor function is again shown in the differential section of the dorsal roots (Twitchell, 1954, *J. Neurophysiol.* **17,** 239). Here you can knock out the exteroceptors, leave the muscle afference intact and find the same sort of thing. The monkey climbs well hand over hand as long as he is permitted vision, deprive him of vision and he cannot do it. In the case of the children with hemiplegia which you referred to I think it is this contact facilitator which is lacking. I have no doubt that their performance could be improved by using the augmented feedback techniques but such children have other problems. They usually have an over-active avoiding reaction, which militates against extension of the arm; their movements, particularly in severe cases, are all biased towards flexion (Twitchell, 1966, *Clin. Orthop.* **46,** 55).

INGRAM: Margaret Jones spent some time with children who had an acquired or a congenital hemiplegia trying to improve their kinaesthetic sensation by training. They were given objects to manipulate and exercises to increase finger movement, at the end of about 18 months no significant improvements were found in either sensory or motor function.

CONNOLLY: I do not think that one can infer from a single study that such change is impossible. What is important is to ensure that the child has feedback, feedback that is which he can utilize.

BRUNER: That is exactly the way I want to put it. I am puzzled by the point which Twitchell is making because vision is being substituted; to begin with both kinaesthesis and vision are operating and it appears that vision can serve for the lot if worked properly. Presumably it would be possible with the right kind of device to convert the position of the limbs into an auditory signal.

TWITCHELL: No, that is not the point.

BRUNER: Well, how do you conceive of that substitution?

TWITCHELL: I do not think that it would help particularly to convert information to another modality. The patients I am talking about all have position sense, they all have intact data for perceiving this sensation.

BRUNER: Why do they need vision then?

TWITCHELL: The motor cortex which is not sensory in the classical sense, is directed by unconscious contact stimulation not perceived contact. So in the absence of such a mechanism movement must be directed by vision. If you knock out the motor cortex you still have the whole mid-brain motor mechanism there, the difficulty now is firing off and this is where vision comes in, vision can serve to direct or facilitate the movements.

KAY: I should like to bring this into relation with something which we were discussing the other day about an anaesthetized limb, such as when a person is operating under conditions of extreme cold. One cannot get tactile cues from an anaesthetized limb and therefore vision must be used. The point I want to bring out is how artificial the movement is under such conditions. There appear to be two temporally distinct sequences which are out of phase. Visual monitoring is slower, as may be illustrated by a simple example. If we ask a person to hold a sharp instrument between two fingers he cannot press it because he would prick himself but he must hold it firmly or it will drop. Now, without using tactile cues this task cannot be done, vision is not enough where there is no limb movement. Fine manipulations of this kind do require somaesthetic information if they are to be performed adequately. The interesting feature about somaesthetic and visual cues is that the sequence of signals is a little out of phase, the normal person is used to this and can cope with it.

INGRAM: Is vision necessary to initiate movement merely or is it necessary for the completion as well as the initiation?

TWITCHELL: There are several interesting experiments which may be important in this context; there is a paper by Gilman and Denny-Brown (1966, *Brain* **89**, 397) and another by Sprague *et al.* (1963, *Arch. ital. Biol.* **101**, 225). In the Gilman and Denny-Brown experiment the dorsal columns of the spinal cord in monkeys were sectioned and in Sprague's experiment lesions were made in the medial lemniscus of cats. Both investigations reported a profound effect on motor performance. There also appears to be a disturbance of spatial behaviour resulting from interference with the lemniscal fibres; both reports make a point of this. Denny-Brown has a rather neat explanation for it in terms of cutting down input into the parietal cortex and as a consequence effectively producing parietal lobe dysfunction.

The Importance of Vision in Control

BRUNER: I was trying to think of anything in the literature which would indicate an instance of where the provision of full information to the visual modality aided the child in carrying out some skilled act which could not have been achieved otherwise. Nothing comes to mind.

INGRAM: A case of mine a few years ago may be relevant. This was a child who had severe refractive errors which had not been previously detected. Providing the child with spectacles, and thus binocular vision for the first time, resulted in the most striking improvement. In other words, this child was doubly handicapped, first by not having binocular vision but suffering refractive errors and secondly by a congenital ataxia. The child began to walk within a few months of being fitted with spectacles. Although this is not experimental evidence I found the improvements astonishing.

CONNOLLY: If I take a cup and pour some water into it, I can walk along carrying this cup and probably hold a conversation at the same time without spilling the water. I could probably even do it with my eyes closed. If I fill the cup to the brim then in order to avoid spilling it I must look at the cup as I walk along. When you watch young children carrying things or carrying out fine manipulations they visually monitor their performance. I think they have to.

BRUNER: This is Eleanor Maccoby's (1964, paper in APA symposium on the development of attentional processes) point that with the young child picking up new patterns they require much more redundant information. I agree that would seem to be something which characterizes both the dissolution side and the developmental side.

PRECHTL: Is it not simply that visual output control is required by the young child because the proprioceptive information is not sufficient. Thinking of it in terms of a control system then I would say that the internal feedback systems are not in themselves enough to maintain control, vision is therefore used in addition. I do not think that there is anything very unusual about this nor would I regard it as intersensory.

BRUNER: In order that vision should aid the internal systems they have to be correlated initially, do they not?

PRECHTL: Yes, but in the case of Connolly's example this seems to me very simple.

HINDE: I think this is the point that Held is making. When Prechtl says this is simple, Held asks the question, why is it that a slight visual discrepancy just matches up with a slight proprioceptive discrepancy or an efferently copied discrepancy? I do not think it is simple. You gloss over the complexity of the problem by saying that these are two sensory systems acting in parallel. The point is that they are co-ordinated and these visual displacements are somehow matched up with the activity in the proprioceptive system. How that equation is made is the crucial issue.

PRECHTL: By simple I merely meant something which is not mystical. It is actually a complex servo-system.

BRUNER: I think that what Hinde means is that there is some connection between these two systems, otherwise they would not be able to operate in parallel. I agree with him that this is not a simple point, it takes us right back to the question about how the sensory modalities relate to each other so that they may serve in this way.

HINDE: In insects there are examples of motor patterns which are independent of practice: the classic case is the dance of the bee when it transposes from orienting with respect to the sun to orienting with respect to gravity. These cases appear to be independent of any particular intersensory development.

A Model

LEFFORD: Now that the problem of what ties the modalities together has been raised I wonder if Held's experiments provide the answer? They would suggest that it is the response itself which established the connection.

WHITE: Yes, this is fundamental.

CONNOLLY: Fundamental yes, but we must be careful not to make it the whole explanation. Remember, after all the deprivation which these animals have been subjected to, the response develops very quickly when normal conditions are restored. There must be something to account for this speed of relearning.

In their monograph Birch and Lefford (1967, *Monog. Soc. Res. Child Develop* **32,** 110) argue that developmental improvements in cross-modal transfer tasks and in perceptual skills are due to a greatly increased liason between the senses rather than to an improved ability to make intra-modal discriminations. I think they are correct in arguing that if we are to understand the mechanisms underlying the emergence of skilled performance we need more detailed knowledge about the relationship between visual and kinaesthetic processing. We recently carried out some experiments on intra-modal and cross-modal judgements on groups of children of different ages. Because of the difficulties of obtaining a good metric for shapes we had subjects judging the length of lines. They inspected a standard and then made judgements about a variable. There were four experimental conditions as follows:

>visual–visual match v–v
>kinaesthetic–kinaesthetic match k–k
>visual–kinaesthetic match v–k
>kinaesthetic–visual match k–v.

The experiment was basically quite simple and the details have been published elsewhere (Connolly and Jones, 1970, *Brit. J. Psychol.* **61,** 259). The results, which were examined in terms of absolute errors and variances, show that performance on the tasks improves with increasing age. Intra-modal performance was more accurate and less variable than cross-modal performance and the v–v condition was less variable than the k–k condition. An interesting feature of the results was a marked asymmetry between the two cross modal conditions at all age levels, k–v performance was more accurate and less variable than v–k performance.

In our discussions of integration we have talked so far as if the different input channels were equivalent. I think these findings with respect to the asymmetry of cross-modal matching cast some doubt on this. In order to account for these findings Jones and I proposed a formal model accounting for the observed developmental changes and for the

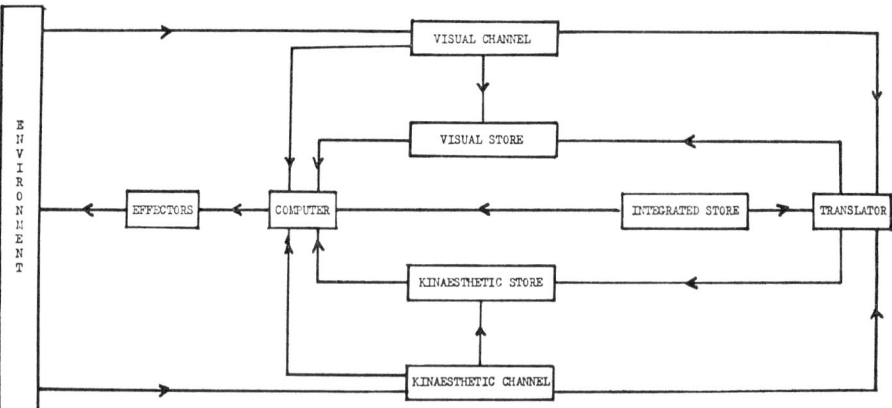

FIG. 2. Diagrammatic model for intra-modality and cross-modality matching. Inputs for the integrated store are shown in Fig. 3 (from Connolly, K. and Jones, B. 1970. *Brit. J. Psychol.* **61,** 259).

asymmetry in cross-modal performance. We assume that visual and kinaesthetic information is held in separate short term storage systems and that translation between modalities is dependent on an integrated long term store, Fig. 2. There is evidence in the literature indicating that visual storage is more efficient than kinaesthetic (Posner, 1967, *J. exp. Psychol.* **75,** 103). An essential feature of the model is that the translation of information between modalities takes place prior to its being put into short term store. In the case of the v–k task the visual information is translated into kinaesthetic code and stored before being reproduced kinaesthetically, and similarly with a k–v task. The greater susceptibility of the kinaesthetic store to decay increases the variability of v–k performance over that of k–v. Translation between modalities is performed on the basis of information held in a long term integrated store which contains some internal representation of the relationship between visual and kinaesthetic information. The additional process of translation which a cross-modal match requires serves to increase the variability of cross-modal over intra-modal performance.

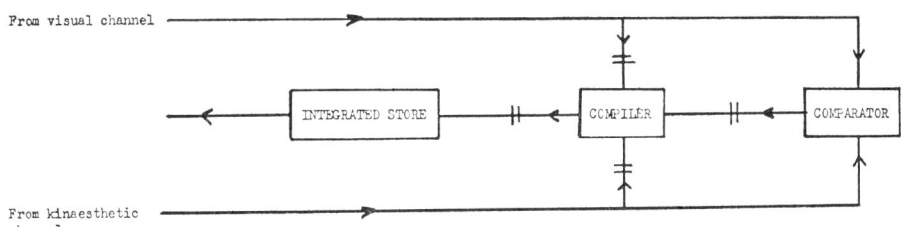

FIG. 3. Compiler unit embodying error-correcting system; the double bars refer to the switch mechanism (from Connolly, K. and Jones, B. 1970. *Brit. J. Psychol.* **61,** 259).

Developmental changes in intra-modal performance may result from improvments in the short term storage system or from an increased efficiency on the part of the computer, which issues commands to the effector processes on the basis of comparisons which it makes. The compiler, Fig. 3, serves to collate visual and kinaesthetic inputs and transfers the results into long term store. By analogy the visual and kinaesthetic inputs may be thought of as English and French dictionaries, the compiler is then responsible for collating a French–English dictionary, the integrated long term store. The comparator is responsible for detecting mismatches between the inputs. A mismatch serves to activate the compiler which re-samples the visual and kinaesthetic inputs, calculates new relationship between the two and switches a new mapping function into store.

We have checked independently (Jones and Connolly, 1970, *Brit. J. Psychol.* **61,** 267) that translation occurs before storage by examining the memory properties of intra- and cross-modal matches after varying time delays. The results lend support to the model.

HOWARD: That is a very interesting experiment. Can I just clear up one point? You say that you found greater variance in the visual to kinaesthetic condition. If the standard were presented to the modality with the least variance then clearly you would be cutting down on the task variance in the initial stages of processing, but if the standard were presented to the modality with the greater variance then there would be no way of compensating for the information loss. I wonder if you could account for the asymmetry in terms of the variance of the encoding modality?

CONNOLLY: I do not think the results can be explained in that way. We spent a long time trying to account for the results in terms of what we called the resolving power of the different modalities and we assumed that the accuracy of the visual system would be greater than that of the kinaesthetic system. However, if this were the reason for the asymmetry one would predict that the difference in variance between the two cross-modal conditions would be reversed, k–v matches should be less accurate than v–k matches.

HOWARD: Yes, I see the point. Howarth and Fisher (Cited in Howard and Templeton, 1966, *Human spatial orientation*, Wiley, London) have done some interesting experiments in the same field. You may remember they had two hypotheses. The first was that the variance of inter-modal judgements would represent the sum of the variances of the intra-modal judgements, this was called the additive variance hypothesis. The experimental arrangement involved the subject in making a judgement about the position of a sound in relation to a previously perceived point of light, in addition there was a visual–visual condition. However, I think that they overlooked the importance of the neck in the feedback loop. To my knowledge no one has repeated this experiment and I certainly think that it needs doing again. The second hypothesis was that constant errors for the different modalities are algebraically additive. The lack of visual–kinaesthetic symmetry in your study does not support this hypothesis.

LEFFORD: In the model there is a component labelled computer. Do the properties of this component change as development proceeds?

CONNOLLY: Yes, this is assumed to be a self organizing system and is probably responsible for the changes in intra-modal matching which we observed to be correlated with age.

KAY: If I understand you correctly you are saying that improvements in a child's skilled performance can be partly explained in terms of an error correcting process which produces a closer representation of the relationship between information from different sensory modalities. Am I right?

CONNOLLY: Yes, exactly, but this is not to deny that development also relates to many other factors. The child becomes better at attending to and selecting the relevant information from the display.

An Evaluation

Concluding Remarks

KEVIN CONNOLLY

University of Sheffield

To SUMMARIZE THE papers which have been presented and our discussions around them, dealing as they do with a range of diverse methods and concepts, is an almost impossible task. However, it is possible to identify some issues where there are common threads running through our thinking and these I shall try to bring out. In planning the study group it was our intention to adopt an interdisciplinary approach. We felt that the nature of the mechanisms underlying the development of motor skills could only be tackled sensibly by an approach at several levels. By bringing together people from different disciplines we formed a multi-disciplinary group and in so doing gained something of the flavour of the methods and concepts of specialist fields other than our own. However, the inter-disciplinary approach was not always apparent, indeed it is arguable that in order to achieve an inter-disciplinary position we must each learn something of the other's specialist field. Perhaps if we were to reconvene in 5 years time we could move from the multi-disciplinary position to a truely inter-disciplinary one where we are more able to integrate levels of explanation and ask the right question of anothers speciality. For the experimental psychologist to know something of the underlying neural substrate with which he is dealing and its physiology should make him better equipped to formulate questions which are more meaningful biologically. Similarly I have no doubt that the neurologist and paediatrician would benefit from an understanding of the methods and findings of contemporary experimental child psychology.

Skill and movement are not synonymous. When we speak of simple (because they are common) skills such as throwing a ball, building a tower of bricks, drawing with a crayon, we are talking of activities which require the co-ordination and regulation of whole sequences of movements. Motor skills involve many psychological processes; perception, attention, selection and movement to name but some. The manner in which these processes are deployed and the way in which they are inter-linked towards the achievement of a goal characterize skilled behaviour. Earlier attempts to explain the co-ordination of sensory information and its integration with muscular respones leaves much to be desired. The notion of skill acquisition as the formation of stimulus response chains was challenged by goal directed theories of behaviour and the inadequacy of the Hullian S-R model was exposed by Lashley (1951). From a developmental standpoint the inadequacies of a chaining model are apparent both from Kay's paper and from Bruner's.

The analysis of adult performance has placed great emphasis on the concept of feedback. Feedback tells the system what it is doing and provides it with a means whereby it may maintain its output in a state of dynamic equilibrium. A system which is sensitive to its own product has greatly increased flexibility which is an important feature of behaviour which we describe as skilled. In addition cognitive features further facilitate flexibility. Indeed once a strategy or technique has been mastered it may be used in a range of situations; it appears to embody a principle of transfer. In the introduction I mentioned the molar versus molecular approach to motor skill. The molecular approach sees the individual as an information processing device; in order to function efficiently he must encode and interpret information continuously and he must compute and execute responses in accord with some strategy or programme which guides him towards his goal. Bruner's experiments indicate how an infant develops strategies for using information intelligently in order to choose among modes of responding and to change his mode of responding. My own experiments on information processing in older children show quantitative improvements as a function of increasing age and reveal also certain qualitative changes which take place. It is important that we recognize qualitative changes and accommodate our model of skill development accordingly. The child is not a smaller and more rudimentary version of the adult, and development is only a smooth progression if examined with a crude instrument. Similarly, although there are superficial resemblances between the behaviour of infants and adults the neurology of the infant is not simply a primitive copy of the adult.

For skilled motor activity we can stipulate certain minimum logical requirements. There must be an output mechanism (effector) to be regulated and a source of control which defines the intended action. In addition there must be a receptor mechanism which registers the course of the action and some means whereby the output can be compared to the plan. Finally there must be an error correcting process which converts the discrepancies between the plan and the outcome into regulatory signals. Skills then consist in an organized framework of co-ordinated serial movements which correspond to a pattern which, within limits, is predetermined. What has emerged from our discussions is an emphasis on the cognitive features of skill; notions of programmes and analysis by synthesis and on the components of performance rather than an overriding concern with a learning theory framework.

In dealing with the problem of serial order and the modularization of skill Bruner and I independently used the concept of a sub-routine to identify a functional unit. We were both concerned to develop a means of discussing and investigating the assembly of components into an integrated, planned activity. Kay dealt with similar questions and developed the ideas of a macro-strategy and the micro-structure of a skill. These notions are of course inter-related. The macro-strategy demands a continuous interaction between input and output monitoring which matches the varying demands of the two sources of information. Where the units are large the amount of switching between the two sources will be reduced, grouping material or the establishment of sub-routines will therefore serve to reduce the load. In the course of our discussions these concepts found favour as heuristic devices, whether they can be operationalized and so be of value empirically remains to be seen. A further important point which emerged is that for the child almost everything in the environment is information, in the sense that it is uncertain. Redundancies must be established and in order to accommodate to the environment the child must learn something of the contingencies of certain events. In discussion Bruner and Kay differed over how this was achieved; for Bruner the child was learning rules whereas Kay spoke of learning probabilities. On reflection I suspect that they are both right and that the difference between them is partly semantic. When does a knowledge of probabilities merit the description of a rule, perhaps when it can be modified to meet changing circumstances when in fact it is not too situation specific. If rules and transfer functions are established they are presumably based upon the child's experience of contiguities and the probability of a given outcome. Knowing which features of a display are redundant in a given context implies the ability to predict the important cues.

A point touched on by several members of the group but which we made little of in discussing how responses are co-ordinated and built up into larger serial units, is the notion of anticipation (Bartlett, 1958). Little is known of the role of anticipation in the development of sensory-motor skills though it is presumably important. A distinction between rules and probabilities may emerge at this point. On one occasion I spent an afternoon in the University gymnasium playing with a 3-year-old. One of the games which we played was chasing a hoop; I would roll a hoop down the gymnasium and the little girl would chase and try to capture it before it fell down. After rolling about 30 feet the hoop would lose momentum and begin to describe an ever decreasing circular track until it finally fell. The child would dash after the hoop and pursue it round its circular track, almost catching it but never quite doing so. For an adult it was easy to catch the hoop, one simply had to cross a sector of the circular path in order to grab it. The 3-year-old never showed anticipation, in Poulton's (1957) taxonomy perceptual anticipation. Anticipation of this kind depends on the emergence of some organized pattern. Kay expressed the view that the developmental approach had much to contribute to the understanding of adult skills and I think the emphasis on cognitive features may be one such important contribution; we appear to be dealing with the expression of some internal programme rather than the acquisition of specific responses. Whilst not disputing the old adage that "practice makes perfect" we must remember that practice improves something which one can already do. Logically practice cannot account for the initial appearance of a skill.

Hinde's paper on the development of bird song provides an interesting example of a motor skill particularly in relation to the role of performance in learning. Although bird song, viewed as a skill, lacks an orientation to the environment it resembles other skills which we discussed in that its acquisition involves both learning the nature of the task and how to carry it out. Further studies on the development of motor skills in animals may help clarify the notion of a motor programme and may indeed throw some light on the underlying processes. Hinde also pointed out that some quite complex and finely adjusted movements may be independent of experience. This directs our attention to biochemical and physiological questions regarding the development of anatomically correct nervous connections (Sperry, 1951).

The reafference principle developed by von Holst and Mittelstaedt (1950) has had a considerable effect on the direction of research on sensory-motor skill, the work of Held and Hein (1963) being perhaps the most obvious example. The problem of how a child assembles his body schema and how this accords with his spatial environment is of fundamental importance. The tying together of the different sensory systems which this implies can be usefully studied, as Abercrombie showed, by examining the childs performance in drawing. Drawing provides a good example because it has all the points of difficulty associated with a motor skill; there must be a stimulus analysing system, perceptual discrimination both kinaesthetic and visual, a guiding programme and an error correcting system. Drawing and copying, matching and discriminating perceptual and motor patterns implies not only the existence of programmes but also the importance of the modified signal (feedback) as a basic unit. (Implicitly we were all concerned about the nature of our units and at one point the problem was made explicit when someone confessed that the term response did not describe a unit at all.)

On the whole a child has to monitor his motor outputs more than an adult and he often needs vision to tell him where his hand is or where he must place his foot on a staircase. Gradually visual cues are required less as proprioception takes over some of the monitoring functions of vision. In the case of adults learning a new skill there is evidence indicating an increased dependency on proprioception as the skill improves (Fleishman and Rich, 1963). Such developments serve to reduce the load on the visual system which if freed from some tasks can take on others. The degree of integration between sensory modalities will therefore impose some limiting factor on skill development. In matching the internal and external worlds the child must correlate his perceptions of the external environment (and changes in these perceptions) with the feedback from his own movements. In copying a simple geometric form such as a triangle there must be a mechanism which analyses the visual display and one which transforms the visual pattern into kinaesthetic code so that a whole pattern of movements may be co-ordinated in order to reproduce the figure.

Little is known of developmental changes in the functional efficiency of the proprioceptive mechanisms. However, it is improbable that they will not show improvements as growth proceeds. Adams and Creamer (1963) obtained evidence indicating that proprioception is important in the temporal co-ordination of actions; they found that varying the speed of proprioceptive feedback upset motor performance. Temporal factors are of fundamental importance. For the smooth performance of skilled actions it is essential that the sub-units involved in the attainment of a goal be linked together with great precision, as is evident from ball games. We urgently need more information about the child's ability to time and integrate sub-skills. Reaction time studies have played a major role in the experimental analysis of skill but so far as I am aware there are no data available from investigations where the child himself determines the beginning of a sequence as distinct from responding to an external signal. It seems necessary to ask how well a child can synchronize simultaneous or successive responses.

The emphasis in most of our discussions was on input mechanisms and central processing, with little mention of effector mechanisms. Howard's ideas about the introduction of perturbations into the motor system brought us back to the output mechanisms. By introducing transformations into the motor system we can explore the extent to which a child is able to make compensatory adjustments. One way in which this might be profitably investigated was advanced by Kay who suggested that we study tool using abilities in children and systematically change the properties of the tools. Howard also made an important point about children having to learn the physical characteristics of their own limbs and accommodate continuously to changes as growth proceeds. Although a good deal of information is available on somatic changes (Meredith, 1947, 1950) there are gaps in our knowledge. Do hand proportions, for example, change significantly in the first 2 or 3 years?

Hefferline provided us with a thorough and clear review of his work and that of others on the conditioning of single motor units. In reply to the suggestion that single motor unit work appeared to have little relevance to skill development Hefferline suggested that the technique may provide a method of building up a complex skill by welding together the underlying substrata of behaviour. Whilst I am not clear how this might be accomplished, work with single motor units does provide a means of studying the fundamental components of the motor system. It might also be used to develop a model of proprioception and should certainly be exploited further. We have touched upon the motor handicaps associated with the cerebral palsies and we are all aware of the urgent problems of the physically disabled. The application of single motor unit training to myoelectrically controlled prostheses offers many possibilities because of the greatly increased number of trigger sources and control sites which become available. Motor unit work might also be exploited in physiotherapy. Judging from the work in other applied areas we may expect some valuable theoretical spin-off from work directed towards practical problems.

Lefford's elegantly simple experiments provide a link between developmental psychology and neuropathology. The development of a schemata of the fingers bears some relationship to the dissolution of such schemata in pathology. There are many pitfalls in likening the effects of distortion to development and great caution must be exercised since behavioural similarities do not necessarily arise from the same mechanism. However, Lefford's speculations with respect to left–right disorientation, acalculia and agraphia suggest that it may be possible, by examining such conditions, to look at the genesis of action programmes. Lefford's paper also served to remind me of the essential unity of psychological processes, which our analytic bias often leads us to lose sight of.

Twitchell's paper on the role of grasping and avoiding reactions in the development of prehension provided us with an example of the kinds of hardware changes which are involved in motor development. Were it not for such changes manual skills as we have defined them would not be possible. Although we did not fully come to grips with the problem of the shift from reflexive to voluntary control we at least appreciated the need for further studies at the neurological and neurophysiological level. Work on the properties of individual neurones has so far provided no inkling of how these mechanisms relate to co-ordinated, skilled behaviour. Investigations of the kind reported by Twitchell and those discussed by Denny-Brown (1966) are therefore of great concern to us in thinking about physiological explanations of skill development.

An important feature of both Twitchell's and White's work was the care taken to provide a detailed description of the behaviour they studied. There are moments when I feel that psychology has lost sight of behaviour and become involved only in extending and developing highly sophisticated measuring techniques. Whilst I take Hinde's point that description and analysis go hand in hand studies which provide detailed descriptions of behaviour in a "natural" context are rare. The question of *how* a child accomplishes a particular task is as interesting as how well he can do it, measured in terms of time required and error produced. Bruner mentioned the power and precision grips which Napier (1956) has studied in the adult organism but we know little of their development and expression in natural settings. In tool using the configuration of the hand may profoundly effect the outcome of the action (Connolly and Elliott, 1971).

Science progresses not only by solving problems but by finding better ones. In the course of our discussions we have solved very little but we have I think made some progress towards finding better problems. We have clarified certain conceptual confusions and perhaps most importantly we have made the first step towards an inter-disciplinary attack on the mechanisms which subserve the development of motor skills.

REFERENCES

ADAMS, J. A. and CREAMER, L. R. 1963. Proprioceptive variables as determiners of anticipatory timing behavior. *Human Factors* **4**, 217–222.

BARTLETT, F. C. 1958. *Thinking, an experimental and social study.* Allen and Unwin, London.

CONNOLLY, K. and ELLIOTT, J. 1971. The evolution and ontogeny of hand function. In N. Blurton Jones (Ed.), *Ethological studies of child behaviour.* Cambridge University Press.

DENNY-BROWN, D. 1966. *The cerebral control of movement.* University of Liverpool Press.

FLEISHMAN, E. A. and RICH, S. 1963. Role of kinesthetic and spatial-visual abilities in perceptual-motor learning. *J. exp. Psychol.* **66**, 6–11.

HELD, R. and HEIN, A. 1963. Movement-produced stimulation in the development

HOLST, VON E. and MITTELSTAEDT, H. 1950. Das reafferenzprinzip. *Naturwissenshaften* **37**, 464–476.

of visually guided behavior. *J. comp. physiol. Psychol.* **56**, 872–876.

LASHLEY, K. S. 1951. The problem of serial order in behavior. In L. A. Jeffress (Ed.), *Cerebral mechanisms in behavior: the Hixon symposium.* Wiley, New York.

MEREDITH, H. V. 1947. Length of upper extremities in *Homo spaiens* from birth through adolescence. *Growth* **11**, 1–50.

MEREDITH, H. V. 1950. Body size norms for children four to eight years of age. *J. Pediatrics.* **37**, 183–189.

NAPIER, J. R. 1956. The prehensile movements of the human hand. *J. Bone Jt. Surgery* **38B**, 902–913.

POULTON, E. C. 1957. On prediction in skilled movements. *Psychol. Bull.* **54**, 467–478.

SPERRY, R. W. 1951. Mechanisms of neural maturation. In S. S. Stevens (Ed.), *Handbook of experimental psychology.* Wiley, New York.

Author Index

Numbers in italics refer to pages where References are listed at the end of each article.

A

Abercrombie, M. L. J., 308, 309, 310, 312, 315, 318, *323*, *324*
Adams, J. A., 12, *14*, 379, *382*
Adrian, E. D., 273, *275*
Alexander, D., 308, *324*
Allin Smith, W., *133*
Annett, J., 281
Amatruda, C. S., 4, 8, *15*, 98, *133*
Ames, L. B., 8, *14*
Amy, M., 339, *351*
Archer, E. J., 174, *187*
Archer, W., 174, *187*

B

Bamber, D., 264, *276*
Barlow, W., 322, *324*
Bartlett, F. C., 66, *91*, 377, *382*
Basamajian, J. V., 266, 273, 274, *275*
Bassett, E., 12, 14, *15*, 147, *150*, 198
Bateman, D. E., 246, *277*
Baver, J., 36, *37*, 344, 348, *350*
Bayley, N., 8, *14*, 139, *150*
Bax, M., 51
Beintema, D., 48
Bekhterev, V. M., 246, *275*
Bender, L., 330
Benton, A. L., 216, *217*
Berman, A. J., 264, *278*
Bernstein, N. A., 52, 67, 69, 70, 90, *91*, 151, 201, 236, *241*
Bernuth von, H., 47
Bersh, P. J., 250, *278*
Bickford, R. G., 248, *275*
Biederman, I., 174, *187*
Bilodeau, E. A., 187, *187*
Birch, H. G., 11, *14*, 213, 218, 322, *324*, 353, 367

Birch, J. D., 253, *275*
Black, A. H., 253, *275*
Bossom, J., 116, *133*
Bousfield, W. A., 6, *14*
Brash, J. C., 251, 266, *275*
Brian, E. R., 12, *15*
Bridgman, C. S., 6, *14*
Broadbent, D. E., 174, 178, *187*
Brody, S., 113, *133*
Bronk, D. W., 273, *275*
Brown, K., 12, 14, *15*, 147, *150*, 198
Brown, P. L., 254, 255, *275*
Bruner, B. M., 70, *91*
Bruner, J. S., 70, *91*, 225, *241*
Bruno, L. J. J., 260, *275*
Bryan, W. L., 12, *14*
Bryant, P. E., 11, *14*
Buchtal, F., 273, *275*
Buchwald, A. M., 245, 246, 248, *276*
Bullock, T. H., 7, *14*
Burnham, C. A., 264, *276*
Burns, D. B., 191
Burnside, L. H., 8, *14*

C

Cannon, L. K., 310, *324*
Carmichael, L., 6, *14*, 36, *37*
Casler, L., 113, *133*
Castle, P., 10, *17*, 99, 100, 103, 105, 114, *133*
Cernacek, J., 318, *324*
Chaudry, A. S., 196
Clark, K. R., 100, 101, 102, *133*
Clark, W. E. Le Gros, 13, *15*, 64, *91*
Cody, D. T. R., 248, *275*
Coghill, G. E., 6, 7, *15*, 72, *91*
Cohen, H. B., 347, *349*
Collins, C. C., 339, *350*

Connolly, K., 11, 12, 13, 14, *15*, 147, *150*, 188, 198, 309, *324*, 329, 355, 368, 369, 370, 381, *382*
Court, S. D. M., 309, *324*
Craik, K. J. W., 12, *15*, 146, *150*, *151*, 161, *187*
Craske, B., 344, 349, *350*
Creamer, L. R., 379, *382*
Crossman, E. R. F. W., 10, *15*, 162, 174, 186, *187*, 189, 190
Cumming, W. W., 263, *278*

D

Davidowitz, J., 266, *276*
Davis, F. H., 246, *277*
Davis, J. R., 310, *324*
Davis, R. C., 245, 246, 248, 249, 261, 262, *276*
Davol, S. H., 12, *15*
Dawson, H. E., 249, *276*
De Ajuriaguerra, J., 314, 316, *325*
Denenberg, V. H., 113, *133*
Denny-Brown, D., 25, 35, *37*, 365, 381, *382*
Ditchburn, R., 229, *241*
Doehring, D. G., 249, *276*
Douglas, B., 260, *277*
Dow, G., 19
Dyk, R., 174, *188*

E

Efstathiou, A., 348, *350*
Ehrhardt, A. A., 308, *324*
Eichorn, D. H., 13, *15*
Elampied, N. M., 260, *277*
Elliott, J., 381, *382*
Ellis, E., 309, *324*
Ellsworth, D. W., 260, *276*
Escher, M. C., 320, *324*

F

Falls, J. B., 296
Fantz, R. L., 89, *91*

Faterson, H. F., 174, *188*
Fender, D., 229, *241*
Ferguson, G. A., 117, *133*
Festinger, L., 264, *276*, 310, *324*
Fetz, E. E., 253, *276*
Fink, J. B., 261, *276*
Fisher, G. H., 370
Fitts, P. M., 174, *187*
Fleishman, E. A., 379, *382*
Fletcher, F. G., 255, *278*
Fog, E., 13, *15*
Fog, M., 13, *15*
Forrin, B., 173, 174, *187*
Fortuyn, J. D., 282
Frankmann, R. W., 245, 246, 248, *276*
Freedman, S. J., 11, *15*, 345, *350*
Frostig, M., 311, 312, *324*
Fuller, J. L., 6, *15*

G

Galanter, E. H., 260, *278*
Galbraith, R. F., 248, *275*
Galperin, P. Y., 226, *241*
Gardiner, P. A. G., 309, *324*
Gerstmann, J., 216, *218*
Gesell, A., 4, 8, 9, *15*, 98, *133*, 139, *151*
Gibson, E. J., 295, *295*
Gilman, S., 365
Glickstein, M., 250, *277*
Goldberg, I. A., 253, *276*
Goodenough, D., 174, *188*
Goodenough, F. L., 12, *15*, 173, *187*
Gottlieb, G., 7, *15*
Gramsbergen, A., 282
Grant, D. A., 249, *276*
Greene, M., 348, *350*
Gregory, R. L., 339, *350*
Gruner, G. E., 13, *15*
Gubbay, S. S., 309, *324*

H

Hall, S. B., 345, *350*
Halle, M., 300
Halverson, H. M., 9, *15*, *16*, 32, *37*, 139, *151*

Hamburger, V., 7, *16*
Hamilton, C. R., 345, *350*
Hansen, E., 309, *324*
Hardyck, C. D., 260, *276*
Harford, R. A., 251, 257, *276*
Harris, C. S., 320, *325*, 343, 348, *350*
Harris, J. R., 343, *350*
Harrison, V. F., 273, 274, *276*
Hastings, M. L., 12, *15*
Hay, J. C., 343, *350*
Haynes, H., 100, 106, 107, *133*
Head, H., 212, 217, *218*
Hecaen, H., 314, 316, *325*
Hefferline, R. F., 251, 253, 257, 259, 260, 262, 265, *276*, *277*, 323, *324*, 356
Hein, A., 10, 11, *16*, 36, *37*, 40, 53, 116, *133*, 297, 344, *350*, 378, 382
Held, R., 10, 11, *16*, *17*, 36, *37*, *37*, *38*, 40, 53, 96, 97, 99, 100, 101, 102, 103, 104, 105, 106, 107, 114, 116, 118, 120, 121, 123, 125, 126, *133*, 309, *324*, 341, 342, 344, 348, *350*, 378, 382
Hering, E., 338, *350*
Herrick, R. M., 253, *277*
Hertzmann, M., 320, *325*
Hick, W. E., 141, *151*, 162, *187*
Hilden, A. H., 249, *277*
Hinde, R. A., 293, *295*, 296
Hines, M., 41
Hirsch, J., 6, *16*
Hollingshead, W. H., 273, *277*
Holst von, E., 11, *16*, 67, *91*, 378, *382*
Howard, I. P., 310, *324*, 340, 342, 343, 344, *350*, *351*, 370
Howarth, C. I., 370
Howells, F. C., 65, *92*
Hubel, D. H., 361, 362
Hunt, W. A., 248, *277*
Hunter, W. S., 249, *277*
Hyvärinen, J., 192

I

Illingworth, R. S., 8, *16*, 139, *151*
Immelmann, K., 293, *295*
Inhelder, B., 311, *325*
Irwin, R. J., 260, *277*

J

Jackson, H., 217, *218*
Jacobson, E., 245, *277*, 300, 322, *324*
Jacobson, J. L., 248, *275*
Jakobson, R. C., 300
James, M., 314, *325*
Jenkins, H. M., 254, 255, *275*
Jonckhere, J., 309, *324*
Jones, B., 11, *15*, 368, 369, 370
Jones, F. W., 64, *91*
Jones, H. E., 173, *187*

K

Kahneman, I., 70, *91*
Karas, G. G., 113, *133*
Karp, S., 174, *188*
Karsch, C. S., 343, *350*
Katzman, R., 248, *277*
Kay, H., 144, *151*, 171, *187*, 197
Kaye, H., 6, *16*
Keenan, B., 251, 253, 257, *276*
Kessen, W., 89, *92*
Kimble, G. A., 247, 254, *277*
Kinsbourne, M., 216, *218*, 219, 314, *325*
Kirkpatrick, C., 264, *276*
Klein, D. A., 12, *15*
Kohler, W., 237, *241*
Konishi, M., 291, 923, 294, *295*, 298
Kuo, Z. Y., 6, 7, *15*, *16*
Kupfmüller, K., 196

L

Lacey, B. C., 246, *277*
Lacey, J. I., 246, *277*
Landis, C., 248, *277*
Landmark, M., 316, 317, *324*, 332
Langworthy, O. R., 13, *16*
Lanyon, W. E., 293, *295*
Larsell, O., 19, 119
Lashley, K. S., 7, *16*, 68, 69, *92*, 376, *382*
Lauretana, M. M., 34, 35, *37*
Lecours, A. R., 34, *38*
Lefever, D. W., 311, 312, *324*
Lefford, A., 11, *14*, 213, *218*, 322, *324*, 330, 367

Lenard, H. G., 47
Leonard, A. J., 148, *151*
Leontiev, A. N., 226, 241, *241*
Levine, S., 113, *133*
Lewis, H. B., 320, *325*
Liddell, H. S., 250, *277*
Lindon, R. L., 309, 318, *324*
Ling, B. C., 135
Lippold, O. C. J., 247, 266, *277*
Lowman, A. E., 343, *351*
Luria, A. R., 220, 314, *324*, 361
Luschei, E., 250, *277*
Lynn, R., 248, *277*

M

MacCorquodale, K., 295, *295*
MacKeith, R., 51
Maccoby, E. 366
Macfarlane Smith, I., 323, *324*
Machover, K., 320, *325*
Mackintosh, N. J., 295, *295*
McFie, J., 314, *324*
McGraw, M. B., 5, 8, *16*, 139, *151*
McLaughlin, S. C., 349, *350*
McMillan, D. E., 253, *277*
Maki, N., 320, *325*
Malmo, R. B., 246, *277*
Marcuse, F. L., 250, *277*
Margulies, S., 253, *277*
Marler, P., 294, *295*
Meehl, P. E., 295, *295*
Meier, G. W., 113, *133*
Miller, G. A., 193
Meissner, P. B., 320, *325*
Meredith, H. V., 380, *382*
Merton, P. A., 264, *277*, 338, *350*
Mikaelian, H., 116, *133*
Miller, N. E., 247, *277*
Mintz, D. E., 253, *278*
Mittelstaedt, H., 67, *91*, 378, *382*
Money, J., 308, *324*
Moore, A. U., 250, *277*
Morin, R. E., 173, 174, *187*
Morris, D., 42, 307, *325*
Mortenson, O. A., 273, 274, *276*
Mowbray, G. H., 148, *151*
Muenzinger, K. F., 227, *241*

N

Napier, J. R., 64, *92*, 381, *382*
Neisser, U., 189
Nicolai, J., 293, *295*
Norris, F. H., 266, *277*
Nottebohm, F., 291, 293, 294, *295*, 298
Notterman, J. M., 250, 253, *278*

O

Oldfield, R. C., 241, *241*
O'Meara, D. M., 339, *350*
Ono, H., 264, *276*
Over, J., 317, *325*
Over, R., 317, 320, *325*

P

Partan, D. L., 34, 35, *37*
Patton, R. A., 253, *277*
Pavlov, I. P., 250, *278*
Perera, T. B., 260, 262, *277*, 356
Petrinovich, L. F., 260, *276*
Piaget, J., 37, *37*, 111, 122, *133*, 216, 218, 225, *241*, 311, *325*
Pick, H. L., 343, *350*
Piercy, M., 314, 316, *325*
Poddyakov, N. N., 228, *241*
Poklekowski, G., 196
Posner, M. I., 174, *188*, 369
Poulton, E. C., 378, *382*
Pravdina-Vinarskaya, E. N., 314, *324*
Prechtl, H. F. R., 19, 47, 48, 50
Pritchard, R. M., 229, *241*
Pushkin, V. N., 238, *241*

R

Rapin, I., 248, *278*
Rekosh, J. H., 345, *350*
Retanova, E. A., *241*
Rhoades, M. V., 148, *151*
Rich, S., 379, *382*
Riesen, A. H., 11, *16*, 115, 116, *133*, 297
Riggs, L., 339, *351*
Robinson, D. A., 339, *350*
Rock, I., 320, *325*

Rosenblith, J. F., *133*
Rudel, R. G., 34, *38*
Rumyantsev, D. A., 233, *241*
Ruzskaya, A. G., 228, *242*

S

Salapatek, P., 89, *92*
Saslow, C., 250, *277*
Scheibel, A. B., 13, *16*
Scheibel, M. E., 13, *16*
Schick, C., 339, *351*
Schlosberg, H., 249, *278*
Schneirla, T. C., 6, *16*
Schoenfeld, W. N., 246, 250, 263, *278*
Scott, A. B., 339, *350*
Seyffarth, H., 25, *37*
Seymour, E., 216, *217*
Shackel, B., 310, *324*
Shagass, C., 246, *277*
Shannon, C. E., 162, *188*
Sherman, H. L., 332
Shirley, M. M., 139, *151*
Sidman, M., 255, *278*
Skinner, B. F., 250, 254, 255, *278*
Smader, R., 188
Smith, E. E., 162, *188*
Smith, K. U., 188
Smith, R. W., 250, *278*
Sokolov, E. N., 248, 249, 250, *278*
Solomon, G., 309, *324*
Sperling, G., 233, *241*
Sperry, R. W., 247, *278*, 378, *382*
Sprague, J. M., 365
Stark, L., 361
Stengel, E., 216, *218*
Stevens, S. S., 260, *278*
Stevenson, J. G., 291, 292, *295*
Stoper, A. E., 339, *350*
Stratton, P., 13, *15*
Sutherland, N. S., 295, *295*
Szafran, J., 171, 186, *187*, 190
Szekely, G., 7, *16*

T

Tamura, M., 294, *295*

Tanner, J. M., 13, *16*
Taub, E., 264, *278*
Templeton, W. B., 310, *324*, 340, 342, 343, 344, *350*, *351*, 370
Terrace, H. S., 263, *278*
Teuber, H. L., 34, *38*
Thistlewaite, D., 295, *296*
Thompson, G. G., 6, *16*
Thompson, W. R., 6, *15*
Thorndike, E. L., 246, *278*
Thorpe, W. H., 287, 288, 289, *296*
Tighe, T. J., 295, *295*
Tinker, M. A., 12, *15*
Tolman, E. C., 228, *241*
Twitchell, T. E., 10, 16, 25, 34, 35, 36, 37, *38*, 48, 70, *92*, 353
Tyson, M. C., 308, 309, 318, *324*

U

Uchtomsky, A. A., 227, 241, *241*
Ullet, G., 19

V

Van Lehn, R., 246, *247*
Van Liere, D. W., 248, 249, *276*, *278*
Venger, L. A., 228, *242*
Vereecken, P., 316, *325*
Vergiles, N. Y., 229, 233, *241*
Vlach, V., 51
Volkmann, F., 339, *351*
Vossius, G., 196
Vuchetich, G. G., 233, *241*
Vurpillot, E., 191
Vygotsky, L. S., 65, *92*

W

Waddington, C. H., 7, *16*
Walton, J. N., 309, *324*
Walk, R. D., 295, *295*
Wapner, S., 320, *325*
Warrington, E. K., 216, *218*, 219, 314, *325*
Washburn, S. L., 65, *92*
Weaver, W., 162, *188*

Webster, R. G., 349, *350*
Welford, A. T., 162, *188*
Whatmore, G. B., 260, *278*
White, B. L., 10, *17*, 37, *38*, 96, 97, 99, 100, 101, 102, 103, 104, 105, 106, 107, 114, 115, 116, 117, 118, 119, 120, 121, 122, 123, 124, 125, 126, 128, 129, *133*
Whittlesey, J. R. B., 311, 312, *324*
Wiesel, T. N., 361, 362
Windle, W. F., 6, *17*
Winer, B. J., *133*
Witkin, H. A., 174, *188*, 320, *325*
Wober, M., 321, *325*
Woodworth, R. S., 67, *92*, 249, *278*
Wyckoff, L. B., 262, *278*

Y

Yarbus, A. L., 229, *241*, 309, 314, 316, *324*, *325*
Yarrow, L. J., 113, *133*

Z

Zangwill, O. L., 314, *324*
Zaporozhets, A. V., 226, 228, *242*, 311, *325*
Zazzo, R., 224
Zeaman, D., 250, *278*
Zincheko, V. P., 228, 229, 233, *241*, *242*

Subject Index

A

Acalculia, 216, 217, 381
Action programmes, 74, 75, 77, 85, 90–91, 197–198, 378–379, 381
Agraphia, 217, 381
Anticipation, 66, 142–144, 145, 152, 377–378
Anticipatory instructed conditioning, 249, 250, 262
Anticipatory postural changes, 196
Apraxia, 221, 314
Associated movements, 13, 58, 318–320, 358
   changes with age, 13
Athetotic movements, 32, 43, 70
Attention, 8, 71, 73, 81, 174
   visual, 102–103, 114–115, 121, 122, 124, 126, 127, 129, 232
Avoiding reactions, 25, 30–32, 34, 38, 44–45, 364
   role of, 32–33

B

Behaviourism, 4, 7
Bird song,
   development of, 287–295
   early experience, effects of, 291
   group rearing and, 287–290, 294
   isolated rearing and, 289–290
   reinforcing effectiveness of, 290, 291–292, 302
   restrictions on song learning, 293
   sensitive period for learning, 293, 297
   stereotypy, 300
Brain damage, 222, 320, 353, 356, 358, 359, 361
   copying and, 308, 316–317
   drawing and, 313–314
   motor training and, 353–359

tonic-neck-reflex and, 21

C

Central patterning in nervous system, 7
Cerebral inhibition, 13
Cerebral lesions, 40, 42, 361–366
Channel capacity, 142, 143, 149, 155, 156, 157, 158, 174, 182, 195–196
Classical conditioning, 247, 248–250, 253–256
Clumsiness, 84, 309
Cognitive factors,
   in motor skill, 207–217, 222, 225–241, 376
Computer analogies, 9
Contact body-righting reflex, 27, 28–29, 35
Control capacity,
   limits on, 9
Copying, 307, 311–312, 313, 316, 329–332
   brain damaged children by, 313–314
Corollary discharges, 339, 343
Covert/overt response correlations, 246
Cross-modal matching, 11–12, 362, 370
   model of, 368–370
Cybernetics, 12

D

Defence reaction, 248
Deltawert, 68
Detour reaching, 83–89
   as function of age, 84
Development,
   direction of,
      cephalo-caudal, 4
      proximo-distal, 4
   sequences of, 7

stages of, 8
Developmental diagnosis, 8
Drawing, 307
  by apes, 307–308
  by brain injured adults, 314
  by brain injured children, 308, 316–317
  by children, 308, 311, 315
  diamonds, 315–316, 325, 328–329, 332–333, 334
  difficulties, 309–310, 325–326
  oblique lines, 319, 326, 330

E

Electromyogram, 245, 249, 250, 255, 257, 258, 261, 266, 268, 269, 271, 273, 274
  measurement technique, 251–252, 266–267
Embryo,
  behaviour, 7, 10
  isolated movements, 6
  rhythmical movements, 7
Epigenetic system, 7
Evolution, 9, 72–73
  hand use of, 64
Experience,
  definition of, 7
Exploration,
  tactual, 97, 98
  visual, 97, 98–99, 122
Exteroceptive dominance, 30
Extinction, 252, 256
Eye movements, 93, 154, 229, 231, 238, 240, 309–310, 316, 338–339
  brain injury, 310
  method of recording, 230–231
  of children, 310, 311
Eye position, 339

F

Feedback, 52, 57, 68, 194, 228, 257, 258, 259, 260, 274, 341, 351, 376, 379
  auditory, 42, 284
  augmented, 247, 256–275, 356, 364
  exteroceptive, 246–247

  kinaesthetic, 57, 143, 203, 356
  proprioceptive, 143, 282, 302
  response discrimination and, 260–264
  visual, 203, 281, 282, 284
Feedback loops, 8, 203
Finger–thumb opposition, 9, 33, 34, 207–217
Flexion,
  arm, 28, 30, 48
  finger, 26, 28, 33, 34, 43, 48, 52
  synergistic, 26, 27, 28, 32, 35
  wrist, 26, 28

G

Gamma system, 196
Gaze aversion, 134, 135
Generalized action patterns, 6
Genetic predeterminism, 5
Genome, 7
Gerstmann's syndrome, 215
Grasp,
  adequate stimulus for, 28
  anticipatory, 54–57
  instinctive grasp reaction, 29–30, 33, 35, 42–43, 58
  palmar, 48, 191
  role of, 32
  voluntary, 9, 25, 33
Grasp reflex, 9, 25, 58, 363
  fractionation of, 29, 33, 34
  in prematures, 51
Grasping, 10, 74
  automatic, 10
  developmental sequence of, 9, 26–30
Growth, 4

H

Habituation of conditional stimulus, 250
Hand,
  movements in drawing, 318–320
  proportions, 380
  regard, 97, 98, 111, 114, 119, 123–124, 127, 128–129
  skills, 63
  topography, 212, 217

Hands,
    complimentary use of, 63, 75, 77–88
    neuropathology of, 215
Hand–eye co-ordination, 309, 322, 337
Hand–mouth co-ordination, 47, 73, 74

I

Image, 225, 226, 228
    distortions of, 235
    development of, 232
    invariance of, 236
    memory for, 233–234
    transmission of, 237
Imitation,
    movement of, 207–217
    song, 293
Information,
    flow, 140–142
    integration of, 8
    load, 142, 162
    rate of gain of, 170–172
    reduction, 145–147, 282
    transfer, 152
    transmission, 141, 147, 158, 161, 178, 179, 360
Information processing, 141, 152, 161, 162–174, 194, 197, 376
    as function of age, 162–174, 186
    effects of irrelevant stimuli, 174–178, 179–183, 183–186
Instinctive response, 59
Intersensory,
    discordance, 344
    integration, 11, 154, 213, 322, 330–331, 357, 358, 362, 363, 367–370, 379
Intra-modal matching, 367–370
Istwert, 68

K

Kinaesthetic code, 379
    matching, 368–369
    processing, 367–368
    store, 367, 368, 369

L

Labyrinthine reflexes, 34, 37, 40

Learning readiness, 157
Left–right disorientation, 216–217
Localized movements, 6

M

Manipulation, 89
Manipulative skill, 9–10
Manual intelligence, 63–65
Mass movements, 6
Mass to specific trend, 6, 18
Massed *vs* distributed practice, 12
Maturation, 7
    anticipatory principle of, 36
    of cortical centres, 38
    experience and, 20, 21
    Gesell's principles of, 4–5, 17
    hypothesis, 4–7, 10, 17
    of reflexes, 34
    Schneirla's definition of, 6–7
Molar *vs* molecular approach, 12, 376
Motivation, 17, 256, 281
Motor,
    alphabet, 226–228, 232, 237, 238, 240
    impairment, 219, 281, 309, 353–359, 361, 362, 380
    outflow, 339, 342, 344
    programme, 378–379
    units, 202, 249, 267, 269, 282, 357, 380
Motor cortex, 57–59, 365
    lesions, 364
Motor development,
    stages of, 139, 228
Movement,
    ballistic, 196, 198, 282–283
    of body, 344
    foetal, 6, 7
    speed of, 12–14, 169–170
    symbolic representation of, 213–215
    visual control of, 307
Myelin sheath, 13
Myelination, 12–13, 19
    order of, 13
Myogenic response,
    alpha component of, 247–248
    amplitude of, 253, 260
    beta component of, 247–248, 249–250, 251, 254, 255

evoked, 247, 250
magnitude and conditioning of, 252

N

Nature *vs* nurture, 5, 7, 19–20
Neonate, 6, 8, 30, 195, 296
  generalized movements of, 18–19
  grip of, 26
  tonic-neck-reflex and, 17, 21
Nerve impulse transmission, 13
Neural,
  network, 54
  organization, 5
  programming, 59
Neurological hierarchies, 53
Noise in nervous system, 186, 190–192, 359, 360

O

Ontogenetic organization, 6
Operant conditioning, 247, 250–253
  and shaping, 355–356
  and fading, 278–279, 282, 357
Orientation-search, 226, 227–229, 237
Orienting reaction, 248, 250, 254, 255
Ozeretsky tests, 222

P

Palpebral response, 97, 100, 107–111, 130–131, 132
Perceptual-motor integration, 10–12
Perceptual rivalry, 361
Play, 80
Points of articulation,
  arm, 339–340
  eye, 338–339
  head 339
Posture, 55, 196, 303
  and movement, 282
Power grip, 63, 64, 71, 204, 381
Practice, 197, 378
  massed *vs* distributed, 12
Precision grip, 63, 64, 71, 204, 220, 381

Prehension,
  brain injured children and, 33–35
  development of, 25, 119–121, 124, 381
  reflex substrata for, 34, 363
  visual control of, 33, 36, 54–57, 99
Proprioception, 10, 42, 379
Proprioceptive dominance, 26, 28

R

Reaction time, 140, 141, 148, 173, 174, 187, 189, 355, 379
Reafference, 11, 52, 67, 323, 332, 342, 343, 344, 353, 358, 378
Redundancy, 148–149, 377
Reflexes,
  hand, 47–51, 70
  Moro, 47–48, 50
  tonic-neck-reflex, 5, 17, 21, 27, 28–29, 55, 70, 98, 123, 194
Reflex to voluntary control, 51–54
Reinforcement, 247, 250, 251, 253, 254–255, 355
  negative, 252
  positive, 252, 257

S

Schema, 220, 223, 303, 307, 312, 317
  body, 212, 215, 216, 217, 378
  hand-finger, 212, 215, 220, 380
  proprioceptive, 212, 215
  tactual-kinaesthetic, 215
  visual, 212
Selective filtering mechanism, 14, 174, 175, 178, 179, 185, 186, 189, 190
Self-organizing system, 7
Sensory deprivation, 11
Serial order, 65, 66, 67, 68, 77, 140, 146, 161, 162, 193, 216, 377
Signal to noise ratio, 186, 190
Simultaneous responses, 379
Skeletal musculature,
  control of, 247, 248, 250
Skill
  intention and, 67–70
  macro-strategy of, 144, 149–150, 152, 377

micro-structure of, 144, 149, 377
modular quality of, 66, 68, 70–71, 377
training, 193, 201
Skill development,
role of experience in, 95
Sollwert, 68
Sound spectrogram, 202, 287, 288, 289, 301
Spatial orientation, 216, 323, 337
Speed, 66
speed-accuracy trade-off, 147
changes with age, 12, 188, 198
developmental changes in, 12–14, 161, 186
of muscular movement, 12
Stabilized retinal image, 229–234
and eye movements, 232
method of obtaining, 229–230
Stage dependent theories, 8
Stimulus-response,
chain, 376
compatibility, 148, 173, 175, 186
mapping, 174
Storage and deposit of objects, 75–76
Strategies, 376
Sub-routine, 8–9, 14, 18, 19, 65, 71, 88, 149, 152, 153, 155, 157, 158, 196, 377
Substitution rules, 65–66, 220
Sucking, 6
Swiping movements, 32–33, 55, 73, 119, 122, 124, 134

T

Taking possession of objects, 73–77
Temporal,
sequencing, 161
co-ordination, 379
Timing, 66, 67
Tool use, 63, 64, 92, 200, 381

Tracking of events, 88–91, 93
Traction response, 26–28, 32, 33, 34, 43
in monkeys, 41
in prematures, 51
Trap reaction, 29, 35

U

Units of behaviour, 59, 67, 194, 195

V

Vicarious trial and error, 227–228
Visual,
accommodation, 97, 98, 100, 104–106, 127, 130
avoiding reactions, 134, 135
fixation, 135
groping reaction, 134
pursuit, 97, 133
scanning, 64
Visually directed reaching, 10, 34, 36–37, 38–39, 44, 68, 73, 95, 97, 99, 103–104, 120, 196, 297
Visuomotor,
adaptation, 11
development, 11, 116
performance, 115
Visuomotor system,
basic performance of, 340
components of, 337–340
conditions for adaptation, 341–345
growth and adaptability of, 340–341
site of adaptive change, 345–349

W

Walking, 8